PRIVACY AND DISCLOSURE
OF
HIV IN INTERPERSONAL RELATIONSHIPS

A Sourcebook for Researchers and Practitioners

PRIVACY AND DISCLOSURE
OF
HIV IN INTERPERSONAL RELATIONSHIPS

A Sourcebook for Researchers and Practitioners

KATHRYN GREENE
Rutgers University

VALERIAN J. DERLEGA
Old Dominion University

GUST A. YEP
San Francisco State University

SANDRA PETRONIO
Indiana University–Purdue University

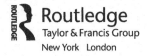

Routledge
Taylor & Francis Group
New York   London

First published by Lawrence Erlbaum Associates, Inc., Publishers
10 Industrial Avenue
Mahwah, New Jersey 07430

Reprinted 2009 by Routledge

Routledge

270 Madison Avenue
New York, NY 10016

2 Park Square, Milton Park
Abingdon, Oxon OX14 4RN, UK

Cover design by Kathryn Houghtaling Lacey

Library of Congress Cataloging-in-Publication Data

Privacy and disclosure of HIV in interpersonal relationships : a source-
    book for researchers and practitioners / Kathryn Greene ... [et al.].
        p. cm.
Includes bibliographical references and index.
ISBN 0-8058-3694-2 (cloth alk. paper)
ISBN 0-8058-3695-0 (pbk. : alk. paper)
1. AIDS (Disease)—Reporting.   2. Privacy.   3. HIV-positive persons.
    4. AIDS (Disease)—Social aspects.   I. Greene, Kathryn
RA643.8.P755 2003
362.1'969792—dc21   2002192838
                                                              CIP

10   9   8   7   6   5   4   3   2   1

For Sandie,
a courageous soul who left us too soon,
and everyone else whose lives are touched by HIV

Contents

Preface   xi

1 Introduction   1
  Worldwide Prevalence of HIV and AIDS   2
  Prevalence of HIV and AIDS in the United States   3
  What is Disclosure?   4
  The Importance of HIV Disclosure   7
  Summary of HIV Disclosure   8
  Chapter Overviews   9
  Interviews Utilized in This Project   15
  Conclusions   15

2 Communication Privacy Management and HIV Disclosure   17
  CPM   17
    Suppositions   18
    Rule Management System   20
  Privacy Rule Management Process 1: Rule Foundations   20
    Privacy Rule Development   21
  Rule Management Process 2: Boundary Coordination   25
    Coordination Operations   26
  Rule Management Process 3: Boundary Turbulence   30
  Conclusions   34

3 Decisions to Disclose or Not Disclose About an HIV Positive   36
   Diagnosis
  Stigma as Risk Criteria Influencing Disclosure Decisions   37
    Perceived Risk Affecting Decisions to Disclose   40
    Motivations Regulating Revealing and Concealing an HIV   45
    Diagnosis

Decisions Leading to Disclosure for Self-Gain   46
Decisions Leading to Disclosure for Other-Gain   49
Decisions Leading to Disclosure for Interpersonal-Gain   52
Motivational Criteria For Nondisclosure of an HIV Diagnosis   55
Decisions Leading to Nondisclosure for Self-Gain   56
Decisions Leading to Nondisclosure for Other-Gain   60
Decisions Leading to Nondisclosure for   62
    Interpersonal-Gain
Summary of Decisions Leading to Nondisclosure   63
Relational Contexts for Disclosure Decisions   63
Anticipated Response to Disclosure   64
Relational Ties   67
Past Discussion of HIV   77
Perceived Relational Quality   78
Discloser's Past Experience   79
Ethnicity and Gender   81
Conclusions   83

4   **Features of HIV Disclosure Messages**   **84**

Mode of Communication   85
Face-to-Face Versus Non-Face-to-Face Disclosure   85
Third-Party Disclosure   90
Contextual Considerations   94
Setting   94
Timing   97
    When to Disclose After Learning Diagnosis   98
    Preplanned Versus Unplanned Disclosure   103
    When to Disclose in a Conversation   105
Message Features   110
Directness–Equivocality   110
Length of Message   113
Message Content   114
Alternative Disclosure Message Strategies   116
Vernacular Tactics   118
Conclusions   119

5   **Consequences of HIV Disclosure and Nondisclosure**   **121**
    Decision Making

Consequences of HIV Disclosure   122
Actual Responses to HIV Disclosure   125
Boundary Coordination Issues with HIV Disclosure   127
    and Social Support

HIV Diagnosis, Psychological Health, and   136
    Identity—Implications for HIV Disclosure
HIV Disclosure and Stigma   138
HIV Disclosure and Close Relationships   142
    Relationship Closeness   142
    Significant Others as Caregivers   147
    Effects of Disclosure on Children   150
    Impact on Safer Sex and Other Risk Behaviors   154
    Summary of Consequences of HIV Disclosure   159
Privacy Protection, Management, and HIV Nondisclosure   160
    Conflicted Feelings About Others' Right to Know   160
    HIV Nondisclosure as Information Control   162
    Breakdown of Information Control   163
    Privacy and Nondisclosure as Psychological Inhibition   168
Conclusions   170

6   Epilogue: Looking to the Future of Disclosure and HIV   172
    HIV and AIDS Treatments   172
    AIDS Vaccine   173
    Changes in Stigma   174
    Relationships   175
    Future Research   176
    Conclusions   180

Appendix   181
Resources for Individuals Living With HIV, Their Significant
Others, Researchers, and Health Professionals
    Personal Exercises   182
    Measures Related to Disclosure and HIV   186
        Other Measures   213
    Additional Resources   214
        HIV and AIDS Related Websites   215
        National HIV and AIDS Associations   217
        National Telephone Hotlines   218
        Other Readings   219
        Social Artifacts   222
    Conclusions   223

References   225

Author Index   251

Subject Index   261

Preface

Human immunodeficiency virus (HIV) is one of the most pressing health issues of this century. HIV also has ramifications for the relationships and daily lives of those infected and affected by the disease. One of the most widely recommended AIDS prevention options revolves around whether or not to disclose about one's HIV positive status to others—particularly to potential sex partners. In this volume, we consider the impact of HIV disclosure for AIDS prevention. Relying on a theory of privacy and communication (communication privacy management theory), we explore the impact of HIV disclosure for a wider range of issues including communication, social interactions, and the development and maintenance of personal relationships.

This book focuses on choices to disclose or not disclose an HIV positive diagnosis. These decisions about disclosure and privacy are critical for how people with HIV live and manage their relationships. Because the book pointedly focuses on disclosure of HIV infection, it is at once unique and yet of interest to a wide variety of related fields of study. The focus of this book is on private, voluntary relational disclosure (e.g., "Should I tell you about the diagnosis?") not on forced or public disclosure (e.g., "Information about my HIV diagnosis was divulged to others by a public health worker"). Disclosure is examined in a variety of social contexts, including in relationships with intimate partners, families, friends, health workers, and coworkers. Of particular interest is examination of decisions to disclose an HIV diagnosis (e.g., reasons for disclosure, stigma, and relational quality), disclosure message features, and consequences of disclosure of HIV infection (e.g., social support, physical health, sexual behavior, self-identity, relationships with family and others in one's social network).

This book has been in progress for several years. During that time, many changes have occurred in the HIV epidemic and in the lives of the authors. As we finish writing this book, the 14th International Conference on AIDS concluded in Barcelona, Spain (July 2002), and researchers continue to report studies of existing and new treatments as well as possible vaccines. HIV-related stigma is clearly still a problem, perhaps inhibiting HIV testing. For example, more than three fourths of young gay men in the United States who tested positive for HIV were unaware of their infection (MacKellar, 2002), much higher than previous estimates. A new rapid (20 minute) HIV test (OraQuick) was approved in November 2002 (see MMWR, 2002). This test is useful to reduce waiting time (previously 2 weeks) but also to address concerns about nonreturns (people who are tested but never pick up results).

Antiretroviral therapies have drastically changed the health prognoses for many with HIV. Although the price for antiretroviral therapies has decreased dramatically, for many (most in many countries) they are unavailable. The majority of those with access to the best treatments (antiretrovirals) live in high-income countries. For example, in the United States treatment for a person with advanced AIDS currently costs more than $34,000 per year.

The report by the joint United Nations Program on HIV/AIDS (UNAIDS) released in July 2002 contradicted prior predictions that the epidemic would peak in many countries around the year 2000. We have, however, not seen a leveling off of infections at this point. In contrast, the epidemic is expanding rapidly, with 95% of people with HIV living in the developing world. The epidemic continues to rise dramatically in Africa, Asia, the Caribbean, and Eastern Europe. In Africa, for example, 2.2 million people died of AIDS in 2001 (Kresge, 2002). AIDS is the fourth leading cause of death worldwide (see UNAIDS, 2001) and the leading cause of death in some countries. It is predicted that there will be more than 65 million deaths in the next 20 years. Thus, there is a call for increased prevention programs.

This book project developed over several years. The people we interviewed about HIV disclosure affected us profoundly. Many who gave their time, energy, and spirit have since died or have advanced AIDS. These people shared themselves, the good and the bad of HIV, with grace and humor. The resilience of these wonderful people serves as a continued inspiration to us. Beyond talking with people with HIV, their partners, families, and friends were also open to describing accounts of struggles with disclosing about HIV. Finally, during this project, we talked with many people who work with those with HIV (e.g., therapists, social workers, and health practitioners) who contributed their experiences.

A word of caution is worthwhile about language used to refer to someone with HIV and/or AIDS in this book. The use of terms related to HIV infection have changed and will continue to change, and this is as much a reflection of social changes as politics. Early epidemic terminology used phrases like "GRID" (gay related immune deficiency) or even "gay plague." Later phrases were developed to focus on "people living with HIV" ("PLWHs") or "people living with AIDS" ("PLWAs") or some combination such as "people living with HIV or AIDS" ("PLWHAs"). Others have taken an approach utilizing "HIV and/or AIDS" to emphasize that some people live with both HIV infection and AIDS, whereas others live with HIV infection but not AIDS. We have consciously adopted phrases such as "individuals with HIV" to refer to all people with HIV (including someone with AIDS) and phrases such as "individuals with AIDS" to refer specifically to people with an AIDS diagnosis. On the other hand, we have avoided phrases such as "persons with HIV/AIDS" because it may incorrectly imply that all persons with HIV also have AIDS. *HIV* (human immunodeficiency virus) is the term used to describe the disease associated with HIV infection, and *AIDS* (or acquired immune deficiency syndrome) is the final stage of HIV-related infection associated with physical symptoms (e.g., recurrent pneumonia, HIV wasting syndrome) of severe immune deficiency. We have also used care with language related to sexuality, choosing to focus on behavior (e.g., men who have sex with men or MSM) rather than identity (gay or homosexual) where possible. We hope this language provides one mechanism for sensitivity to these issues in this book.

The four authors of this book represent different areas of expertise related to HIV and disclosure. Kathryn Greene's research in communication focuses on both disclosure of HIV and risk prevention messages, primarily with adolescent populations. Val Derlega's research in social psychology explores the role of disclosure in relationships. Gust Yep's research in communication focuses on the role of ethnicity in health decision making. Finally, Sandra Petronio's research explores how privacy is managed in everyday life. The multidisciplinary approach to the topic provides a unique way to explore how disclosure is managed in the lives of those with HIV.

Kathryn Greene thanks the many people with HIV and their families and friends who participated in the interviews reported in the book. The HIV service organizations in eastern North Carolina were instrumental in this project (namely Pitt County AIDS Service Organization [PICASSO], Eastern North Carolina HIV/AIDS Coalition [ENCHAC], Pitt County Health Department, East Carolina School of Social Work, and East Carolina School of Medicine Department of Pediatrics). Several departments provided support for my research during this project: East Carolina University Department of Communication, University of Wisconsin–Madison Department of Communication Arts, and my current academic home, Rutgers University Department of Communication. I extend gratitude to my parents, Jim and Judy Greene, who provided guidance and support for my education, and encouragement for my career. I also thank my sisters, Karen Dinicola and Kristen Greene, for their humor and tolerance of my passions about my work. I thank Nancy and Ken Church, who lost a daughter to AIDS early in the epidemic, for sharing their experiences (and they express gratitude to Sheila Kay, Karen Person, Curtis Buttenheim, Archie Hahn, Tom Shell, Mimi Davis, Hollywood Helps, the fourth floor nurses at Midway Hospital, and Elizabeth Taylor for funding a room). I am indebted to Don Rubin, Lynda Walters, and Jenny Krugman, who each encouraged me in a unique way to become a more thorough scholar. Thanks are due to the wonderful friends who have listened tirelessly about this and other projects: Jane and Sam, Marina, Rhonda, Karen, Judy, Harrell, Sandra, Stacey, and Yolanda. I express thanks to the Highland Park crew for their humor and support in exploring ways to enjoy such a terrific place to live. I also recognize and thank those who worked on the book project: Angel, Kelly, Susan, Keith, Karen, and Andrea. While this book was in progress, my spirited companion, Ashley, died; Lucy and I miss her presence.

Finally, I extend my gratitude to my fellow aikidoka for gently encouraging me to explore other paths.

Val Derlega expresses thanks and gratitude to the many persons with HIV who participated in interviews reported in the book and to the HIV service organizations in southeastern Virginia (Tidewater Aids Crisis Task Force, Full Circle, Candii House, Peninsula AIDS Foundation, AIDS/HIV Service Group of Charlottesville, Virginia, Fan Free Clinic, and International Black Women's Congress) that have provided assistance in many ways. In particular, thanks are due to Ramona Smith, Gloria Valentine, Jim Spivey, Irma Hinkle, Al Torres, Chris Wilson, Vega Ova, Vann Massie, Alicia Devine, William Devine, Andrew Sterling, Charles Ford, Mitch Rosa, Willliam Ka Agyei, Jimmy Vines, and Reverend Jim Downing. I also express thanks to the faculty and staff at the Center for Comprehensive Care of Immune Deficiency at the Eastern Virginia Medical School, including Edward C. Oldfield III, Sharon Hopson, LuAnn Gahagan, M. Randy Smith, Julie Turner, and Mary Virginia (Ginny) Sealey-Bobby. I also extend thanks to Xiushi Yang at Old Dominion University and for financial support provided by Grant R01DA13145–01A1 from the National Institute on Drug Abuse of the National Institutes of Health. Thanks are also due to Anita Barbee at the University of Louisville's Kent School of Social Work. Gratitude is also due to Robert B. Hays for his generosity and interest in our research. Robert Hays was a brilliant researcher on the social ramifications of living with HIV. Robert Hays passed away recently. I also thank my family, Barbara Winstead, John Derlega, Ann Winstead-Derlega, and Christopher Winstead-Derlega, and the folks in the West Belvedere neighborhood who have given much support and encouragement, particularly Iva Robinett and Bill Robinett. During the time period of working on this book, much good and some pain occurred in my family, including the passing of a gracious and loving person, Lois Winstead.

Gust Yep expresses the following thanks. Many people contributed to my commitment, knowledge, and experience about the daily realities of people living with HIV and AIDS. Because the disease is still a highly stigmatizing one, I do not name them individually. I thank the people on the San Francisco Noe Valley meal delivery route. As a volunteer for Project Open Hand, I brought meals and groceries to you every Monday night for over a year, and you generously shared your lives and stories with me. You made HIV and AIDS very real. Through these visits I learned about the struggles, suffering, joys, courage, and love of people living with this disease. I wish to thank Mark, Emma, Beth, Karen, Amy, and other members of my "family of choice," and Cindy Yep. Your support and love make my life and my work real and meaningful. Finally, I thank Michael, a friend who has lived with HIV for more than 15 years, for showing me how to live with grace, optimism, humor, peace, and love in spite of physical challenges and social adversities. You are truly a role model.

Sandra Petronio wishes to acknowledge a number of people for their thoughtful insights to this volume. Books are written with the knowledge that scholarship from others helps shape and influence the ideas by considering, questioning, and digesting their work. My colleagues have recognized many of those people. I would like to contribute the name of Irwin Altman whose work gave me foundational concepts for the theory of Communication Privacy Management. A hearty thanks to the graduate students I have been fortunate enough to work with over the years at the University of Minnesota, Arizona State University, and Wayne State University. A number of these valued students are now professors in their own right using the CPM theory and illustrating its worth. Dawn Braithwaite at the University of Nebraska, Mary Claire Morr at the University of Denver, Susanne Jones at the University of Wisconsin, Milwaukee, and Jack Sargent at Kean University. Current students who are using CPM at Wayne State University include Laura Andea, Mihaela Gherman, Peggy Reganis, and Jeffrey Younguist who are finishing their PhD degrees. These professors and students are just a few who have contributed to the ideas in found in CPM theory. I would be remiss if I did not thank my friend and husband, Charles R. Bantz for his perceptive and astute comments and my daughter, Kristen E. Petronio who always keeps me anchored. Finally, I am indebted to all of those who have applied CPM theory to significant problems like HIV/AIDS and continue to illustrate that this theoretical base gives us a practical way to approach an understanding of privacy management.

The authors would like to recognize the staff at Lawrence Erlbaum Associates, Inc., in particular Linda Bathgate, the acquisitions editor, for her commitment to this project. We also recognize the contributions of three anonymous reviewers who provided helpful and detailed feedback on drafts of this book. A not so anonymous person who provided feedback on the manuscript with his usual insightful style and wit was Bill Elwood. Jenny Mandelbaum also provided helpful input for chapter 4. Kathryn Greene thanks her friends (Mark, Ben, Yolanda, Eugenio, Stacey, Jan, Judy) for their patience and careful editing. Finally, Kathryn Greene would like to thank her co-authors for their thoughtful insights to this volume.

—*Kathryn Greene*
—*Valerian J. Derlega*
—*Gust A. Yep*
—*Sandra Petronio*

CHAPTER ONE

Introduction

The HIV epidemic has now entered its third decade. Being diagnosed with HIV in 2003 is not the same as in 1983 or even 1993 (e.g., Vázquez-Pacheco, 2000). There have been many changes in the medical management of HIV since the outbreak of the epidemic (e.g., Catz & Kelly, 2001; Sepkowitz, 2001), including the introduction of new combination therapies with promising effects (Bartlett & Gallant, 2001; Hammer, 2002). Yet there is still no vaccine available in the immediate future (Haney, 2002). Individuals infected with HIV with access to combination drug therapies have increased life-span estimates when compared with early epidemic figures, but these drugs may have serious side effects, do not work for all patients, and are not widely available in many countries (Epstein & Chen, 2002). This book is particularly relevant in describing what occurs in countries where the combination therapies (including protease inhibitors) became widely available in the mid to late 1990s and as a consequence where there has been a significant decline in AIDS deaths and reduction in physical symptoms associated with HIV disease. Despite these encouraging medical advances, an HIV diagnosis creates significant anxiety and distress about one's health, self-identity, and close relationships (e.g., Chesney & Smith, 1999; Holt et al., 1998; Winstead et al., 2002).

The profile of persons with HIV has changed, but stigma linking HIV to groups such as men who have sex with men (MSM) and injection drug users (IDUs) continues to persist despite changes in the profile of the epidemic and extensive educational campaigns addressing transmission (Herek & Capitanio, 1999; Herek, Capitanio, & Widaman, 2002). Today, most HIV infections in the world derive from heterosexual transmission, "a fact that is still overlooked by many" (Sepkowitz, 2001, p. 1765). Academic research and health outreach efforts have turned to the personal relationships of people with HIV and to their social interactions with others (see Derlega & Barbee, 1998a; Derlega, Greene, & Frey, 2002; Greene, Frey, & Derlega, 2002). This research and outreach work certainly connects with existing educational campaigns, for example, those targeting transmission routes and stigma, but it differs importantly in its focus on the quality of the interpersonal relationships of those with HIV (see Derlega & Barbee, 1998a; Greene & Serovich, 1998).

One key feature that needs to be understood to address HIV issues is the process of disclosing about an HIV diagnosis. People report great stress around disclosure decisions (e.g., Holt et al., 1998), and the actual revelation itself can become an added trauma (Limandri, 1989). Vázquez-Pacheco (2000) described the dilemma:

> So when exactly do you bring it up? When do you talk about serostatus? Is there ever a good time to talk about it? ... When to have that disclosure discussion remains one of the most difficult decisions for an individual to make in this epidemic. (p. 22)

Not all people with HIV disclose their infection (see chap. 3), but failure to disclose has potential to harm the self, others, and close relationships. Disclosure of HIV status is crucial for both the individual's health and broader health prevention efforts. The goal of this book is to bring together a wide spectrum of information from research literature and organize it into a cohesive framework to generate new questions and identify critical issues about HIV disclosure. One way to provide an organizational structure is to use a theoretical formulation to synthesize research findings in a systematic fashion. We depend on the theory of communication privacy management (CPM) in this book to give us a way to understand the choices that people diagnosed with HIV make about disclosing this information to others (Petronio, 2002). Using a theoretical foundation gives us a way to organize existing information in a more meaningful way to establish additional paths for new research endeavors and more fully understand the existing information. By doing this, we can help those with HIV and those who try to help people with HIV come to some understanding of practical approaches they might take to cope with this disease. This introduction reviews HIV and AIDS statistics, addresses what constitutes disclosure, describes the importance of disclosure, overviews the chapters in the book, and finally reviews the interviews used for the book. First, we turn to a profile of the epidemic worldwide and in the United States.

WORLDWIDE PREVALENCE OF HIV AND AIDS

The United Nations Program on HIV/AIDS (UNAIDS) and the World Health Organization (WHO) reported that through the end of 2001 there were an estimated 40 million people living with HIV around the world (UNAIDS/WHO, 2001). The majority of these HIV cases are in developing countries (95%). There were nearly 3 million AIDS-related deaths estimated in 2001, with nearly 22 million people worldwide who have died from AIDS (Sepkowitz, 2001). Despite earlier estimates predicting the HIV epidemic would peak by 2000, the latest calculations announced at the XIV annual Conference on AIDS in Barcelona, Spain in July of 2002 indicated AIDS will cause an additional 65 million deaths by 2020.

This figure is more than three times the number who died in the first 20 years of the epidemic, reflecting the underestimate of rapidly expanding HIV in many developing countries.

AIDS is the leading cause of death in sub-Saharan Africa, and HIV infection is rapidly increasing in both South and Southeast Asia (particularly China), Europe (particularly Russia), and the Caribbean and Latin America. In some countries, more than 30% of adults are infected (UNAIDS, 2001). There is great diversity in how countries are affected, some with more than 10% of their population with HIV, but many countries with less than 1% seroprevalence. The differences in location or specific populations at risk vary by country. However, there is similarity in infection in young people ages 15 to 24 in most countries. The profile of those infected currently highlights dramatic increases in infection in Asia and Africa and is roughly equal by sex (48% of adult infections worldwide are in women). The U.S. HIV/AIDS profile differs significantly, as we describe next.

PREVALENCE OF HIV AND AIDS IN THE UNITED STATES

This book focuses primarily on experiences with HIV in the United States. Statistics related to HIV change rapidly. Currently, the two best sources for HIV statistics information are available at www.cdc.gov/hiv/pubs/mmwr.htm (MMWR-Morbidity and Mortality Weekly Report) and www.cdc.gov/hiv/stats/hasrlink.htm (HIV/AIDS Surveillance Reports). We highlight recent figures here but encourage people to review updated figures. Sepkowitz (2001) provides two useful tables describing the chronology of the AIDS epidemic in the United States.

The U.S. Centers for Disease Control and Prevention (CDC; 2002) revealed that a total of 816,149 AIDS cases had been reported in the United States through December 2001. AIDS-related deaths in the United States total 467,910. To put this in perspective, this number is more than the total number of Americans who died in World Wars I and II combined (see Sepkowitz, 2001). AIDS cases have decreased dramatically since 1996 (when highly active antiretroviral therapies, or HAART, were introduced), but the rate of decline has slowed considerably in the past 2 years (HIV/AIDS Surveillance Report, 2002). As a note, these cases are for AIDS, not HIV infection, as criteria for HIV reporting to the CDC varies by state. The demographics of these reported AIDS cases in the U.S. included 82% men and 1% children under age 13. Among those who have been diagnosed with AIDS, 42% are White, 38% are Black, 18% are Hispanic, and lower percentages from other ethnic backgrounds. Of the people known to have AIDS, 45% were men who were infected when having sex with another man (MSM); 25% were infected by sharing needles when engaged in injection drug use (IDU).

The face of the HIV epidemic in the United States changed dramatically in the 1990s (CDC, 1999). Specifically, data indicate a growing proportion of HIV cases among Blacks and Hispanics and in women and a decreasing proportion among men who have sex with men. There are also trends indicating increasing infections in adolescents. Specifically, persons aged 13 to 24 accounted for 15% of reported HIV cases in 1999. There has been a sharp decline in perinatal transmission in the United States in the 1990s, possibly linked to increased testing in pregnant women or new delivery protocols for women with HIV or both. Particular attention has also been focused recently on new infections in minority women. Women accounted for 32% of HIV cases reported in 1999 (CDC, 1999), with Blacks and Hispanics comprising 77% of cases in women and 59% of cases in men. Thus, the U.S. profile shows increases in adolescents and minority (especially Black and Hispanic) women, with continued infection in MSM and IDUs.

These figures alone, worldwide and in the United States, indicate many people are affected and will be affected by HIV. One significant issue these people must confront is whether and when to share this information. This book focuses on that process, often labeled *disclosure*.

WHAT IS DISCLOSURE?

These alarming figures both in the United States and worldwide illustrate the obvious need for a better understanding of ways to assist people with HIV in coping with the disease and to stop the spread of HIV. One prominent public health recommendation for people with HIV is to disclose or tell others about their diagnosis, especially their sexual partners (see Rothenberg & Paskey, 1995). This longstanding disclosure recommendation has not been without controversy. In particular, many states have adopted laws encouraging or mandating notification of sexual partners (see Burris, 2001; Rothenberg & Paskey, 1995), and this is a major component of the public health response to the HIV epidemic.

People do not indiscriminately reveal private information, however, because doing so would make them feel too vulnerable (Gilbert, 1976; Petronio, 2002). People more than likely calculate how much they want to tell, when they want to tell, and who they want to tell for the very reason that the information is risky (Petronio, 1991, 2002). Often, when people consider disclosure of HIV status, they are dealing with a decision to allow access to the information to someone and to deny access to others. Consequently, when people refer to "private information," they mean that the information is based on facts and feelings to which others would not normally have access (Derlega, Metts, Petronio, & Margulis, 1993). CPM theory (Petronio, 2002) helps one see that regulating access is important because people often think about private information as something that belongs to them, and in conjunction with the possibility of feeling vulnerable, they want to control who else is privy to the information. When people disclose private information, they may do so by giving complete access through making a full disclosure, giving partial access (selectively disclosing), or restricting access by keeping the information secret (Bok, 1984; Kelly, 2002). It is useful to note here that information about the HIV diagnosis may be considered either private or secret. Private information refers to information about oneself that others might not normally have access to but that is not actively hidden from them, whereas secret information is actively withheld from most others. In this book, we use the term *private information* as an overarching concept that includes secrets (see Bok, 1984; Derlega et al., 1993; Kelly, 2002; Petronio, 2002).

The privacy and disclosure process consists of at least two individuals engaged in a social interaction, each with her or his own feelings, beliefs, attitudes, values, and expectations, and the behavior of both persons is affected by the social, psychological, relational, and physical context. Personal or private information is shared by one person to another specific person or persons. This distinguishes self-disclosure from public disclosure. In public disclosure, for example when the tennis star Arthur Ashe[1] announced via a press conference that he had AIDS (Ashe & Rampersad, 1993; Winston, 1992; Wright, 1999) or Mary Fisher (1992, Fisher is an AIDS activist) announced that she had AIDS at the Republican National Convention, the recipient of the information is difficult to identify (the "general public"). These public disclosure decisions are broad and sweeping, with little control over who knows the information. Self-disclosure, on the other hand, involves intentionally sharing one's private or intimate information with another person (or several people; Dindia, 1997). Disclosure is also generally considered voluntary, that is, a person makes a choice to tell another (without undue threat, coercion, deception, reading a diary, overhearing, etc.). *Disclosure* or *nondisclosure*, as we use the terms, focus on people choosing to share or not share personal information with others.

Disclosure may be relatively infrequent in naturally occurring conversation (Dindia, Fitzpatrick, & Kenny, 1997), yet it carries tremendous relational consequences and is crucial in relational development and maintenance (e.g., Dindia, 2002; Omarzu, 2000). For relationship development, disclosure serves to help get to know another person, and for relational maintenance disclosure allows people to "catch up" with one another. Self-disclosure was originally seen as a trait (e.g., Jourard, 1971); that is, some individuals simply like to share personal information about themselves with others more and some less. An alternative view is that self-disclosure is affected by situational and social contextual factors (e.g., Altman & Taylor, 1973), such as the place where people are interacting (at home or in a public setting), community or cultural attitudes about appropriateness of disclosure, as well as the type of relationship between the discloser and the potential disclosure recipient (e.g., friends, lovers, parents and children, coworkers, health professionals and their clients). Although we do not want to underestimate the possible

---

[1] In the early 1990s, after Magic Johnson announced his HIV infection, tennis star Arthur Ashe went public with his infection. For some time after his diagnosis, Ashe told only those close to him (to avoid any stigma for his family, particularly his young daughter). In 1992, Ashe discovered that *USA Today* was planning to run a story about his HIV infection and he went public at that point. This case, different from Magic Johnson and Mary Fisher, focused on mode of infection. Ashe received blood transfusions during heart bypass surgeries in 1979 and 1983 (prior to mandatory testing of donated blood that began in 1985). In 1988, Ashe went in for further surgery and discovered his HIV infection.

impact of traits and temperament on self-disclosure (see Kelly, 2002), we emphasize in our book the role of situational and social contextual factors affecting HIV
disclosure.

The content of disclosure can reflect a direct message (e.g., "I have AIDS") or
more indirect messages (e.g., "I'm sick," or leaving medical reports for another to
see; Derlega et al., 1993; Petronio, 1991; also see detailed discussion in chap. 4).
Disclosure of private information can include what medical professionals may
term "disclosing a diagnosis," specifically, physicians telling patients about their
condition. However, the nature of disclosure in the physician's case has to do with
revealing a diagnosis by someone who is not personally affected by the disease.
Consequently, although the physician tells the patient pertinent information that
is more relevant to the patient than to the physician personally, the information
belongs to the patient and not to the physician. A medical disclosure of this type
poses a unique situation in which the information actually belongs to the patient,
but the physician is included because he or she is instrumental is making the patient aware of the condition (Petronio, 2002). Many times people share information that is relevant to others personally. As a result, although these people are
messengers, they know something private about others and people with HIV
want them to help control further dissemination. To do that, people typically rely
either on implicit professional expectations about doctor–patient confidentiality
or explicitly negotiate privacy rules for revealing and concealing medical information such as HIV status. Although this type of disclosure condition occurs with
people who have HIV, much of our discussion about disclosure focuses on how individuals manage their own telling about the diagnosis or collectively work with
friends and family to manage other people knowing their diagnosis.

With advances in the treatment of HIV using protease inhibitors and combination therapies (e.g., Bartlett & Gallant, 2001), there has been a sharp drop in the
number of people dying from AIDS-related illnesses. As a consequence, people
with HIV (and their loved ones) are focusing more on how to maintain close relationships and to initiate new relationships with others. This increased focus on
close and personal relationships is reflected in an upswing in research on close relationships among individuals living with HIV (e.g., Derlega & Barbee, 1998a;
Greene et al., 2002; Kalichman, 2000; Winstead et al., 2002). This book integrates
literature on disclosure with relationships of people living with HIV. The distinctive role of HIV disclosure, which involves whether or not to disclose to others
about a potentially life-threatening disease that is often associated with stigma and
prejudice, is the central topic of this book. This book captures the distinctive role
of HIV disclosure and offers some insights into the way researchers can address a
critical need for those infected by the virus and those affected by people with HIV.
As such, this book exclusively concentrates on disclosures about an HIV positive
diagnosis and not about disclosure issues of people who are diagnosed as
seronegative after testing. The latter topic also is important and there is a lot of decision making about this sort of HIV disclosure, too. However, this book is about
living with HIV and its disclosure ramifications.

THE IMPORTANCE OF HIV DISCLOSURE

HIV disclosure as a research and media topic has received increasing attention over the last decade. First, there are possible advantages to the person with HIV and to significant others associated with choosing to disclose.

- Individuals living with HIV who disclose to selected target people may gain access to social support. To receive assistance (e.g., access to money for medication, child care when ill, or transportation to a physician's office), it may be necessary to disclose. Beyond these instrumental or tangible support needs, an individual with HIV also may want to talk about the illness or plan for the future, and disclosure is necessary to obtain this support as well. Hence, by having others to confide in, infected individuals can build a social support system (Remien, Rabkin, Williams, & Katoff, 1992; Serovich, Brucker, & Kimberly, 2000).

- In the case of sexual partners, HIV disclosure can provide others with information that allows both the person with HIV and his or her sexual partner to make choices that could lower the risk of HIV transmission. There are instances in which not knowing a person's HIV status could put another at risk. For example, if a sexual partner (current or potential) were told about the HIV diagnosis, then one or both parties could use condoms (or dental dams, gloves, finger cots) or choose to modify sexual risk behavior. Following HIV disclosure, the sexual partners might also choose not to be sexually intimate, not to engage in specific behaviors, or not to share needles.

- Disclosure can provide direct health benefits to the discloser. People with HIV are at greater risk for contracting sexually transmitted diseases due to compromised immune systems (Kalichman, 2000). Thus, if disclosure of HIV status results in condom use (or other protective behaviors), this provides direct health benefits for the person with HIV as well. Even couples in which both partners live with HIV can infect each other with modified strains of HIV (Kalichman, 2000). Also, if others are aware of an individual's HIV status, they may be able to warn the infected person about potential health threats such as possible exposure to someone who has chicken pox or another virus.

- People who disclose their HIV diagnosis may also obtain more appropriate medical treatment. People who have not told medical personnel about their HIV status may complicate medical management of other illnesses. This can even extend to not sharing what medications are taken with all physicians, with possible drug interaction effects (Bartlett & Gallant, 2001).

- Disclosing an HIV diagnosis could potentially reduce stigma associated with HIV and AIDS. To date, changes in public perception of the epidemic have been slow at best. Many people still report not knowing anyone with HIV (e.g., Greene, Parrott, & Serovich,1993, reported that less than one fourth of their sample of college students, parents of young children, and parents of college students, indicated personally knowing a person with HIV), although most likely they do know people with HIV and are unaware of it.

• A person could decrease his or her stress by disclosing to a trustworthy confidant. Keeping secrets may be stressful (Lepore & Smyth, 2002; Pennebaker, 1995), and worrying about to whom and when to disclose about the HIV diagnosis may be an additional psychological and physical burden. HIV disclosure to supportive disclosure recipients, other things being equal, has the possibility of increasing life span and improving mental and physical health (e.g., de Vroome, de Wit, Stroebe, Sandfort, & Griensven, 1998). This idea is based on research suggesting that holding in thoughts and feelings might lead to chronic stress and in turn to weakened immune system functioning (e.g., Booth & Petrie, 2002; Cole, Kemeny, Taylor, Visscher, & Fahey, 1996; see also Lutgendorf & Ullrich, 2002).

• Disclosing may bring the person with HIV into a closer relationship with others. Although there are possible risks associated with HIV disclosure, someone who is told about the diagnosis might feel trusted, bringing him or her closer to the person who disclosed. People who are not told may view HIV nondisclosure (once they find out the information) as a violation of the relationship (especially family, friends, and intimate partners; see, e.g., Greene & Faulkner, 2002). People who find out about the diagnosis may also feel they should have been told earlier. The overlap in concerns about HIV disclosure and close relationships is explored throughout this book.

SUMMARY OF HIV DISCLOSURE

Although reasons for HIV disclosure may be compelling, there are also possible disadvantages (and risks) to the person with HIV and to significant others associated with HIV disclosure (Derlega, Lovejoy, & Winstead, 1998; Derlega, Winstead, Greene, Serovich, & Elwood, 2002; Greene & Serovich, 1996; Kelly, 2002; Petronio, 2002). Documentation of risks (including discrimination, violence, and rejection) for people who disclose their HIV diagnosis is extensive (e.g., Leary & Schreindorfer, 1998), and many individuals with HIV report negative responses to at least some of their disclosures. Table 1.1 presents a list of some reported negative and positive consequences of disclosing HIV status. This list is derived from interviews described later in this chapter and from other research.

Because it is clear that those who do not disclose and still participate in sexual and drug related risky behavior can spread HIV to others, one way to further prevent the spread of HIV and possibly increase life quality for individuals with HIV is to understand why people are reluctant to reveal their status (or not disclose). For some persons with HIV, there is a code of silence around HIV (Elwood, 2002; Vázquez-Pacheco, 2000) in which some do not want to know their HIV status (and would not know what to do if positive) so they even avoid HIV testing (or disclosing if they are infected with HIV). Numerous factors contribute to the reason people may seek to withhold information about their HIV diagnosis from others. The difficulty arises when protection of a person's status potentially contributes to the spread of HIV and can also threaten the infected individual's health. In both cases, there are risks and benefits to consider, and many individuals report great

TABLE 1.1

Some Reported Negative and Positive Consequences of Disclosing an HIV Diagnosis

Negative	Positive
Ostracism	Relationship became closer
Physical violence	Educated others
Blaming	Others were tested
Relationship ends (also divorce)	Practiced lower risk behaviors
Cannot see children, nieces, nephews	Able to talk about stresses
Lost housing, evicted	Reminded to take medications, eat well
Fired from job, not hired	Others prepared meals, helped around the house
Lost insurance	Assisted with child care
People do not speak to you	Financial assistance (rent, meals, medication)
Asked to leave church (and other groups)	Met others with HIV
Disowned (by parents/family)	Received help with filling out forms, using Internet
People will not eat food prepared	Joined support group, visited AIDS service
Do not want to burden other	organization

Note. These descriptions are derived from interviews reported in this book and other research (e.g., Derlega et al., 1998; Greene & Faulkner, 2002; Greene & Serovich, 1996; Hays et al., 1993; Marks et al., 1992; Marks, Cantero, & Simoni, 1998; Serovich, Kimberly, & Greene, 1998; Simoni et al., 1995; Winstead et al., 2002).

distress around decisions to conceal or reveal their illness (e.g., Greene & Faulkner, 2002; Holt et al., 1998; Winstead et al., 2002). Thus, disclosure is a critical issue to investigate, as this book illustrates.

CHAPTER OVERVIEWS

After this introductory chapter, the second chapter presents an overview of CPM theory (Petronio, 2002). The third chapter examines predictors of disclosure or what variables influence decisions to disclose or not disclose an HIV positive diagnosis. The fourth chapter describes the features and content of the HIV disclosure messages along with examination of timing and setting of these disclosures. The fifth chapter explores the consequences of HIV disclosure and nondisclosure decisions. The sixth chapter is the epilogue, which looks to the future of HIV disclosure issues. The appendix provides exercises, measures, and practical applications of disclosure research for individuals with HIV and those working with clients with HIV and their families.

Chapter 2: CPM and HIV Disclosure

In this chapter, the theory of CPM is presented (Petronio, 2002). As a practical theory, CPM is used in this book to organize the existing research literature on disclosure and HIV. Given the disparate nature of the research, this theory provides a core set of concepts from which new ways of understanding the problems associated with HIV disclosure emerge. This theory is predicated on the notion that people believe private information is something that belongs to them. Individuals want to control the flow of that information because they perceive that they own it, and revealing private information often has the potential to make them feel vulnerable. Consequently, we can more easily think about this information if we first use a boundary metaphor to illustrate the parameters that people set around their private information. Next, if we consider that people regulate the flow of their information through privacy rules, or what CPM calls a rule management system, we are able to see the way that people control that flow to others. Cast in this way, we can begin to envision how people with HIV tend to manage the dialectical tensions of privacy and disclosure by the way they control revealing to or concealing their HIV status from others.

Chapter 2 articulates the fundamental structure and processes of the CPM rule management system. Because the rule system is the key to grasping the decision criteria for telling HIV status or concealing it, knowing the underlying judgment heuristics people use when they develop privacy rules is critically important. In this chapter, we learn how privacy rules are formulated, adjusted, and changed when they are no longer function. For many who learn of their HIV status, the rules used to judge the level of privacy they wish to maintain often change. They may no longer feel comfortable talking to their partners or spouses about their health. Consequently, they may need to change an old rule (they always tell their partner about health problems) to a new privacy rule that limits what they tell their partners or spouses about health issues. We also learn that the theory provides a way to understand the fact that when individuals disclose private information, they link other people into their private boundaries. Doing so means that individuals make others co-owners of the information. As such, they need to negotiate or coordinate which privacy rules they will use to regulate third-party disclosures or which rules are used to restrict others from knowing.

Boundary coordination takes place once people disclose and others are linked into the privacy boundary. Coordination represents the process of negotiating privacy rules. When successfully agreed on rules become synchronized among the co-owners, the coordination process to run smoothly. However, we do not live in a perfect world; as a result, we also face boundary turbulence. Turbulence reflects situations when the negotiation of privacy rules managing the boundaries around private information fail to work. This failure may occur because co-owners or confidants violate a trust, mistakenly use the wrong rules, have difficulty because the rules are ambiguous, the original disclosers believe that confidants are capable of keeping confidences (and they are not), confidants misjudge the rules, or they completely ignore their agreement to abide by mutually negotiated privacy rules.

Boundary turbulence suggested by CPM has significant consequences for both the owner of private information and the confidant. Particularly when we examine the communicative interactions between individuals diagnosed with HIV and family members, partners, and/or friends, finding themselves in a turbulent situation regarding the disclosure of their HIV status can be traumatic. This chapter acquaints the reader with CPM theory as it is applied to the disclosure process for people with HIV. The theory offers a way to grasp how individuals grapple with regulating the revealing and concealing of their HIV diagnosis.

Chapter 3: Decisions to Disclose or Not Disclose About an HIV Positive Diagnosis

This chapter explores what predicts or explains decisions to disclose (or not) about the HIV infection to another. These explanations reflect the tension and uncertainty (whether or not to tell someone, how to tell someone) about finding out about the HIV diagnosis. Disclosure of HIV status is a complex communication event involving high levels of vulnerability and risk, and these decisions are processed carefully.

We first explore how HIV-related stigma affects HIV disclosure decisions. The perceived risk from HIV stigma stems from perceptions of possible negative emotional reactions, fear of infection and contagion, disapproval, and failing to contribute. For any of these aspects of stigma, if individuals with HIV anticipate a stigmatizing response, they likely will not choose to disclose.

The next portion of the chapter explores differences in motivations for disclosure based on self-, other-, and interpersonal-gain. People often disclose to gain some benefit for themselves. In the context of HIV, self-gain motivations include catharsis and seeking help. However, people also disclose based on what the other might gain. For individuals with HIV, other-gain motivations include duty to inform and educating others. People also disclose based on interpersonal considerations. Interpersonal motivations include testing others' reactions, establishing emotionally close and supportive relationships, and common experiences. These self-, other-, and interpersonal-based criteria can serve as motivations to disclose, but people also have motives for nondisclosure or maintaining privacy. Decisions to disclose an HIV diagnosis also include privacy protection. Hence, we explore motivations for nondisclosure including third-party leakage, self-blame or self-concept difficulties, fear of rejection or being misunderstood, and protecting others.

The final section of the chapter examines the relational influences on disclosure decisions. First, anticipated response can explain disclosure decisions. If people think a recipient may respond poorly to a disclosure, they would be less likely to share an HIV diagnosis. Next, strength of relational ties might explain disclosure. That is, the role may be important in deciding whether to disclose. Chapter 3 describes disclosure decisions in eight specific targets or roles: partner or lover, parent(s), siblings, children, friends, family, coworkers, and health care workers. Disclosure decisions may also be affected by past discussion of HIV in which a person who has discussed these issues previously might be more inclined to share an HIV diagnosis. Individuals with HIV may also choose to bring up the general topic of AIDS to see the reaction before they decide to disclose. Perceived relational quality may also influence disclosure decisions beyond strength of relational ties. People who are close to their mothers may be more likely to disclose a diagnosis to them sooner because they are close, beyond simply the mother's role as a parent. The discloser's past experience with sharing the diagnosis may also affect decisions. If people had difficult episodes in the past (e.g., a bad reaction such as violence or gossip), they may be less willing to disclose. Finally, culture may influence disclosure decisions, specifically gender and ethnicity.

Chapter 4: Features of HIV Disclosure Messages

In this chapter, we focus on the actual disclosure process and messages once a decision has been made to share the HIV diagnosis. We explore both verbal and alternative disclosure messages. The major areas covered in this chapter are mode of communication, context, and message features.

We first examine the communication mode or channel. These include differences between face-to-face and non-face-to-face disclosure. Specifically, people may disclose in person in the same room or they may send a letter, e-mail, and so forth. These choices of mode affect the message itself and how the recipient can respond. Additionally, this chapter examines third-party or indirect disclosure, both voluntary and not. For instance, perhaps a person's sister revealed the brother's diagnosis to their mother, and this could have been requested or not.

Next, the chapter looks at contextual considerations, specifically effects of the setting and timing on HIV disclosure. The setting (such as the physical context of the disclosure) affects perceptions of privacy and appropriateness, and the discloser may select a more equivocal message in public but a more direct message in private. Timing of disclosure can also be a factor in disclosure messages. For instance, disclosing about HIV status on a first date may be perceived as appropriate or inappropriate, but in another situation it might be a practical assessment of relational potential. Three aspects of timing are explored: when to disclose after learning a diagnosis, whether it is spontaneous or preplanned, and when within a conversation to disclose.

The chapter then examines specific HIV disclosure message features including directness, length, and content. The directness section includes discussion of the level of specificity or abstractness of the disclosure message. Messages can also vary in length from extremely brief to long and involved. Finally, the disclosure message content may contain information in addition to the HIV diagnosis, such as unknown sexual partners, sexual orientation, or drug use. That is, a person may share that he or she was diagnosed with HIV but also choose to share past sexual history in addition to the diagnosis.

The last section of the chapter explores what may be modes beyond verbal disclosure for revealing one's HIV diagnosis to others. The chapter discusses, for instance, the role of body language (e.g., physical symptoms such as "wasting") or of providing environmental props (e.g., leaving medications in view in the bathroom or refrigerator) to disclose about the HIV diagnosis.

Chapter 5: Consequences of HIV Disclosure and Nondisclosure Decision Making

The decision to disclose or not to disclose to others about the HIV diagnosis can have numerous outcomes. The chapter begins by summarizing reports of actual responses to HIV disclosure. Many of the responses to disclosing an HIV positive diagnosis may be helpful and supportive, yet there may be adverse social consequences of self-disclosure of the HIV diagnosis. Individuals—or their loved ones—may be shunned, discriminated against, or blamed for what happened. In some cases, individuals with HIV may be subject to verbal and/or physical abuse (see van der Straten, King, et al., 1998; Vlahov et al., 1998).

Next we examine the relation between disclosure and social support by looking at types of social support, coping, satisfaction, support groups or activism, and identity. One's role in a social network is significant for both physical and mental health. One possible outcome for those who disclose is accessing this social support to assist in coping with the disease; however, not all support is helpful.

We then turn to one especially difficult outcome of HIV disclosure: stigma. Many people with HIV report experiences with stigma, although the extent of these experiences varies a great deal. For some individuals, stigmatizing responses (including being treated differently) are the dominant outcome of disclosing, but for others these responses are more isolated (see Alonzo & Reynolds, 1995; Derlega et al., 2002; Fife & Wright, 2000; Greene & Faulkner, 2002). Our discussion of HIV stigma examines outcomes based on misinformation, group bias, and courtesy stigma.

The final section on consequences of HIV disclosure decisions looks at the outcomes of disclosing on close relationships. First, we look at how HIV disclosure affects relationship closeness, as disclosing can increase, decrease, or have no affect on the quality of the relationship. Then we look at how significant others can be caregivers, including promoting medication adherence and providing daily assistance. Next, we explore one specific relationship consequence—relationships with children after HIV disclosure. Finally, we examine how HIV disclosure affects safer sex and other risk behaviors in intimate relationships.

Although much of this chapter focuses on the impact of disclosure for persons with HIV, we also consider the impact of the decision to disclose or not disclose on others. People also choose to maintain privacy or not disclose, and this has consequences. Individuals with HIV report conflicted feelings about others' right to know the diagnosis. They may also see nondisclosure as a form of informational control, and this control at times breaks down if others share the diagnosis. Finally, nondisclosure can be a form of psychological inhibition.

Chapter 6: Epilogue: Looking to the Future of Disclosure and HIV

This closing chapter looks to future issues that involve HIV disclosure. For example, new drug combination therapies have potential to affect disclosure decisions. If there is a change in perception of HIV from a terminal to chronic illness, there may be more willingness to disclose. Additionally, with changes in the demographics of the epidemic, it is important to continue to assess changes in cultural attitudes about HIV and HIV-related stigma. Public perception of the epidemic in the United States still focuses on homosexuality and injection drug use, even though adolescents and women of color are now the fastest growing infection groups. As Herek et al. (2002) reported, stigma has decreased in some areas (e.g., support for quarantine) yet increased in others (e.g., inaccurate beliefs about some risks of casual social contact and belief that people with HIV deserve their illness). Also, the development of a vaccine to prevent HIV infection—if and when it happens—would change disclosure and relational issues in ways that are difficult to anticipate.

Appendix: Resources for Individuals Living With HIV, Their Significant Others, Researchers, and Health Professionals

In this appendix, we discuss many of the potential applications of the theory and research findings that we have presented throughout this book. Understanding the why, what, when, and how of the disclosure process can assist health care providers, mental health professionals, public policy specialists, health campaign planners, public health message designers, community volunteers, public advocates, behavioral researchers, and anyone who is involved in the HIV and AIDS epidemic to communicate more appropriately and sensitively, and ultimately, more competently.

The appendix examines issues that could be used, as appropriate, to empower individuals in making the decision about whom to tell or not to tell about the HIV positive diagnosis. We do not prescribe that everyone (or even anyone in one's social network) must be told about the diagnosis. However, we illustrate the benefits and costs of this decision making. We illustrate via social-skill building techniques how individuals might actually disclose about the HIV diagnosis to others. These illustrations are based on knowledge acquired from interpersonal skill training and the actual experiences of people with HIV who felt successful in disclosing about the diagnosis to particular others. Overall, this assumes individuals must assess what their goals are for disclosure and nondisclosure and have the confidence and social skills to act on these decisions.

Next, we present a number of research tools (measures) such as a questionnaire focusing on the reasons for and against self-disclosure. These questionnaires might be useful to individuals with HIV, health professionals, and researchers in understanding the pros and cons of disclosure–nondisclosure. These measures are presented so an individual could easily fill them out, but we also present information about past use and how to score the measures. Finally, we present a summary of HIV-related resources that may be useful such as magazines, books, Web sites, telephone numbers, and academic journals.

INTERVIEWS UTILIZED IN THIS PROJECT

Accounts about HIV disclosure for this book project came from a combination of three groups of projects, all semistructured or directed interviews. Quotes from these interviews are used extensively and set as extracts throughout the book to illustrate concepts discussed. Where quotes are presented in chapters in this book (unless specifically cited), they came from interviews described here. The procedure and samples for some of the interviews we reference here.

Initial interviews were conducted with men and women with HIV living in Virginia in the early 1990s (Derlega & Barbee, 1994). The sample and procedure for these interviews is described in detail in Barbee, Derlega, Sherburne, and Grimshaw (1998). Another set of interviews (Derlega & Barbee, 1998b) was conducted among women living with HIV in the late 1990s in Virginia (see Winstead et al., 2002, for method details).

The second set of projects began in the latter 1990s in North Carolina. These 10 initial interviews with African American adolescents infected with HIV are described in Greene and Faulkner (2002). These interviews were supplemented by additional interviews using a similar interview guide between 2000 and 2002 in North Carolina, Wisconsin, and New Jersey/New York. These supplemental interviews included an additional 27 individuals living with HIV and 23 of their family members, partners, or social network members. The supplemental interviews were more specific in questions about disclosure message content, timing, and setting (see chap. 4). The third and final project was comprised of interviews conducted by G. Yep in San Francisco from 1997 to 1998.

CONCLUSIONS

We focus in this book on decisions of whether or not to disclose about the HIV positive status, its antecedents, consequences, and how it is done. We acknowledge that there is more to HIV disclosure than whether or not others are told about the diagnosis. For instance, disclosing about the HIV diagnosis may include a description of one's feelings about having this disease, a description of behaviors that may have put one at risk of infection, as well as a description of how the person with HIV (as well as loved ones) will "move on" now with medical management of the disease, relationships, family, work, and life generally. Also, once someone is told about the diagnosis, people with HIV may go back to that person from time to time, often, or never with further information about how one is coping or adjusting to the diagnosis. These are all important aspects of HIV disclosure that deserve research attention. Nevertheless, a unique contribution of this book is that we show how people with HIV cope with the complex set of problems and range of issues affecting who, when, and how to tell someone about the HIV positive diagnosis itself. We present a synthesis of information and through using the frame of CPM theory (Petronio, 2002), we are able to identify new directions and needed research that can get to the heart of many persons' concerns surrounding HIV disclosure.

CHAPTER TWO

Communication Privacy Management and HIV Disclosure

People who are HIV positive must confront a series of difficult decisions when they consider disclosing their HIV status. This chapter offers a theoretical map that lays a foundation to understand when people choose to reveal their HIV diagnosis, when they refrain from making that status known to others, and the consequences of these choices. To study how and why people conceal or reveal their HIV status, we apply Petronio's (2002) theory of *communication privacy management* (CPM) to understand the decisions people with HIV make about disclosing or concealing their illness (e.g., Greene & Faulkner, 2002; Greene & Serovich, 1996; Petronio, 2000a; Petronio, Reeder, Hecht, & Mon't Ros-Mendoza, 1996; Yep, 2000).

Focusing on the CPM theory gives us a heuristic to illustrate the interconnection between opening up and disclosing about the HIV diagnosis or withholding information. People are social beings with needs to connect as well as needs to separate from others. In many ways, this is the paradox of the HIV dilemma. There are conditions that justify withholding information about a person's HIV status from others. Colleagues at work might disengage interpersonally if they know, family members might find it difficult to cope with the knowledge, and friends may not understand how to help. For example, MSM may conceal their HIV status when others do not know their sexual orientation (e.g., Marks et al., 1992). Yet, to obtain the much needed social support or because others may be affected, disclosure is necessary. The key to navigating the markers between private lives and shared ones is people's decisions to open up completely, partially, or keep their privacy boundaries closed. However, every decision has a consequence that may complicate future privacy maintenance depending on who is told, when someone is told, how much is told, and what is told about the diagnosis.

CPM

CPM is a practical theory that is applied to understand the way that people manage the dialectical tensions of disclosure and privacy of an HIV diagnosis

(Petronio, 2002). The theory can be understood by considering two domains: suppositions that underpin the theory and a rule management system that together represent the way people regulate privacy and disclosure (Petronio, 2002). Figure 2.1 proposes the relations among the elements of the CPM theory.

Suppositions

There are five suppositions that form the basis of the theory (i.e., privacy dialectics, privacy boundaries, private information, control/ownership, and privacy rules). Because these suppositions are interrelated, thereby giving the theory its base, they are discussed as an integrated whole.

To understand CPM theory, it is useful to recognize that Petronio (2002) assumes neither privacy nor disclosure stands separate from each other. Rather,

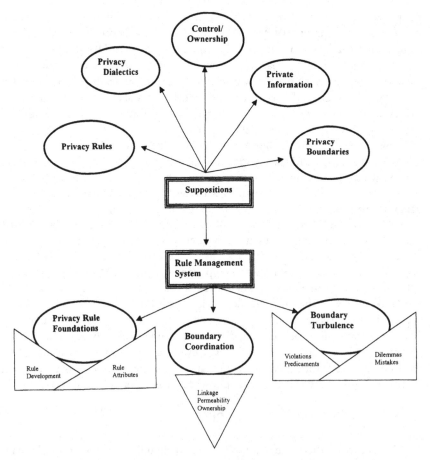

FIG. 2.1   Communication privacy management theory.

they are viewed in dialectical tension with each other. Consequently, the theory does not argue that to have one you have to give up the other. Because disclosure and privacy are defined as dialectical tensions, it is difficult to imagine disclosure without privacy. Likewise, we cannot see the reverse because when you reveal something, you still maintain some measure of privacy.

In addition to this fundamental idea, CPM uses a boundary metaphor to illustrate how people mark private information (Petronio, 2002). Boundaries serve as a useful metaphor to exemplify the way the management process functions for people (Derlega & Chaikin, 1977; Petronio, 1991, 2002). Given the dialectical tensions between making private information known to others and keeping it hidden from view, the notion of boundaries makes it easier to comprehend the choices to make private (and possibly secret) information public and keep it hidden from view. The extent to which something is private or secret depends on the level of control people wish to have over the information. CPM argues that the more risky the information, as we find with secrets, the more need for boundary control.

In general, privacy boundaries can shift and change over the life span, growing to accommodate responsibility for more private information. Boundaries may also shrink when private information is necessarily given up, for example, when older people in nursing homes need to disclose a great deal about their personal information to secure medical attention (Petronio, 2002) or a person with HIV must tell a provider to coordinate medical care. Typically, people manage two types of privacy boundaries: personal and collective. In other words, CPM argues that people develop personal boundaries around information that they see belonging to only them. However, because people do disclose, private information that is shared becomes collective in nature (i.e., two people know the information). Further disclosure of the information can extend the boundary to include more than two people evolving into a larger collective boundary. Consequently, people may manage personal, dyadic, group, family, or organizational privacy boundaries.

As this discussion illustrates, not only is the boundary expanding to incorporate more people, the nature of the private information also fundamentally changes. Along with the expanding boundary lines, CPM theory argues that private information can be "owned" by one person (i.e., personally private information). However, when it is disclosed, the original owner shares responsibilities for managing the privacy boundary with someone else and it becomes co-owned (even if we do not necessarily define it that way—the other person knows the information).

The early work on self-disclosure is most illustrative of the meaning given personally private information (Derlega et al., 1993). However, CPM proposes that disclosure (even about the self) is a process and private information is what we reveal. Consequently, we can own private information about ourselves such as an HIV diagnosis; however, when we tell others, they take part in managing revealing and concealing, making it co-owned. Thus, when private information is the provenance of one person (personally private boundary), the individual determines the rules to control disclosure. However, when the information is shared or becomes collectively co-owned, all people who know the information are expected to negotiate the rules that control the level of revealing and concealing. The reason rule negotiations are critical is all people within the collective privacy boundary are held accountable for following those revealing and concealing rules.

In addition, rules help the people within the privacy boundary feel they have control over the information defined as belonging to them or for which they have some level of responsibility. Rules give a sense of control, an essential element because not only do people see the ability to manage private information as their right of ownership but also even partial disclosure of their information may result in feelings of vulnerability, particularly important with HIV-related stigma.

To understand the dynamic nature of privacy management, the level of access or protection of private information for both personal and collective boundaries varies across a continuum. CPM proposes that rules regulate privacy boundaries in ways that allow for complete access to the private information (full disclosure), partial access (selective disclosure), or restricted access/full protection (secrets) (Petronio, 1991, 2002).

Rule Management System

The rule-based system that CPM theory proposes to manage the dialectical tensions of privacy and disclosure consists of three management processes (Petronio, 2002). The first management process focuses on the foundations of privacy rules. The second management process concerns the way privacy boundaries are coordinated between and among people. The third management process involves situations in which people are unable to regulate their privacy boundaries in ways that are useful. This process is called *boundary turbulence*.

PRIVACY RULE MANAGEMENT PROCESS 1:
RULE FOUNDATIONS

Privacy rule foundations incorporate both the way that rules are developed and the attributes they possess (Petronio, 2002). To understand how people with HIV handle the management of concealing and revealing, it is useful to know the criteria on which they formulate the rules used to judge whether they should disclose or keep their diagnoses private. In addition, investigating the rule attributes, such as how individuals come to use these rules, whether the rules are routinized (become ingrained through repeated usage), and the sanctions employed if their rules are violated, also contributes to understanding the communicative choices people with HIV make to regulate their privacy.

Privacy Rule Development

CPM proposes five criteria used to develop privacy rules for managing the disclosure and concealing of private information such as being diagnosed with HIV. These criteria include culture, gender, motivation, context, and risk–benefit ratio (Petronio, 2002). Chapter 3 features decision making about revealing HIV status using several of the criteria articulated in CPM. Most of the conditions used to develop privacy rules serve important functions in guiding choices about disclosure of HIV status.

Cultural Criteria. Cultural considerations are paramount in coming to understand the choices people make about disclosing or concealing their HIV status because cultural values are fundamental to privacy rules for individuals (Altman, 1977; Moore, 1984; Spiro, 1971; Yep, 1992, 1993, 1995, 2000). Yep (1992, 1993, 1995) has repeatedly found that culture plays a significant role in the way that Hispanic, Asian and Pacific Islander populations and the transgender and transsexual communities develop rules used to regulate their privacy boundaries according to cultural expectations. For example, Yep and Pietri (1999) suggested in their study of transgender and transsexual individuals that the use of the proper personal pronoun (e.g., "she") might make it more likely that individuals feel able to disclose to a health care worker because the cultural sensitivity to this need is seen as a necessary criterion for revealing. Using incorrect forms of address (e.g., "sir") conveys a lack of understanding about the cultural expectations that transgenders or transsexuals use as a community. This usage may be seen as a marker for deciding to disclose about HIV status because the usage indicates a cultural expectation being met by a health care provider.

Gendered Criteria. Gender and sexual orientation serve as criteria on which people judge whether to reveal or conceal their health status to others. Hence, gender plays a role in the construction of rules managing the level of disclosure and protection of private information. For those with HIV, the issues of gender and sexual orientation are essential factors in making disclosure decisions. For example, although HIV is not a gay man's disease, those men who are gay and HIV positive often depend on criteria for privacy management that are affected by their gender (e.g., Collins, 1998; Marks et al., 1992). Sometimes there are compounding issues of gender expectations and stigma for gay men that also influence disclosure decisions.

Decisions to protect HIV status may stem from a previous stressful experience with coming out and revealing one's sexual identity. Plummer (1995) wrote that "the most momentous act in the life of any lesbian and or gay person is when they proclaim their gayness—to self, to other, to community" (p. 82). In the same vein, "coming out" as a person with HIV may have a similar impact. Consequently, to tell about their HIV status, some individuals may use the same kind of criteria they did in disclosing about their sexual identity to judge whether to reveal. For example, one man recalled his HIV disclosure to his parents:

> It was like coming out all over again. I came out to my parents when I met my first "serious" boyfriend right after college. I remember agonizing about how to tell them ... that the person I was dating was not a girl from Hawaii but a guy from Hawaii. They took it very well and invited K [his boyfriend] to spend Christmas with us. My parents have been great and they know that I am happy. Then, about a year ago, I was diagnosed with HIV. When K and I visited last summer, I decided to tell them [the HIV diagnosis]. I knew that they were okay with my homosexuality, but now this. ... I rehearsed every line a million times before I told them ... just like I did when I came out to them.

For heterosexual men, revealing their HIV status may be a different challenge because people have come to associate the disease with one particular sexual identity (see Devine, Plant, & Harrison, 1999; Herek & Capitanio, 1999; Leary & Schreindorfer, 1998). Thus, deciding to reveal one's health status may not always take into account the extent to which others are linking the disease with being a gay man. For example, one heterosexual man described the following experience about disclosing about his HIV diagnosis to his father:

> When I told my father I had AIDS, all he did was scream about "my son, the faggot." I've never seen him go off like that. Instead of talking about my illness, all I could do was repeat over and over, "I'm not gay." How do you prove you're not gay? Like that was really the important issue. I still don't think he believes me, but we don't talk much any more after that.

The gender issues for lesbians are no less problematic or significant in determining rules for privacy protection or disclosure (Harney, 1999). Unfortunately, lesbians tend to be more invisible with less research conducted on how they contract or cope with HIV (Mays, 1996). One woman who has sex with women described the difficulties being a lesbian with HIV:

> I started out telling people, to help educate. But sometimes it's too complicated, with all the questions. So many people cannot get that I am a lesbian with HIV. Period. A lesbian, not a heterosexual woman. And other lesbians are almost as bad, they think they are just immune, like HIV only targets gay men.

This woman's experiences with stereotypic responses to disclosing her HIV diagnosis were frustrating and led to remaining private more often. Consequently, we know less about how women who have sex with other woman transmit HIV to others and how they cope with the disease.

For all women, there are additional factors of race, class, and poverty that converge to make a very complicated decision package for determining whether to protect the information about their HIV status or tell others (e.g., Cline & McKenzie, 1996; Greene & Faulkner, 2002; Kimberly, Serovich, & Greene, 1995; Weeks, Grier, Radda, & McKinley, 1999). For example, one woman reported how she felt her family did not understand (in fact, her family assumed she used drugs). She stated, "I told my family one day [parents and brothers] about the HIV. Moreover, they said, 'only those gays and crack heads get that.' Ever since then, they keep after me about 'Do you use drugs?,' 'Do you sleep around?' They can't get that I just got AIDS, got it from a boy they know." Not only do cultural and gendered expectations affect the development of rules used to reveal or conceal, but individuals' motivations are also critical.

Motivational Criteria. Motivational criteria have a bearing on the development of rules used to judge disclosure or privacy protection (also explored in chap. 3). CPM proposes that the goals people want to achieve and needs that they have influence the rules used to judge decisions about revealing and concealing (Petronio, 2002). For example, this type of criteria is seen in considerations of reciprocity and striving for desired outcomes such as preserving a relationship.

Because disclosure of HIV status may and sometimes does result in loss of friends and family relationships, people with HIV are keenly aware of this possibility. Of course, the dilemma that individuals with HIV often face is the need to tell but the reluctance to experience the aftermath. Thus, the motivation to tell is often moderated by a need to preserve a relationship. Consequently, those with HIV may use a number of strategies to achieve both goals simultaneously. For example, one gay man stated the following about revealing his HIV status:

> This is not something you bring up on your first date! When I eventually do, I talk about something in the news related to AIDS to see how my date reacts. If he makes comments like, "Those people deserve to have it!" or "Those people really piss me off," then I will not say anything about being HIV positive. If he seems cool about it, then maybe I would tell him if we start to "get serious."

As this example shows, the person with HIV may test the viability of reaching both goals (telling and starting a relationship). This example illustrates a strategic measure used in other similar circumstances to fulfill motivational criteria. For example, in a study of child sexual abuse, Petronio et al. (1996) found that children who wanted to disclose about the abuse yet were afraid that they might compromise their relationship with the confidant or experience negative feedback chose to use "incremental disclosure" as a means of testing the viability of revealing to that person. Strategies like this one help define the rules for reaching the goals and fulfilling complex needs.

Contextual Criteria. Contextual criteria represent a decision base that accounts for changes in the situation (see chaps. 3 and 4 for more information). CPM suggests that in addition to culture, gender, and motivations, people take into account the situation to formulate rules for managing, revealing, and concealing private information (Petronio, 2002). Two elements serve as a basis for contextual criteria: the social environment and the physical setting. The social environment includes such factors as the appropriateness of the topic, timing of revealing and concealing, and the changes in the situation that call for altering or revamping the rules.

In the following account, a man mentioned the significance of the physical setting to judge revealing his HIV status:

> My mother came to visit and asked me how I was doing when we were having a nice dinner at a popular restaurant. I said, "I'm generally alright but let's talk more later." When we got back to my house, I told her, "Now that we have more privacy, let me tell you [I'm HIV positive]."

The physical environment can make a difference in decisions to disclose. For this man, the publicness of the restaurant did not feel like the appropriate place in which to make a disclosure about his status. He wanted control over the environment and assurance that no one else could overhear the information. The need to select the physical environment is similarly found with disclosure of other types of traumatic events such as sexual abuse (Petronio, Flores, & Hecht, 1997).

Timing of a disclosure is another factor found in the contextual criteria (Derlega et al., 1993; Petronio, 2002). For instance, a man with HIV described his decision rule using timing about revealing his health status to others:

> When the time is right, like when Linda was sharing with me about sex with her husband. The time was right for me to share my message, you see. And then when I shared with Louise, the time was right because being 82 years old, she could die tomorrow.

Timing is an important issue because being forced to reveal violates a person's ability to maintain the needed sense of control of the information. People have to feel that they can make these decisions to disclose HIV diagnoses because they have to live with the consequences of the revelations.

Risk–Benefit Ratio Criteria.   Finally, risk–benefit criteria also play a part in developing decision rules to disclose or maintain privacy (Petronio, 2002). Given that control over private information is important to people, the rules that people develop weigh the level of vulnerability they feel with the expected advantages from disclosing and concealing. Consequently, people evaluate the risks and benefits of disclosing and protecting their privacy (see Table 1.1 and chaps. 3, 4, and 5 for more details). One man reported the following:

> I tell on the first date and advise everyone to do so. I mean, what's the point of waiting if he's going to react badly? Why waste the time to go on another date when he

has a problem with my HIV status? I usually try to slip it into our conversation, like, "My drug cocktail does not interfere with my meals now," and see what he says.

For this man, the risk of not disclosing seems more problematic than making his health status clear from the beginning. Of course, in some situations the opposite is true. The way people assess the risks and benefits matters in terms of the rules that they use to decide whether to disclose, how much to disclose, or the extent to which they might wish to conceal their health status.

Summary of Rule Development Criteria. Understanding the ways these five criteria provide the background for rule production is important because learning about the diagnosis often means that previously developed rules on which people may have come to depend must change (Petronio, 2002). Consequently, if people previously depended on routinized rules, for example (i.e., rules for disclosure that had typically been used to regulate revealing and concealing over time), they might not find them appropriate or helpful for coming to terms with managing disclosure about HIV. For instance, perhaps before learning about the HIV diagnosis, a person was characteristically very open, but after learning the change in health status, the person suddenly realized that being open could result in negative consequences. As a result, this person's situation has changed and so too must the privacy rules used to manage revealing and concealing. Thus, privacy rules are revamped, changed, or altered in some way to accommodate new situations.

RULE MANAGEMENT PROCESS 2: BOUNDARY COORDINATION

CPM argues that because disclosure is a communicative process, the act of revealing links people into a privacy boundary that becomes collective (Petronio, 2002). In other words, telling someone personally private information (typically thought of as self-disclosure) makes confidants co-owners of the information, drawing them into a privacy boundary around that information, and they also become responsible for the information. Thus, the private information becomes collective because two or more people are expected to take responsibility for the information. Typically, the original owner sets the rules that guide access to the information. However, once told, co-owners might also negotiate who, when, where, and how much is told to others outside the privacy boundary. As CPM contends that individuals own and co-own private information and that the private information is not just about oneself, the theory moves the historical idea of self-disclosure beyond information about one individual and opens it up to include managing information about which a person is privy (Petronio, 2002). In this way, people have both personally private boundaries and collectively private boundaries that they manage. The personally private boundaries can move to become collective, but the collective boundaries rarely shrink back to solely personal. This is because, just like in all communicative situations, telling others private information makes

the information co-owned and cannot be taken back from a confidant once revealed. Both parties collectively become responsible for the information even
though it originally belonged to just one person.

Co-ownership of the information does not mean that everything is known.
However, that which is shared becomes the mutual responsibility of all parties
who know the information. Boundaries may expand to include co-ownership of
dyadically private information (e.g., two people manage private information),
group private information (e.g., three or more people are within the privacy
boundary), family private information (e.g., all family members manage private
information), organizationally private information (e.g., proprietary information
belonging to the corporation), or societally private information (e.g., information
belonging to whole societies such as government top secret security issues). As
more people become privy to the information, the co-ownership also increases.
Co-ownership calls for developing management rules that are mutually held by all
individuals in the know. To do this, people within the privacy boundary need to
coordinate the rules for information management. Coordination means that people negotiate privacy rules and agree on common ways to regulate the flow of the
shared private information. Coordination leads to synchronicity between and
among the co-owners.

For example, when a person with HIV decides to tell someone else, the information shifts from being personally owned to being the responsibility of the infected person and the individual he or she tells. If, for instance, a son tells his
mother about his HIV diagnosis, the mother becomes a co-owner of the information. As such, she must "take care of" the information because it has the potential
to make her son vulnerable. If she tells someone who could do harm to her son,
she risks his well-being. Because there is the possibility of risk when there is
co-ownership, those involved need to coordinate a set of rules to maintain control
and regulate the privacy boundary around this information. Thus, coordination
with others after the information is disclosed becomes as important as the decision making to reveal in the first place.

Based on research conducted using Sensitive Interaction Systems Theory
(Barbee & Cunningham, 1995; Barbee et al., 1998; Derlega, Winstead, Oldfield, &
Barbee, in press), it is known that distressed people have a sense of how they want
others to help them. This expectation is a likely explanation for why individuals
with HIV assume that others will respect their desire to set the parameters of
co-ownership and third-party disclosure through mutual negotiation of rules that
regulate the boundaries established with others regarding their status.

Coordination Operations

CPM proposes three interrelated coordination operations (Petronio, 2002). The
three coordination operations include linkages, ownership rights, and permeability (Petronio, 2002). These operations represent the way that privacy boundaries
are managed when personally private information has been shared and becomes

collectively held. Understanding these operations is important because the kind of relational quality experienced often depends on the ability to effectively coordinate boundary rules. Thus, it is useful to identify the coordination process in which collective rules are formed to manage disclosure about HIV status among those who are considered confidants. These operations consequently reflect the system used to regulate the flow of information to third parties when the boundaries are collectively held. We examine boundary linkages first.

Boundary Linkages. For CPM theory, boundary linkages are connections that form mutual responsibility for information (Petronio, 2002). In other words, if people are brought into (linked into) a boundary surrounding private information through disclosure, although they may be "reluctant confidants" (see Petronio, 2000b), an expected alliance is formed between the confidants and disclosers around the private information that becomes the responsibility of both parties. Linkages may arise in many ways, for example, linking through topic selection, timing, overhearing a disclosure, or through being a confidant. The manner in which linkages take place has the possibility to influence the level of commitment those joined into the boundary have toward negotiating rules and following them. For instance, if people overhear a disclosure about a person's HIV diagnosis, they may feel less inclined to responsibly protect that information than if they were considered a confidant. In addition, if a person with HIV discloses to strangers to help educate them, the recipients may not be concerned about third-party disclosure or telling additional people. In other words, the strength of the linkage often depends on the nature of the relationship the recipient has with the discloser (Petronio, 2002).

On the other hand, if the confidant is a person trusted by the discloser, he or she is more likely to feel responsible and judiciously protect the HIV diagnosis information according to the specifications of the person with HIV. In each case, the definition of the relationship matters in the way that people define the linkage and subsequently take responsibility for the private information that has been shared. Thus, linkage brings others into a personally private boundary around, in this case, information about HIV status and changes that boundary into being collectively held by one or more individuals who are privy to the information. Because more people are "in the know" and responsible for managing the information, they have to negotiate collectively held rules so that the level of vulnerability of all parties is controlled.

Boundary Permeability. In CPM theory, the concept of boundary permeability represents the degrees of revealing and concealing private information (Petronio, 2002). Levels of boundary permeability range from open access (loosely held, thin boundary walls) to closed access (tightly held, thick boundary walls). When boundaries are closed, protection rules prevail, keeping the information secret and the informational walls impenetrable. Some people find it difficult to reach out and talk about their HIV status. They keep the information secret, however, as several of the chapters in this volume illustrate, building thick boundary walls around HIV status can be problematic not only for a person's physical health but also for his or her emotional well-being.

HIV carries so many possible associations that even when people do reveal, they may not completely disclose to everyone. Hence, individuals with HIV more likely have thick, impenetrable boundaries with some people and open up their privacy boundaries to some degree with others. As Squire (1999) pointed out, "with HIV ... you are never entirely out; you carry the closet around with you" (p. 126). Thus, people may fully reveal making the boundaries completely permeable or partially disclose rendering the boundary semipermeable. People may also choose to make privacy boundaries impermeable, remaining completely secretive and closing off the possibility of revealing their HIV status.

Boundary Ownership.   In CPM theory, boundary ownership rights refer to the privileges of sharing in someone else's private information and expectations for taking responsibility to manage that information in a way agreeable to the original owner (Petronio, 2002). In the following example, a mother relays her reaction to learning about her daughter's HIV status:

> It was at Thanksgiving that I first learned of Sandie's HIV. It was the first time she didn't come home for Thanksgiving and we couldn't reach her on the phone. She came home the next day and I could sense that something was wrong but waited for her to tell me about it. I will never forget it. She was sitting in my chair in the living room and started crying, so I went over and just cradled her as she told me. We cried, rocked, and hugged for quite some time. Talked about what it all meant. The young man that she had been with told her she should be tested because he was HIV positive. ... I was so mad. When it comes down to it, it was the same as murder as far as I'm concerned. To have unprotected sex when he knew he was HIV positive is unforgivable. We kept the news just between the two of us until after she left. She didn't want to be there when I told [husband/father]. She didn't want to see the hurt on his [her father's] face. We [the parents] chose not to say anything to anyone for a while.

They eventually told some members of the family but not others, and the mother and daughter managed the information together along with selected family members.

Because both the discloser and recipient become mutual owners to one degree or another, coordination is predicated on negotiating which rules are used for access and protection, how much of the information is protected or revealed, who else might know, and when they might know. As this narrative illustrates, the mother and daughter decided on rules for keeping the information within their collective boundary and away from others. They also agreed to make the mother a "privacy spanner" (Petronio, Jones, & Morr, 2003). Privacy spanners are those individuals who bring collectively held private information outward to link others—in this case, the father. The daughter did not want to tell her father directly so the mother functioned as the conduit bringing the father into the boundary.

As this narrative also illustrates, ownership or co-ownership of the information is not static. In other words, boundary lines may extend to include others or become more rigid to exclude others from knowing the information or those who know from gaining subsequent information (Petronio, 2002). Telling a third party extends the number of people who know and complicates the task of negotiating permeability rules regulating further inclusion of others. A decision to include or exclude others may depend on a prediction of how a recipient is able to handle the information. For example, one person with HIV stated the following:

> When I tell others about my HIV status, I usually think about whether I have the emotional energy to take care of them after I tell them. I mean, the last few times I disclosed that I have AIDS, the others started crying hysterically and I had to calm them down and reassure them that I am not going to die tomorrow.

Although it is useful to reveal about HIV status, there are hidden costs of expecting co-ownership (Petronio, 2002). Considering the way people react helps us understand certain cautions people with HIV take when they do disclose. Even when individuals try to anticipate how someone will react, they may not be prepared for the actual response. One man described telling his partner about his HIV diagnosis. He noted, "Of course I remember what I said. I'd been leading up to it for weeks, had every last word picked out. And then nothing went like I'd planned, and I can't forget the look on his face." This man expected his partner to willingly become a co-owner and responsible party for his information. However, his predictions failed him and so did his partner. Assuming others will be open to a disclosure about HIV status may not always be an accurate view of those selected to be confidants.

As this discussion underscores, the nature of co-ownership is complex and often difficult to maneuver. Nevertheless, many people extend their boundary by linking it with others in the hopes that they can benefit from disclosing information that is a burden to them. However, people selected to be confidants do not necessarily wish to know or if they do may not routinely negotiate privacy rules to keep the information in a manner that is amenable to the person making the initial disclosure.

For example, one person interviewed noted that she decided to tell the family. Among the individuals told was a brother:

> I went over there one day after [a daughter] went to school to talk to [the sister] about something and my neighbors across the street. ... When I pulled up in front of the house, they were doing yard work; I went over to talk to them. My brother was home at the time and my sister and parents were at work so I was talking to

the neighbors for a little while. Then I went into the house and my brother said, "So, what were you talking to the people across the street for?" I said I was talking to them, and asked why. He said, "I hope you're not going around and telling the whole neighborhood that you are HIV positive." I just looked at him and said, "Is there something bothering you that you want to talk about concerning this?" [Did not wait for a response and then] I said, "Whom I choose to tell about this is my business, you know."

This example illustrates several points about co-ownership. First, having been told about the sibling's HIV status, the brother became a co-owner of the information giving him some sense of responsibility. Second, as a co-owner the brother felt he had some rights to contribute to the development of privacy rules managing the boundary around the information. Third, being privy and because it was his sibling with HIV the brother wanted to institute a rule prohibiting disclosure to anyone outside the family. Fourth, because the sibling was still trying to maintain primary control over the information, given the information was about her, the two siblings enter into a negotiation about the rules for third-party disclosure and rights over the information.

Although the parameters for each of these coordination operations have been presented individually, it is clear that linkage, permeability, and ownership are interdependent aspects of boundary coordination (Petronio, 2002). When boundary coordination is achieved, these operations work in a synchronized fashion. The outcome is a smooth series of communicative interactions that manage private information in a mutually accommodating way for all parties involved. Although synchronicity in boundary coordination is the goal, the complexity of trying to orchestrate linkages, permeability, and ownership for two or more people suggests that there will be times when the coordination will break down (Petronio, 2002). When breakdowns occur, the boundary system is in a state of turbulence.

RULE MANAGEMENT PROCESS 3: BOUNDARY TURBULENCE

CPM proposes that because people manage both personal privacy boundaries around information they individually own and they manage collective boundaries with others, the complexity of coordinating privacy rules can lead to lack of symmetry (Petronio, 2002). Both disclosers and confidants may experience obstacles in boundary coordination by intentionally or inadvertently violating expectations, using the wrong privacy rules, misunderstanding expectations, or being caught in privacy dilemmas.

Disturbances in the coordination process can be both positive and negative (Petronio, 2002). They are positive because disruptions force the individuals to reconsider their needs and expectations for privacy rules. Hence, these disturbances may lead to a better understanding of the way people define their privacy and management of revealing and concealing. On the other hand, breakdowns in the coordination system may mean conflict and unpleasant interactions with others. Nevertheless, turbulence encourages individuals to attempt to correct the problem and in so doing integrate new information into the rule system so they may preserve some level of coordination to manage their privacy.

There are many cases of boundary turbulence when examining the way people with HIV try to manage their privacy and disclosures. There are a number of reasons that privacy boundaries become turbulent. Sometimes people mistreat private information that belongs to someone else. Expectations can be violated, making people feel that they have lost control over their private information. For example, some people may have learned about their HIV diagnosis from a health worker over the phone (currently not a practice employed by most HIV testing sites, which require "in person" visits to obtain test results). Test site personnel have extensive training in counseling people who receive a positive test and now generally deliver this news in person, face-to-face. People tested may have chosen to call for results for expediency or because they may have more confidence in the anonymity of a phone call compared to an in person visit. Yet learning about one's HIV diagnosis by phone (as opposed to in person) and from someone they did not know is not the way many persons expect to be told such sensitive information about themselves. Being told traumatic information in this way can violate expectations of how private information should be handled. In this case, others (health care workers) are linked into the boundary around this private information without the person (whose information it is) having the opportunity to control how the information about the diagnosis is conveyed. This presents an odd paradox. The health care worker (a stranger) is telling this person something extremely personal, which may become highly secretive information. Given the circumstances, the individual owning the information about health status has little control over the information. Some reactions show that people have different rules for managing privacy boundaries, preferring to learn about their HIV status in a different manner, perhaps in person.

In addition to personal information being controlled by others, sometimes boundary coordination is cut short because those whom a person wants to draw into a privacy boundary reject the option. Many examples illustrate cutting off the process of linkage through recipients refusing to accept the entry into the boundary around the private information about a person's HIV status. For example, one person who wanted to tell immediate family about a recent HIV positive diagnosis explained the following:

> I said, "Well, I need to tell you something that's kind of serious" and she said, "What are you talking about?" I said, "well, it has to do with my health" and she said,

"What's wrong with your health?" I said, "Well, this isn't easy to say, but I need to say it." I basically told her that I'm HIV positive, and she didn't say anything. Just looked at me. I didn't get a whole lot of feedback from her at all.

This person also told other family members and was unsettled that "ever since I've told them, nobody will talk to me about it. It is like they choose to ignore it." This person invited the family to be linked into the privacy boundary around the diagnosis and they refused the invitation, making coordination difficult and causing this person to feel upset.

When someone opens a privacy boundary to others, they expect those selected as confidants to accept the responsibility of knowing the information. In addition, disclosing to family members often has a built-in expectation that they will offer support. Violating this expectation is hurtful and at times frustrating. There are many reasons family members might reject an invitation to be linked into a privacy boundary belonging to another member. For example, denial of the diagnosis is one possible explanation. One mother reported difficulty accepting the fact that her daughter had HIV. The daughter stated the following:

When I told my mom that I was HIV positive, she was like, "So. Can you still walk? Is your heart still beating?" and I was like, "Yeah, mom." And then, we never really talked about it thereafter. ... She was basically in a state of denial. She would not talk about me dying.

The daughter was upset about the mother's reaction to her disclosure. The mother's reluctance to talk about the daughter's health status hampered the daughter's ability to gain the support she needed. In addition, the mother's unwillingness to respond implied that her daughter's request to belong to this privacy boundary was somehow inappropriate. The only reaction of the mother initially was to tell her daughter that she should have faith and it would pull her out of this situation. By not jointly sharing the privacy boundary, the mother brought into question the legitimacy of the daughter's problems or choice to share.

Difficulties when married couples' expectations are violated is another example of boundary turbulence. CPM suggests that couples often define certain information as dyadic (two people), to be shared with each other (Petronio, 2002). When one partner does not comply, the other partner may feel that they have the right to know information that affects them and the family. One person illustrated the difficulty of this scenario for individuals with HIV:

The day I found out, I was in a state of denial because I said "There's no way." I've never done IV drugs, I've never had a blood transfusion, I've not been promiscuous, there is no way, and I don't fall into any category for this disease. So, I went to the hospital and I said, "You guys have to check me again." They did, and I came back positive. They said, "We're sorry, we hate to tell you this but, this is the way it is."

And then three days after that I found out that my ex-husband came back positive, too. That night, he told me he had gotten it through a homosexual relationship.

This woman was angry that her husband had not told her about his sexual activities and hurt that he had acted irresponsibly. The process of discovery also contributed to the difficulty. At first, her husband told her that he was drunk and raped by someone. Only after she overheard him talking to a friend where he admitted he was gay did she learn the truth. She asked him, "How could you do that, if you knew when you were 16, you had no right to marry me when we were 21."

Likely, this woman believed that she should be privy to her husband's private information about his sexuality. However, just as likely her husband defined his sexual behavior as information belonging to only him and not to be shared with others. From the data it seems the wife felt deceived by the husband. The husband no doubt found it difficult to disclose this information, keeping it secretly hidden away from the family.

There is boundary turbulence because of the inconsistent definition of ownership. The wife stated that the husband should have shared it with her making it dyadically private, whereas the husband defined the information as solely personally private. With two opposing definitions of the information, the possibility of smoothly coordinating the information was unlikely. Unfortunately, the inconsistent definitions of ownership resulted in devastating outcomes.

Another example of boundary turbulence proposed by CPM occurs when family privacy rules are violated (Petronio, 2002). Often families develop rules that function within the family to keep private information out of public view. Parents teach their children about privacy rules they want them to follow to manage information belonging to all family members. The following example illustrates the way one mother identified privacy rules for her daughter regarding disclosure about her HIV status to people outside the family:

I told her, I said, "You know, if you want to talk about it, that's fine." I said, "But, you have to understand, although we talk about it openly at home and we're very comfortable with it, not everybody else is that way." I said, "There are gonna be times when, if you tell somebody that Mommy's HIV positive, they may say something hurtful to you or they may do something that hurts your feelings. And, if that happens, you just have to walk away and come home and we'll talk about it." I said, "There's really not a whole lot you can do." I said, "Because people are afraid."

CPM argues that when a novel situation arises, people have to change their privacy rules to accommodate the different circumstances that surround the management of private information (Petronio, 2002). For the most part, this family functioned according to a certain set of privacy rules to regulate information that was private to the family. However, when the mother contracted HIV and the daughter was old enough to interact with people outside the family, this situation triggered the need to change the parameters of the rules to fit the new challenges. Consequently, it was necessary for her to identify the rule expectations for ways to handle the privacy boundary around her mother's HIV status. The mother explained that the information should be kept within the family and not disclosed to outsiders. She justified this rule by describing why it was better to keep the information within the family and the possible ramifications for not following this rule. The mother's point about talking freely within the family also underscored their routine orientation to family private information yet highlighted the need for making a distinction with outsiders.

CPM proposes that families often have two sets of rules for private information (Petronio, 2002). One governs how private family information is regulated to those outside the family. In this case, the rules were being identified for the child. A second set of rules families typically have is those governing disclosure within the family (e.g., "Don't tell Uncle Joe"). For this mother and daughter, the internal rules remained the same. The mother noted the following:

> Since it's [HIV status] always been a part of our lives, since they were very young, I never tried to hide it from them. It's always been direct and up front, and we've talked about it in the house and when I come back from the doctor. We talk about it; I talk about it ... so they've always known about it. They didn't know what it was until they saw ... [or] learned it in school.

Although the internal rules did not change, the rules for external disclosure changed as the children began to interact with people outside the family.

Many types of boundary turbulence conditions erupt as people try to coordinate their privacy expectations. Several examples have been suggested, however, others may be found throughout the book. This chapter presents an overview of the communication privacy management theory to understand a wide array of information on HIV and disclosure (Petronio, 2002). CPM theory helps organize research findings about who receives, when they receive, and how people disclose about the HIV diagnosis and it allows researchers to generate a new set of questions and directions for future studies.

CONCLUSIONS

This chapter gives the reader an overview of CPM theory that is used throughout this book to explain disclosure within the context of HIV (Petronio, 2002). CPM is a practical theory that is applied to HIV disclosure and regulation of privacy. As such, CPM offers a heuristic to understand the way that people manage revealing and concealing an HIV diagnosis. This chapter demonstrates assumptions held by CPM theory that we have both personal and collective private information belonging to us alone or that we own with other people. CPM uses a boundary metaphor to illustrate the notion that we imagine a marker identifying the border for information that we guard within a privacy boundary.

Although private information is that which we reveal, to grasp the process we use to decide to tell or keep something from others requires a management system. CPM argues that the management system people use depends on privacy rules to choose whether they will tell about their HIV status. Because choices to reveal or conceal HIV status have significant repercussions, using CPM as a way to comprehend a decision heuristic for telling or protecting privacy gives us a way to talk about the difficulty people with HIV often face.

When a person does disclose to others, confidants become responsible or serve in a guardianship role. They are likely to negotiate collective privacy rules for subsequent disclosures with the HIV positive individual once confidants know a person's HIV diagnosis. In this way, confidants are linked into a co-ownership role with the person with HIV and together they determine mutually agreed upon privacy rules for disclosure about a person's HIV diagnosis. Through boundary linkage, owners and co-owners coordinate the efforts to determine workable privacy rules. CPM affords a framework to aid us in coming to some broader awareness of how complex making decisions to reveal or conceal are not only for the person with HIV but also for family members, friends, and health care workers linked into a privacy boundary surrounding the diagnosis.

Although boundary coordination is achievable, there are times when people are incapable or unwilling to negotiate privacy rules that work for all parties involved. When boundary coordination breaks down, turbulence arises. Boundary turbulence means that the individuals involved are unable to manage the privacy boundaries around the private information. Breakdowns may take place for a wide variety of reasons. However, the central dimension leading to turbulence concerns a breach in coordination of jointly held privacy rules that are used to manage revealing and concealing. For people with HIV, these breaches are not merely uncomfortable, they may well create such havoc in their lives that the breakdowns increase the stress and add to the considerable pressure they already feel. As the subsequent chapters will show, privacy management is often complex yet critical to protect the person with HIV.

Decisions to Disclose or Not Disclose About an HIV Positive Diagnosis

Living with HIV means facing a lifetime of physical, psychological, and social challenges (e.g., Bartlett & Gallant, 2001; Castro et al., 1998; Hoffman, 1996; Nott & Vedhara, 1999; Siegel, Karus, Epstein, & Raveis, 1996). Along with others who have potentially life-threatening diseases, an HIV diagnosis frequently involves confronting a wide range of troubles such as financial and health problems; upheavals in relationships with family members, lovers, friends, and coworkers; in addition to significant physical discomfort (e.g., Bor, Miller, & Goldman, 1993; Chidwick & Borrill, 1996; Derlega & Barbee, 1998a; Greene & Faulkner, 2002; Kalichman, 1995; Miles, Burchinal, Holditch-Davis, Wasilevski, & Christian, 1997; Pakenham, Dadds, & Terry, 1996; Sowell et al., 1997; Thompson, Nanni, & Levine, 1996; Van Devanter, Thacker, Bass, & Arnold, 1999; Winstead et al., 2002). Some difficulties, however, may be unique for people living with HIV. Unlike other diseases, someone who is known to have HIV may become the target of prejudice (e.g., Herek et al., 2002). This kind of reaction is likely to affect the way people living with HIV process decisions to disclose their infection. However, more information is still needed about how HIV disclosure choices are made.

This chapter explores how people make decisions to disclose an HIV diagnosis to another person. Using CPM (see chap. 2), we are able to identify the way certain decision criteria are applied in making the decision to reveal or not reveal one's HIV status. The criteria, therefore, shape the decisions that lead to HIV disclosure and, perhaps, let a confidant divulge private information about the diagnosis to others. Using decision rules, the person with HIV attempts to exercise some control over when, who, and how others know this private information.

CPM argues that when individuals are in novel situations, such as learning about HIV status, typical rules guiding their privacy decisions may become ineffective (Petronio, 2000a, 2002). The most common relational rules are related to keeping confidences and privacy (Argyle & Henderson, 1985; Argyle, Henderson,

& Furnham, 1985). Consequently, people find that they must develop new disclosure criteria to meet their needs. For example, before finding out about having HIV, someone may have been very open with his or her mother about private matters. Learning the diagnosis, this same individual might feel uncomfortable being so open with his or her mother, especially about health-related issues. As a result, the disclosure norms do not function as effectively as they once did in this relationship with the parent. Changing decision criteria is a necessary step to reduce potential vulnerability and to meet the demands of the situation.

When previous privacy rules are reformulated, people depend on decision criteria to develop new guidelines that fit their needs. The available research on HIV suggests that three main issues have been identified as affecting a judgment about disclosing one's HIV status. In this chapter, we first examine disclosure judgments that account for the impact of the stigma ascribed by others to people with HIV. We begin with issues surrounding HIV-related stigma because it underscores the importance of the risk–benefit criterion used to make disclosure decisions. People make rules for revealing and concealing based on level of perceived risk. To protect possible vulnerability, people with HIV are likely to consider risk factors stemming from other people's reactions to having the disease and develop privacy rules accordingly. Second, we look at the motivations that people have to conceal or reveal the diagnosis and the subsequent decisions they make for sharing or concealing the diagnosis. Third, CPM contends that decisions regulating privacy boundaries depend on relational and contextual issues (Petronio, 2002). Being in a particular kind of relationship or being in a specific type of circumstance often influences the choices people make about disclosing. Thus, the criteria people with HIV develop for revealing or concealing may hinge on whether the confidant is able to handle the information, who that person is, and whether the situation is appropriate (Derlega et al., 1993; Greene & Serovich, 1996; Omarzu, 2000; Serovich et al., 1998). As these three decision criteria illustrate, preliminary understanding about the way people with HIV manage disclosure decisions may be achieved by considering the decision criteria used to determine attempts at disclosing to a confidant. We begin our examination of disclosure decisions by exploring the role of stigma.

STIGMA AS RISK CRITERIA INFLUENCING DISCLOSURE DECISIONS

Stigma "refer[s] to an attribute that is deeply discrediting" (Goffman, 1963, p. 3), spoiling, tainting, or making someone seem inferior in the eyes of others partly because he or she may fail to live up to others' expectations. According to sociologist Goffman (1963), a distinction can be made between two types of stigmatizable persons (see also Crocker, Major, & Steele, 1998; Fiske, 1998). A *discredited* person assumes that a supposed undesirable characteristic is visible and known to others. This person's task is to somehow manage the tension associated with having this information known. A *discreditable* person assumes that the undesirable characteristic is not visible or known by others. For this person, he or she may attempt to conceal the information from others or to "pass." Alternatively, the discreditable person who wants close relationships may decide to disclose the information to some people but not to others or the discreditable person may decide to tailor how much to tell about oneself to reduce the possibility of being rejected or hurting others. We know that the level of stigma biases reporting of trauma (e.g., in cases of sexual assault and incest; Russell, 1986). Given the costs of stigma and the fact that someone with HIV may be symptom free half or more of the time they have the disease (Kalichman, 1995), it makes sense to weigh carefully who to tell and who not to tell about the HIV diagnosis. Disclosing selectively is a way to cope with stigma (Siegel, Lune, & Meyer, 1998). Many individuals—sooner or later—disclose about their HIV diagnosis to at least some significant other(s), with attendant risks.

The stigma associated with HIV may result in people with the disease or partners of someone with HIV being ostracized, ridiculed, shunned, discriminated against, or even physically beaten due to negative attributions (see Herek, 1999b; Peters, den Boer, Kok, & Schaalma, 1994). As one scholar described, "stigma is perhaps the primary filter through which society views HIV disease" (Hoffman, 1996, p. 34). Stigma, as such, poses a risk factor for people with HIV because disclosing their HIV status means potential vulnerability. CPM argues that individuals typically consider a risk–benefit ratio in determining privacy rules (cf. social exchange theory; Blau, 1964; Gouldner, 1960; see also Omarzu, 2000). For those diagnosed with HIV, the level of risk may be a significant dynamic in determining boundary rules that protect privacy rather than grant openness.

Prevalence of Stigma.   In the minds of many people in North America, HIV is strongly associated with homosexuality and drug use (see Derlega, Sherburne, & Lewis, 1998; Devine et al., 1999; Herek & Capitanio, 1999; Lemieux et al., 1998). Negative attitudes about homosexuality may lead those not infected with HIV to see the disease as a by-product of socially unacceptable and "dirty" behavior or as "God's punishment" for homosexuality (Pryor, Reeder, & McManus, 1991; Pryor, Reeder, Vinacco, & Kott, 1989). D'Angelo, McGuire, Abbott, and Sheridan (1998) demonstrated that increased homophobia (using the Hudson & Ricketts, 1980, Index of Homophobia) is related to negative perceptions of individuals with HIV (both blame and respect). In D'Angelo et al.'s study, more negative attitudes toward individuals with HIV were associated with sexual (not medical) transmission of HIV. This line of research can be compared with St. Lawrence, Husfeldt, Kelly, Hood, and Smith's (1990) study in which a homosexual man with AIDS was the most stigmatized (compared with heterosexuals and leukemia patients; see also Kelly, St. Lawrence, Smith, Hood, & Cook, 1987a, 1987b).

Some individuals with HIV may internalize these negative attitudes about the "causes" of HIV, leading them to feel personal blame for having contracted the disease (e.g., Bauman, Camacho, Forbes-Jones, & Westbrook, 1997; Clement & Schonnesson, 1998; D'Angelo et al., 1998; Leone & Wingate, 1991; Moulton, Sweet, Temoshok, & Mandel, 1987). The prevalence of AIDS stigma continues today (Herek et al., 2002). Specifically, overt expressions of HIV stigma (e.g., support for quarantine) decreased through 1990s, with the number of people holding such extreme positions being very low by 1999. However, some misinformation about transmission (such as inaccurate beliefs about casual social contact causing HIV infection) actually increased in the late 1990s. Also, the belief that people with HIV deserve their illness increased in the late 1990s (Herek et al., 2002).

Metts and Manns (1996) described how people with HIV are marginalized as a result of a "social climate of fear and hostility" (p. 347). Deviance is enacted through social processes, often involving labeling (Gill & Maynard, 1995). Leary and Schreindorfer (1998) noted:

> Whether their physical limitations are real or only imagined by others, people with HIV may be viewed as peripheral social contributors who drain more emotional, financial, and practical resources from others than they contribute. Unfortunately, such perceptions lead to stigmatization. (pp. 18–19)

Someone with HIV may be seen as requiring expensive medical and drug treatments and as not being able to carry out normal, day-to-day activities. Due to these types of stigma, people with HIV may want to avoid being seen using HIV services at public health departments or at AIDS service organizations (ASOs; Moneyham et al., 1996). Burris (1999) further argued the legal management of HIV stigma may deter HIV testing; laws regarding HIV may function to both protect and reinforce stigma. On the negative side, particularly regarding antigay politics, there is the "Helms Amendment" (see "No Child Left Behind," 2002); people can also be discharged from the military for being HIV positive (see Miller, 1998, for discussion of the "Don't ask, don't tell" military policy and homosexuality), and there has been restriction of HIV education in schools. On the positive side, the Americans With Disabilities Act of 1990 helps protect people with HIV (see also *School Board of Nassau County, Fla. v. Arline,* 1987).

Many studies suggest that HIV-related stigma influences HIV decision making to regulate privacy boundaries (e.g., Alonzo & Reynolds, 1995; Derlega, Winstead, et al., 2002; Greene & Faulkner, 2002; Hackl, Somlai, Kelly, & Kalichman, 1997; Limandri, 1989; Norman, Kennedy, & Parish, 1998; Siegel et al., 1998; Simoni et al., 1995; van der Straten, Vernon, Knight, Gomez, & Padian, 1998). Chesney and Smith (1999) described how stigma can result in delays in both HIV testing and disclosure of the diagnoses.

Linking Disclosure and Stigma.   Stigma affects choices about disclosing (e.g., Herek, 1997; Klitzman, 1999; Limandri, 1989). A study by Derlega, Winstead, et al. (2002) illustrates how HIV stigma is associated with making HIV disclosure decisions. One hundred forty-five individuals with HIV in this study were asked whether they disclosed about the HIV diagnosis to a friend, intimate partner, and parent. A majority of the male and female participants reported that they had revealed the diagnosis to these various target persons after learning about the diagnosis (i.e., HIV disclosure to a friend = 81% of the men, 70% of the women; to an intimate partner = 73% of the men, 63% of the women; to a parent = 76% of the men, 61% of the women). However, the more people perceived that the general public stigmatized someone with HIV the lower the likelihood of reporting disclosure to a parent. For example, general public stigma items included "Most people feel that how you get HIV is something to be ashamed of." The more agreement with these public stigma items (from Bauman et al., 1997) the less disclosure to a parent. On the other hand, there was no association between perceptions of HIV-related stigma and self-reports of disclosure to a friend or an intimate partner. Results indicated that perceptions of public HIV stigma played no role in the endorsement of reasons for self-disclosure. On the other hand, perceptions of HIV stigma increased concerns for men and women about reasons for not disclosing one's HIV status to a parent and to a lesser extent about the importance of concealing one's HIV status from a friend. Specifically, reasons such as self-blame, fear of rejection, communication difficulty, and protecting other correlated with stigma.

Interestingly, in Derlega, Winstead, et al.'s (2002) study, public HIV stigma is associated with privacy as a reason for not disclosing about the diagnosis to a friend and a parent for the men but not for the women with HIV. Men, compared to women, perceive a greater right to privacy as a reason for not disclosing when they perceive high HIV stigma. Hence, the "right to privacy" functioned as a criterion that regulates access to private information for men more than it does for women in this study.

As this discussion illustrates, the judgment about revealing and concealing HIV status is often based on considering the risks versus benefits (Petronio, 2002). However, the risk–benefit ratio is but one criterion used to determine rules that regulate privacy boundaries. Other criteria contribute to decisions for boundary management such as the motivations people have for keeping something secret or disclosing to others (Petronio, 2000a).

Perceived Risk Affecting Decisions to Disclose

The stigma of HIV is a real risk for individuals with HIV. To assess the kind of impact stigma has on how people manage their privacy boundaries, it is useful to consider the basis on which disclosure decisions are made in reaction to stigma risks. The research suggests four related factors contribute to developing concealing or nondisclosing rules resulting from perceived risks to privacy boundaries. These include emotional reactions, fear, disapproval, and negative assessments by others (e.g., Leary & Schreindorfer, 1998; Rozin, Markwith, & McCauley, 1994).

As one might assume, each factor emerges out of a reaction to how others view the disease. Stigma risks, therefore, contribute to decisions that protect HIV infected people from another's negative emotional reaction, their fear of infection, disapproval, and perceptions that a person with HIV is somehow failing to make a contribution to society.

If stigma risks are perceived to be high, it is likely that those with HIV will opt for concealing their status. Hence, instead of taking the chance of opening their privacy boundary and gambling on further humiliation and hurt, a person with HIV is more liable to use protection rules and not disclose (e.g., Alonzo & Reynolds, 1995; Crawford, 1996; Greene & Faulkner, 2002; Greene & Serovich, 1996; Herek, 1999b; Hoffman, 1996; Leary & Schreindorfer, 1998; Rozin et al., 1994; Shilts, 1987; Siegel et al., 1998; Sontag, 1989). Given how others' opinions about HIV are critical to perceiving stigma, the infected person must make an assessment of the recipient's position in deciding to disclose (see also chap. 5 discussion of "courtesy stigma" for how those close to the person with HIV can also be stigmatized).

Being responsible for knowing a person's HIV status often means that the receiver is expected to understand the riskiness of the information. This notion is described in CPM as co-ownership in which responsibility for information is jointly shared after disclosure. Disclosing according to criteria set by individuals with HIV is critical to guard against increasing their vulnerability. When others express fear or disapproval, people with HIV are more apt to put up a barrier restricting access to their status because they may feel a lack of trust. Thus, the emotional reactions, fear, disapproval, and negative assessment of people with HIV contribute to heightening the possibility of protecting privacy boundaries rather than allowing access to their health status. People with HIV are less willing to disclose in these instances. We explore each of these four aspects of HIV stigma next.

Negative Emotional Reactions.   Negative reactions from others often call for certain types of boundary regulation (Leary & Schreindorfer, 1998). HIV causes negative emotional reactions such as hostility in others (Mondragon, Kirkman-Liff, & Schneller, 1991) because it is viewed as an infectious disease that may ultimately cause death. Others may react with discomfort, apprehension, horror, disgust, and even violence toward someone contracting this potentially deadly disease that attacks the body, often with disfiguring side effects. When the person with HIV perceives that others view him or her negatively, the risk of vulnerability is high, leading to enacting protection rules rather than disclosure rules. A bisexual man reported that "I won't ever tell my in-laws. I just know how they'd be, judging and all." This man used his assessment of the responses of his in-laws as the basis of the decision to remain private. Another woman with AIDS described how she thought her sister would react. "She'd cry and carry on. It'd be a big scene." This woman chose not to tell her sister because she did not want to deal with the negative reaction, specifically the emotional response she expected.

If persons with HIV sense potential negative emotional reactions, they may react by changing the topic, remaining silent, withdrawing from the situation, or avoiding interacting with people who pose a potential threat. It is important to remember that these views are perceptions of how another person might respond that affect decisions to disclose, and they may or may not be accurate. One heterosexual woman described how she would "check out" the topic of AIDS with a friend before deciding to disclose:

> I try to watch the news, see movies with HIV, that kind of stuff. Then I bring it up with the person who doesn't know I'm positive. If they act badly, then I won't tell them. Sometimes they go off just at the mention of AIDS, and that tells me a lot.

Thus, HIV stigma about negative emotional reactions appears to function to inhibit disclosure or tighten boundaries.

Fear of Infection and Contagion.   Individuals with HIV are also stigmatized at times because others fear that they might also become infected, believing that HIV is somehow contagious (Leary & Schreindorfer, 1998). HIV causes negative reactions because it is perceived to pose a threat to the health and safety of others. People with HIV do not pose a threat of infection to others during ordinary social interactions such as in conversations, hugging, or sharing dishes with non-HIV infected persons. Nevertheless, the fear of infection and contagion may lead others to shun the person because many people are still uncomfortable with casual contact with an individual with HIV. Rozin et al. (1994) conducted a study asking about contact with a person with HIV (and other stigmatized or nonstigmatized conditions). There was aversion to direct contact with a person with HIV in this study; people reported avoidance for wearing a sweater, sleeping in a bed, or using an auto owned by a person with HIV (see also Pryor et al., 1989).

People with HIV are often sensitive to the fear others have about catching the disease. When a person conveys that fear, the person with HIV estimates a high risk of vulnerability. One woman with AIDS described vividly how her brother's reaction to her HIV disclosure affirmed their relationship. "He just walked over and gave me a big hug, like he wasn't afraid or anything. It was the best interaction I've ever had with him." In this woman's case, another person responded by minimizing his own fear and supported her.

The prediction that another person may be fearful may lead to developing rules that close off interaction to protect the person with HIV. Consequently, people with HIV may find it necessary to remain private and not disclose. For example, people with HIV may use preemptive rules such as offering factual accounts of research about the way others are infected. One man took a pamphlet about HIV transmission to his parents' house because they had not wanted to be physically near him. People may also use defensive rules such as never sharing food with others. One adolescent with HIV took her own glass to others' homes so they would not worry about her infection. Individuals with HIV may also use rules that convey compassion for the fears others might have about contagion. For example, a person might say, "I know you are worried about being infected (or your kids being infected), and I can understand why you'd be afraid. Maybe we can read about this together and try to find out more." Thus, fear of contagion affects disclosure decisions. We turn next to concern about disapproval.

Disapproval. Others may disapprove of the HIV infected person because they assume that she or he has violated some moral code or group standard (Derlega, Sherburne, et al., 1998; Leary & Schreindorfer, 1998). If people with HIV are perceived as bearing responsibility for contracting the disease, especially because of socially disapproved or "deviant" behaviors (such as male same-gender sexual intercourse, promiscuity, or injection drug use), they are likely to be targets of abuse, prejudice, discrimination, and social rejection (Leary & Schreindorfer, 1998). Individuals with HIV are an outgroup that threatens social identity and creates an "us" (uninfected) versus "them" (infected) boundary in perceptions of some (Devine et al., 1999). In this way, the HIV epidemic served as justification of negative attitudes toward people with HIV (Larsen, Serra, & Long, 1990; Lemieux et al., 1998; Rozin et al., 1994). Specifically, more negative attitudes toward injection drug users are related to more AIDS stigma (Capitanio & Herek, 1999), and association of AIDS with homosexuality or bisexuality is correlated with antigay attitudes (Herek & Capitanio, 1999; Herek & Cogan, 1995).

There is some evidence that religious beliefs may affect HIV stigma, but this is in direct contrast to the many religious-based organizations that provide funding, hospice care, and meals for those infected with HIV. Greene et al. (1993) found that conservative religious ideology (items such as "school teachers should believe in God") is associated with less support for HIV-related privacy, which may be linked to negative attitudes toward homosexuality. Thus, there is some association between religious beliefs and attitudes toward HIV (see Greene et al., 1993). As one man stated, "How many times have I heard 'AIDS is God's punishment on homosexuals.' I have AIDS. I'm dying. Who cares why it started?" This man's exasperation with disapproval is echoed in another person's comments about why she would not disclose. As a heterosexual woman described, "No way I'd tell my aunt, she's really religious and judging. Not all church folk are like that, but my aunt. ... There would be some way to say it's my fault." Rose (1998) explored the difficult experiences of African American gay men with organized religion (see also Schaefer & Coleman, 1992, similar findings for White gay men) and church doctrine concerning homosexuality. This topic deserves more attention, but there may be an association between religious beliefs and attitudes toward people with HIV (see Green & Rademan, 1997; this study, conducted in Scotland, found that evangelical leaders are more likely to blame people with HIV for their infection compared to the general population).

The phenomenon of stigma based in disapproval has been described as a "victim continuum" (e.g., Albert, 1986; Treichler, 1988; Watney, 1987). Most individuals with HIV are assigned blame for their infection, but this level of blame is especially pronounced for MSM and IDUs. Interestingly, language for HIV infected newborns (or children) refers to them as "innocent victims" (e.g., they "did nothing to contract HIV") of the HIV epidemic potentially implying there may be "guilty victims" (see also McAllister, 1992, for discussion of AIDS media coverage). Language is a powerful force in shaping social reality, and this reflection of stigma disapproval is crucial in images of people with HIV. Albert (1986) also described media images of children with HIV who are depicted with medical personnel who wear no protective clothing; in contrast, other individuals with HIV are shown next to people wearing masks and gloves.

Graham, Weiner, Giuliano, and Williams (1993) explored reactions to mode of HIV contraction in people without HIV. They utilized Earvin "Magic" Johnson, a professional basketball player who went public with his HIV diagnosis, before he announced how he acquired HIV (through multiple sex partners). In one part of the study, Graham et al. (1993) asked participants to imagine if Magic had acquired HIV in different ways. People who imagined he acquired HIV through a blood transfusion (like Arthur Ashe around that same time) blamed Magic less than participants who imagined Magic acquired HIV through drug use or homosexual sex. The blame was related to attribution of responsibility (see also Devine et al., 1999), specifically perceived responsibility for the HIV infection resulted in more anger and less sympathy.

People with HIV perceive a high risk of vulnerability when others label them deviants (e.g., Weiner, 1993). Being considered responsible for contracting the disease due to "inappropriate behaviors" assumes that the individual intentionally acted in ways that suggest "they deserve what they get" (Devine et al., 1999) or that their infection was "controllable" (Weiner, Perry, & Magnusson, 1988). This reaction to those who are infected suggests that the others may show no mercy or compassion toward the person with HIV. There is little room to gamble on the possibility of disclosing in this case. Perhaps more than other kinds of risky situations, disapproval poses the highest danger. Decisions for this circumstance would completely constrain the possibility of disclosure for fear of reprisal.

Failing to Contribute.   Finally, as the last aspect of stigma, others may convey their perception that the person with HIV is failing to contribute to the welfare of others (Leary & Schreindorfer, 1998). People with HIV may be targets of stigma if they are perceived to have failed in contributing to the welfare of their children, families, or the community. Although others with severe disabilities (e.g., persons with mental disabilities, patients with advanced cancer) may also be seen as not pulling their weight or share (see Braithwaite & Thompson, 2000), this view is not as pervasive as the HIV perception.

Encountering others who believe a person is somehow compromising those around him or her cannot be a pleasant experience. This kind of reaction is menacing to a person with HIV. As a safety measure, if this type of attitude is communicated, the person with HIV has to protect the possibility of others knowing the diagnosis. Boundaries are tightly drawn and behaviors are enacted in ways that attempt to divert others from considering the possibility that the person might be HIV positive. Some people "cover" or try to "pass," saying they have cancer or some other disease to explain any symptoms (e.g., Greene & Faulkner, 2002; Klitzman, 1999). Thus, in these cases disclosing is not seen as a viable option. The opposite is the case. No one believing that an individual with HIV has somehow failed the community could possibly be selected as a disclosure confidant. The difficulty is in knowing ahead of time (see discussion of anticipated response later in this chapter). One man with AIDS reported that his brother said to him:

> "Why don't you get a job? You sit around here all day, doing nothing, watching TV, wasting my tax money." What the hell does he mean? I sit around all day hugging the toilet, throwing up from these meds, how am I going to work through that?

The person is struggling with another who cannot see how he is coping with the disease and only focuses on how he does not "pull his weight," and he regrets that this brother knows his diagnosis. Although stigma that leads to these reactions is acknowledged by people with HIV, it is sometimes difficult beforehand to protect against negative consequences. When others obviously communicate negative feelings, it is easier to not disclose or to keep the boundaries closed.

For each of the four aspects of stigma discussed, when known, the person with HIV may make disclosure choices to avoid negative consequences found with this stigma. However, many times people with HIV are uncertain about the way others feel. These circumstances require more levels of assessment and other criteria to judge decisions that allow the person to seek help or gain feedback from disclosure about their status while simultaneously protecting their privacy boundary when necessary. People with HIV may not reveal if they are afraid of the implications of being stigmatized. Stigma often inhibits disclosure, but there are other motivations that influence decision making about HIV disclosure beyond these perceptions of stigma.

MOTIVATIONS REGULATING REVEALING AND CONCEALING AN HIV DIAGNOSIS

The reasons for concealing or revealing one's HIV positive status vary from individual to individual. Some people have a high need to tell others because it helps them cope with their illness. Others find it difficult to disclose because they may not be able to tackle dealing with their illness or because they are in denial about their condition. Consequently, they conceal their status from others. Thus, when people with HIV are afraid to reveal, they draw their boundaries tightly. When those with HIV want to disclose, they regulate their boundaries more loosely, allowing some or a great deal of access to their private information. Hence, people are motivated to disclose or keep the information private because of different needs. There are a number of issues that provide insight into disclosure decisions that depend on people's motivations to reveal or conceal. We look first at reasons for revealing an HIV diagnosis based on self, other, and interpersonal criteria and then at reasons for nondisclosure.

People's motivations for HIV disclosure can be broadly categorized in three ways (see Derlega & Winstead, 2001; Derlega, Winstead, & Folk-Barron, 2000). First, they have personal needs to fulfill. Second, people are also motivated to disclose based on others' needs (Derlega, Winstead, Wong, & Greenspan, 1987). Third, people disclose to fulfill interpersonal needs, for the sake of the relationship they have or want to have with another person. These decision motivations—self, other, and interpersonal—are discussed separately.

Decisions Leading to Disclosure for Self-Gain

There are at least two main reasons people decide to disclose their HIV status that are based on a motivation for fulfilling personal needs. They include striving for catharsis and seeking help. Each of these issues sets the stage for ways that individuals with HIV may use disclosure to their own advantage. We examine each of these self-based motivations to disclose next.

Catharsis.   When one considers the reasons why people disclose, individuals with HIV may express concerns about holding this information inside. Catharsis is often a motivation that, in turn, sets the parameters for disclosing rules. In a different context, Allman (1998) described how physicians "confess" as a reason to disclose their medical mistakes. Limandri (1989) suggested that HIV disclosure may be a form of "venting," a "desperate need to tell someone" (p. 74; see also Klitzman, 1999). People may experience relief in letting this HIV secret out, allowing them to begin the coping process and to facilitate self-acceptance (Holt et al., 1998). One bisexual woman in her 40s described feelings that guided her decision to finally talk about the diagnosis with someone. "Well, at first, I was very distraught. And I was still in a degree of shock. It became so overwhelming that I had to share it with someone." She "held in" the secret for several months before sharing.

Although this research is complex (see Kelly, 2002), there is a great deal of evidence that keeping secrets may take a considerable toll physically and psychologically on people who harbor emotionally sensitive information (Lane & Wegner, 1995; Lepore & Smyth, 2002; Pennebaker, 1995). The types of HIV stigma previously discussed may substantially increase stress. Telling someone else may relieve this burden and take some of the weight of the secret off the person with HIV. The desire to do so initiates the development of decision criteria that regulate the person's privacy boundary. For instance, one person reported that he told a cousin about the diagnosis, stating, "The benefit I would get would be not having to carry that information around." For this person, keeping the information secret was a burden too heavy to continue holding and led to the decision to disclose. Another man stated succinctly, "I was tired of holding it all in."

Keeping secrets is often more of a liability for people than telling (Lane & Wegner, 1995). People with secrets have to remain alert about who knows and who does not know, whom they have told, and whom they wish to keep in the dark. They cannot let the information out of their consciousness because they will violate their own rules for who should know; therefore, people maintain a constant vigilance about the HIV diagnosis. This constant monitoring is draining, so much so that one man sought therapy to help deal with the stress of tracking who knew his HIV diagnosis:

> At first, I really didn't tell anyone, but then all this pressure built up and I couldn't take it. I thought I was going to explode. But I wanted to be so careful about who I told. Now, I need a damn score card to remember who does and does not know. It's *soooo* complicated.

This man decided not to tell about the HIV diagnosis initially but finally shared the information with some friends and family to relieve his stress; paradoxically, keeping track of who did and did know may actually have increased his anxiety in the end. Thus, there comes a point when individuals need to release the weight of the information to someone else (Hays, Turner, & Coates, 1992; Lepore, Greenberg, Brunjo, & Smyth, 2002; Lepore, Ragan, & Jones, 2000; Pennebaker, 1995).

One may think about catharsis as a complete and unbridled flow of information about a person's HIV status, but catharsis may not occur quickly after a person is diagnosed with the disease. Instead, the need to talk for some may take time to build (Stevens & Tighe Doerr, 1997). Only after people have lived with the knowledge of the diagnosis for a period of time might they be able to come to grips with the situation by talking to others. Thus, some individuals may be slow to disclose to anyone or they may prefer to not disclose about the HIV diagnosis when they have just been informed themselves about the diagnosis. The effect of several aspects of timing of disclosure messages, including time after learning the diagnosis oneself, is discussed in chapter 4.

The management of privacy and disclosure can be seen clearly in the personal struggles of someone with HIV who is dealing with catharsis. The tension between needing to seek relief from this devastating secret and yet being petrified at the prospect of letting others know makes it clear that people calculate the pros and cons of allowing their private information to become public. Someone with HIV does not let the information become too public or tell others without attempting to estimate the reactions of others for their own protection and safety (Greene, 2001; Greene & Faulkner, 2002; Hoffman, 1996; Holt et al., 1998; Kalichman, 1995; Kelly, Otto-Salaj, Sikkema, Pinkerton, & Bloom, 1998).

Seeking Help.   Besides disclosing to relieve the burden of holding in sensitive information, people may also disclose to seek help to deal with their personal difficulties. To achieve this goal, people with HIV share the information, albeit selectively. For example, Holt et al. (1998) described how people disclose their HIV diagnosis for both practical and emotional support (see also Klitzman, 1999). Because there is a tangible need to depend on others for medical assistance or social support, people with HIV often find themselves in a dilemma of having to disclose but not truly wanting to reveal. Nevertheless, to gain help from others, they have to tell, but carefully. Agne, Thompson, and Cusella (2000) reported that 57% of motivations described by participants for HIV disclosure to health care providers were due to health reasons. One woman with an AIDS diagnosis described how, during a time when she was sick, she told employees at a supermarket about her diagnosis to get more rapid assistance in obtaining food stamps (also so she would not have to stand in line in the cold rain and risk infection). In this example, the HIV disclosure was pragmatic, telling the information to achieve a goal of seeking help. Her description provides insights into the criteria she used to manage the privacy boundary around her HIV status.

Some decisions to seek help are based on pragmatic reasons, trying to fill specific instrumental and concrete needs. One man described his need for a loan:

> I gotta take the medication, sometimes it's hard to get help from the state. So I told my aunt so I could borrow money for the drugs. I paid her back when it got sorted out, but I had to tell her or skip. I didn't know any other way.

In this case, the man would not have told his sister except for this specific need. Another woman in her 20s needed assistance with children. "My mother knows because I have two young children. When I have appointments at the hospital, I need her to watch them. I wonder sometimes if I would have told her [otherwise]. Maybe, but certainly not as soon." For this woman, the need for child care changed at minimum the timing of her disclosure choice.

As these examples illustrate, the motivation to seek help does not necessarily mean that people tell about their HIV status indiscriminately or that they necessarily make a full disclosure to everyone. Instead, individuals with HIV develop rules that are often in reaction to a particular situation (Petronio, 2002). In the examples previously cited, the need for help predominately influenced the choices for disclosure. However, seeking help is manifested in a variety of circumstances with the need for different kinds of assistance. Once told, the person may be expected to assist in ways determined by the person with HIV. Clearly, health professionals have to be told about the diagnosis when seeking medical treatment. There are also cases in which a relative or friend who has a medical background is told about the diagnosis to access information about HIV drug regimens or the side effects of medications. This is different from seeking help that is emotional in nature such as "I just wanted someone to listen to me, maybe remind me to take my medications."

Disclosure decisions depend on the person with HIV's assessment of a confidant's ability to meet the level and kind of need required. For example, one recently diagnosed woman reported, "I can't read the damn things [pamphlets] the Health Department gives me. I had to tell my sister so she'd help." This woman decided to reveal for a pragmatic reason—she needed help understanding a health pamphlet (the same was true about the written instructions for taking her mediations). In this case, one sees that the outcome is important in making choices about telling others and giving access to privacy boundaries.

We have noted how decisions to disclose for self-related reasons are motivated by two factors: catharsis and seeking help. These factors emphasize personal reasons for HIV disclosure. However, people with HIV may also factor in others' needs and characteristics in HIV disclosure decisions. Thus, individuals with HIV take account of other-related issues as they factor in the other through duty to inform and desire to educate.

Decisions Leading to Disclosure for Other-Gain

Although people with HIV are motivated to disclose so they can achieve positive outcomes for themselves, they also consider how their disclosure would affect others. They must balance self versus other considerations in their disclosure decisions (cf. Derlega et al., 1987). Consequently, persons with HIV often feel that they have a duty to inform or educate others even if they are reluctant to disclose.

Duty to Inform. Someone with HIV may disclose out of a sense of duty to inform another person, or the person with HIV may believe that another has a "right to know." Agne et al. (2000) reported "duty to inform" as a reason people with HIV gave for disclosing to health care providers. Klitzman's (1999) participants reported a duty to inform primarily HIV negative partners, feeling they had the right to know. A prospective or current romantic or sexual partner may also be told about the diagnosis to emphasize the importance of taking protective measures for safer sex, possibly to share responsibility for safer sex (see Holt et al., 1998; Nimmons & Folkman, 1999). For instance, a gay man told his boyfriend about the HIV diagnosis because "it was becoming physical, and I felt that I had to let him know." Undoubtedly, disclosing to the boyfriend was done out of a moral obligation to that selected other. However, doing so also obligates the recipient so that he (in this case) is expected to protect the information from others.

There may also be a perceived duty to inform past sexual or drug-using partners to encourage them to be tested for HIV. For instance, one heterosexual man said, "I told her [a former sexual partner] because she was my baby's mother. I just wanted her to be aware of it. She went out and got the test." Perhaps by doing so, persons with HIV may be seeking vindication, especially if they believe they are at fault. By informing others, those with HIV may consider it their responsibility and hope that others forgive them if they are the source of infection.

Relatives might also be informed so that the information does not come as a surprise to them later on (Greene & Faulkner, 2002). People with HIV may want to prepare family members for the final phase of the illness. For instance, a man told his mother because "she had the right to know. In case something did happen I didn't want to wind up on her doorstep, or [to have] somebody call her and say, you know, your son's got so and so." In another case, a man told his roommate about the diagnosis to anticipate possible health problems. He said that "the reason why [I told him] is I am living there and if something should happen to me he had to know what to do." Although disclosing this information fulfills some sense of obligation and therefore is the motivation for disclosure, it is still difficult to enact. Consequently, individuals may not tell everything in one disclosure episode. Thus, people may tell bits and pieces of information at different times that lead up to full knowledge (also see chap. 4 in which we discuss incremental disclosure). Although people with HIV who consider disclosing may perceive a duty to inform, they may initially hint at the information to measure the way others might respond to knowing about the HIV diagnosis.

Even if there are problems in telling someone about the HIV diagnosis, the sense of obligation, or duty to tell, may be increased by a perception that the significant other would expect disclosure (see Greene & Faulkner, 2002). For example, one woman with HIV stated, "My mother had to know. This would have put my life in total chaos if my mother did not know, because I knew she would have really put me through it if I did not tell her." At the core of obligation may be a sense of self-preservation, especially when parents, relatives, and partners are deemed targets of this disclosure. Participants in several studies (e.g., Derlega, Lovejoy, et al., 1998; Greene & Faulkner, 2002; Greene & Serovich, 1996; Serovich et al., 1998) used phrases such as "owed it to her," "had a right not know," and "the right thing to do" when describing this duty to inform through disclosure, but they were not always able to articulate why they felt this duty other than the other person's role (X is my lover, parent, friend, etc.). Thus, perceived duty to inform focuses on the other and increases the likelihood of disclosing.

Educating Others. Besides feeling a duty to inform, someone with HIV may disclose to educate or inform others about the "true facts" regarding infection, similar to findings of goals to educate others about disabilities (Braithwaite, 1991). They may also wish to explain, from their own experience, what is involved in living with the disease. The following statement by a man with AIDS illustrates the rationale of this decision criterion. He stated, "I told him [the friend] so that he could be aware of the fact that this disease is really serious, and it can get anybody. You can look really healthy and still live with it and have it."

Many people with HIV have a strong need to make the lived experience of HIV clear to those who do not have the disease (Winstead et al., 2002). However, if a recipient is a reluctant confidant, the person may not be cooperative about containing information or keeping it confidential (Petronio, 2000b, 2002). Therefore, they may be "educated" but may not respond in ways that the discloser expects. Obviously this may lead to some awkward situations that are not necessarily positive for either party. However, for some individuals with HIV there is a sense of responsibility to make sure others become knowledgeable about the disease and recognize the critical importance of respecting those who are positive.

Individuals with HIV who have told someone about the diagnosis may also be asked about how they became infected. This request for information may be used to educate others about the disease. For instance, a mother was asked by her son to describe how she contracted the disease. She described her conversation with him:

> He [my son] was about nine. He asked me how did I get HIV. I told him that I didn't know exactly how I got it, but that it was before I met his father. I had other partners and some of these partners were IV drug users. They probably came in contact with the disease because they had different [sexual] partners or from using drugs. So, they may have infected me. He said, "If I had not known anyone before his father, then you would probably not have this disease." I said, "That is probably true." That is why now we are very open about sex. I tell him to abstain from sex. And when he is going to have sex, it is with a woman he loves. This is how I hope to make sure that it is his only relationship. Not just to fool around. It was not safe in my time and it is surely not safe now. So, I explain it because he is a preteen. You know he is going to experiment. He will be a teenager pretty soon. I felt like he needed to know exactly what he was wondering about. And I hope that he might learn from my experience.

This mother used disclosure to talk with her son about his safety and dating. She saw this as an opportunity and took advantage of it. Other education motivations are specifically to reduce stigma. One family discussed the pros and cons of telling a particular uncle, and the woman with HIV wanted to be sure that he was told "because he's prejudiced and thinks only gays get it."

Thus, many infected people who cite education or public service as a reason for disclosure mention talking with high school or university students, or appearing on radio or television, to describe their personal experiences living with HIV (e.g., Derlega, Lovejoy, et al., 1998; Wiener, Heilman, & Battles, 1998; Winstead et al., 2002). Siegel et al. (1998) included public education efforts in their description of proactive HIV coping strategies. For example, one heterosexual man interviewed for this book pointed out that:

> When I am speaking at a seminar, they can hear my experience and what I went through. And, maybe it will motivate them to go and get tested if they are sexually active with numerous partners. Maybe they will realize the danger of what they are doing. Maybe it will make them stop their high risk behavior.

The rationale or motive for speaking out and revealing his status was for a larger public good rather than self-focused like catharsis or seeking help described earlier. A person mentioned, "I speak at colleges. It helps me to sleep at night knowing that I may have stopped one person from getting it. They need to be taught." Other examples include "poster kids" (see Wiener, Heilman, et al., 1998) or families with a child with HIV who have "gone public" in efforts to educate the public.

HIV disclosure for educational reasons may not always be a personal decision. Instead, people may be placed in the role of educator by the needs of others who perceive a person as an HIV disease expert. For instance, one woman described how she had told a neighbor, who was lesbian, about her diagnosis. They often talked about HIV-related topics, including sexual transmission of the disease. The neighbor in turn periodically asked the woman with HIV to talk to lesbians in her circle of friends about transmission of HIV and safer sex practices. Thus, the result is the same, but a person can choose or be asked to educate others. Regardless, being willing to function as an expert requires a change in criteria used to manage privacy. The boundary has to expand to accommodate an ever-growing number of people who know about the person's HIV status. It may be more difficult to manage and contain information about HIV when in the role of educator and a person with HIV gives talks and does not know who is in the audience and what they will do with the information (including the identity of the person with HIV). Unknown persons may also see these educators at a later date, affecting disclosure decisions. One woman who lectured on AIDS was grocery shopping with a new acquaintance who did not know her HIV status:

> We were in the middle of Food Lion [a grocery store], and this young man walks up and says, "I heard you talk the other day, and, well, I, it changed my mind about using condoms with my girlfriend. Thanks for coming to the school, and I hope the medication keeps working." Well, what do I say to this friend with me? She was confused, and I had to tell her at that point.

Some people choose to educate others and disclose in this way. This special case has unique potential consequences and may affect other disclosure decisions. We have noted how decisions to disclose for other gain are motivated by two factors: duty to inform and educating others. These factors emphasize other- or recipient-focused reasons for HIV disclosure. However, people with HIV may also factor in interpersonal needs and characteristics in HIV disclosure decisions. Thus, individuals with HIV take the relationship into account and they also factor in the relationship through testing others' reactions, establishing emotionally close and supportive relationships, and common experiences or similarity.

Decisions Leading to Disclosure for Interpersonal-Gain

Although people with HIV are motivated to disclose so they can achieve positive outcomes for themselves and others, they also consider how their disclosure would affect the relationship. They must balance self, other, and interpersonal considerations in their disclosure decisions (cf. Derlega & Winstead, 2001; Derlega, Winstead, et al., 2002; Derlega et al., 1987). These motivations for interpersonal gain include testing others' reactions, establishing emotionally close and supportive relationships, and common experiences or similarity.

Testing Others' Reactions. Living with the HIV diagnosis makes establishing some new relationships complicated. One of the most problematic issues for people with HIV is determining whether another person is willing to be in a dating relationship with them. There are many ways in which individuals with HIV cope with this problem. For example, given concerns about rejection, the person with HIV might develop criteria that call for disclosing about their illness up front or soon after meeting someone. In this way a person with HIV can test the other's reaction about being in a relationship. If the other person decides then to end the relationship, this rejection occurs at a point when there is (hopefully) a relatively small investment in the relationship. This situation reflects an aspect of disclosure decisions relatively unique to HIV.

People initiating new relationships may not reveal private information until they have established some common ground (cf. social penetration theory; Altman & Taylor, 1973, or incremental exchange theory; Levinger & Snoek, 1972). However, the crucial nature of the circumstances in which HIV is involved makes it important for the infected person to change the system that regulates disclosure. The needs of managing the illness trigger changes in the typical boundary rules found in initiating new relationships. As self-protection, many of those infected may not want to "waste time" skirting around the issue. On the other hand, it may be more likely that those with HIV choose to conceal their status until they feel that the person is truly interested in them. Of course this means that the person with HIV either skillfully managed not to have any sexual encounters (or to limit certain behavior) or possibly exposed the other person. Clearly, the up-front strategy is the most preferred if there is any possibility of HIV transmission. However, it is not clear what instigates a choice to tell up front or wait until sexual relations have been established before people with HIV disclose. The role of timing in HIV disclosure is discussed more in depth in chapter 4.

This concept of testing others' reactions is not limited to dating relationships (Miell, 1984). A person might test friends or family members. It is possible to see how close a relationship is by seeing how the other reacts to knowing about an HIV diagnosis. People might use disclosure to test if they want to continue to invest in a relationship such as with a friend or family member. If a person is not able to deal with the information, the discloser may choose not to make efforts to maintain the relationship, such as visiting, calling, or spending time together. People may do this type of testing through discussion of AIDS or related issues, as discussed later in this chapter.

Establishing Emotionally Close and Supportive Relationships. Another motivation for disclosure primarily focuses on relational issues, such as feelings of closeness, caring, and trust (e.g., Derlega, Lovejoy, et al., 1998; Greene & Faulkner, 2002; Mason, Marks, Simoni, Ruiz, & Richardson, 1995). Self-disclosure is often used to accelerate relationship development and to foster intimacy (Gilbert, 1976). People make disclosure decisions so they can protect themselves by depending on people they trust and feel close to as friends and family members. However, the choice of confidant does not necessarily have to be someone with whom the person with HIV has had a previous long-term relationship. Closeness is defined in a variety of ways, as we see with the following example. This woman described how closeness with another woman at church influenced her decision to tell her about the HIV diagnosis:

> The first person I told was one of my church sisters because she and I are very close. ... I think I told her because she is like a big sister to me, and we are very close. ... I knew in my heart she would understand [about the HIV diagnosis].

For this woman, the level of relationship was significant in her disclosure decision. Agne et al. (2000) reported one reason for HIV disclosure to health care providers was a previously established relationship, similar to Klitzman's (1999) finding that a close or trusting relationship with a partner was a reason to disclose. Trust is a complex feature of relationships. It is also related to the quality of relationships and anticipated response to disclosure discussed later in this chapter.

Common Experiences or Similarity. Individuals may disclose to others who have shared a common background or who have similar health problems (Derlega, Lovejoy, et al., 1998; Derlega & Winstead, 2001). There are numerous cases in which the thread of similar experiences forms the basis for deciding to disclose. The following are just a few examples to illustrate this point. For instance, one man told his lover's brother:

> Because he was dying of AIDS and he was open with it. I had no one to go to who was actually in that situation. And to me, to talk to someone who was dying, in the same boat that I would sooner or later be in, was the most important thing to me.

In another case, a man told someone he met at an HIV clinic: "We were both there. He felt like he could share with me, and I could share with him. We discussed our medical problems." Finally, this woman disclosed to her sister before any other family members because the sister had prior experiences in coping with HIV and no doubt seemed a safe choice because she understood the problem:

> The first person I told in my family was my sister. And the reason why I told her was because she had already dealt with dating a guy both of whose parents were positive and he [the sister's boyfriend] lost his mother to AIDS.

As these cases exemplify, the person with HIV often relies on the comfort of knowing that the confidant has some knowledge about the disease that came from a similar experience. Because they have common experiences, these people are generally expected to react better.

Why might someone with HIV disclose their diagnosis to another who is perceived as similar? It may be due to the perception that the other person is likely to be supportive or less likely to be rejecting. Another reason is that social comparison with someone who has undergone similar experiences (whether the similarities are based on sexual orientation, drug use, lifestyle, or living with a life threatening disease) may help in reducing uncertainty about how to cope with the HIV infection (Buunk & Gibbons, 1997; Festinger, 1954; Helgeson & Mickelson, 1995; Stanton, Danoff-Burg, Cameron, & Snider, 1999; Taylor & Lobel, 1989). We note though that it is not inevitable that persons with HIV disclose to others who are perceived as similar. A woman we interviewed mentioned how she had been a cocaine and heroin addict. She noted how "over 50% of the people I used to hang out with, they had died from AIDS and we never discussed it." For this woman, shared similar experiences that would generally make a safe situation for disclosure had not resulted in her sharing. This is important to remember, as similarity or shared experience does not always result in a person choosing to disclose an HIV diagnosis.

Consistent with the importance of similar backgrounds and experiences as a reason for disclosure, MSM with HIV are more likely to disclose to someone about the diagnosis who shares their sexual orientation. MSM with HIV are more likely to disclose about their HIV status to a homosexual or bisexual close male friend or employer compared to a heterosexual male friend or employer (e.g., Hays et al., 1993; Marks et al., 1992; Simoni, Mason, & Marks, 1997). The same may be true of hemophiliacs or injection drug users who would share an HIV diagnosis with another hemophiliac or drug user. The common bond of shared experience or similar situations (and perhaps possible source of infection) may make disclosure more common.

Thus far, we have discussed motivations for disclosing an HIV diagnosis based on self, other, and interpersonal criteria. We first examined two reasons people disclose for self-gain. Next, we turned to two reasons people may disclose for other-gain. Finally, we examined three reasons people may disclose for interpersonal-gain. Although we have discussed motivations for disclosing an HIV diagnosis based on self, other, and interpersonal criteria separately, these types of motivations are not mutually exclusive. Instead, there is often considerable overlap among these motivations for HIV disclosure that need to be considered when studying decisions to disclose. We turn now to motivations for nondisclosure of an HIV diagnosis, or how people make decisions to maintain privacy.

MOTIVATIONAL CRITERIA FOR NONDISCLOSURE OF AN HIV DIAGNOSIS

Disclosing is only one option in decisions about sharing an HIV diagnosis. There are many occasions when individuals are less disclosive and wish to maintain more of their privacy. The decision to preserve a more tightly controlled privacy boundary is motivated by a number of issues. For example, people may feel more uncertain about a disclosure outcome and exercise caution because the risks are more potent for these people. Thus, they opt for concealing their status instead of revealing it to others. Someone with HIV may also feel guilty or blame themselves for their disease. These unhappy feelings often lead to restricting who knows about their status. In addition, fear of rejection contributes to nondisclosure and preservation of privacy. Some individuals may find it difficult to articulate the fact that they have the disease. To protect themselves, they remain closed and do not disclose. Concealment may also be motivated by a desire to shield others who might be hurt by the knowledge of a person's HIV status. Thus, the person may confine the communication of their heath status for many reasons.

The decision not to divulge information about the diagnosis may serve to express one's autonomy and independence (by claiming a right to privacy and ownership over information about the self) as well as a defense against the spread of information about the diagnosis to unwanted others. Some perceive it as "none of their business" (Wilson, Roloff, & Carey, 1998). Hence, those infected perceive higher risks and use many strategies to control the information. Consequently, people who are diagnosed with HIV are actively engaged in regulating their privacy boundaries (Greene, 2000; Greene & Serovich, 1996; Yep, 2000). Because of their need for control, it is not surprising to find that they often express a greater right to or need for privacy than noninfected persons, particularly when asked how much others should be privy to someone's HIV test results (Greene et al., 1993; Greene & Serovich, 1996). Further, the focus on concealment for those with HIV holds true whether the target person is family (e.g., a spouse, lover, parent, child) or nonfamily (e.g., a coworker or neighbor). Next, we explore reasons people are motivated to maintain privacy: third-party leakage, self-blame, fear of rejection, protecting others, and superficial relationship (see Derlega & Winstead, 2001). Self-focused motivations for nondisclosure include third-party leakage, self-blame, and fear of rejection. Protecting others is an other-focused motivation for nondisclosure. Finally, we examine superficial relationship as an interpersonal motivation for nondisclosure. To begin examination of these motivations for nondisclosure, we turn to self-focused motivations.

Decisions Leading to Nondisclosure for Self-Gain

Some decisions to not disclose are based on self-gain or protecting the self. These include third-party leakage, self-blame, and fear of rejection. We begin with apprehension about third-party leakage, that is, unwanted others knowing about their diagnosis leads to nondisclosure.

Third-Party Leakage. Anxiety about privacy derives in part from concern about the extent to which others might misunderstand, breach, or otherwise divulge the HIV diagnosis to unwanted third parties (Derlega & Chaikin, 1977; Greene & Faulkner, 2002; Kelvin, 1977; Petronio, 2000a; Rawlins, 1983). CPM describes these problems with coordination and co-ownership. Because individuals with HIV often worry about whether the disclosure recipient is willing or able to take responsibility for the knowledge of their HIV status, they are concerned about the degree to which their information is safe with the recipient or if the recipient will keep the confidence (Derlega, Lovejoy, et al., 1998; Greene & Faulkner, 2002; Kimberly et al., 1995; Moneyham et al., 1996; Simoni et al., 1995). For instance, one man stated:

> I wouldn't tell a friend that I went to school with [about the diagnosis] because he is a crack user and [an] alcoholic. I don't want him to advertise to the world when he is in one of his drunken states that I'm positive.

In this case, the individual decided against telling this friend because he was not consistently trustworthy, especially when he was using drugs or alcohol. Thus, the friend was unable to be responsible about maintaining the privacy boundaries around the diagnosis.

In another case, a man refused to tell anyone in his family about the diagnosis because, he stated, "if you tell a member of the family, then when you see them again the whole family knows. I wanted it [the information about the HIV diagnosis] to be private." In this circumstance, the man with HIV understood the parameters of information that was introduced into a family privacy boundary. Although the diagnosis was his information, once disclosed to a family member that person would treat it like information belonging to everyone in the family instead of keeping it confidential between the infected person and himself or herself. This example illustrates the problem often encountered when other people presume ownership over private information (cf. Vangelisti & Caughlin, 1997). Often families have rules assuming when one family member knows something like a person's HIV status, all family members should be privy to that information. This is not really considered gossip; instead, the members share a sense of concern for their relative. In families in which there are rules for interfamily openness, all members expect to be told. Because the person in this example wished to keep the information confidential, he chose to conceal it from any relative rather than risk everyone in the family knowing his diagnosis. Although this choice keeps his status secret, it also compromises the possibility of gaining needed social support from certain family members. This point illustrates the difficulty of containing the dissemination of a person's HIV status and underscores the decision criteria people consider when they are judging the way to cope with their disease through disclosure.

One final type of third-party concern is the dissemination of information through databases, an emerging issue. In one study, individuals with HIV were concerned about their name being in a computer database (Moneyham et al., 1996), and this affected decisions to disclose. To date, there is little research on this issue, but with changes in insurance (e.g., HMOs), concerns about privacy

violations by inappropriate access to computer data bases is an area for exploration, especially if this concern inhibits disclosure to health care providers (see
Health Insurance and Accountability Act [HIPAA], Rada, 2002, for discussion of
new regulations). We also explore using a third party in disclosure messages in
chapter 4.

Self-Blame and Self-Concept Difficulties.   People may also not disclose because
they are motivated by feelings of shame, the second self-focused motivation for
nondisclosure. In other words, people with HIV may feel that they have done
something wrong or that they are tainted (recall earlier stigma discussion; cf.
Bauman et al., 1997) and consequently feel it is necessary to keep the information
concealed from others. One woman described how she did not disclose to anyone
after she learned about the HIV diagnosis because she felt tainted and dirty. She
stated, "I think you feel like you're a bad person when you are diagnosed with this,
or obviously there was something you could have done to prevent this." The decisions to conceal rather than disclose depend here on feeling humiliation of having
the disease, as if more should have been done to control and prevent contracting
the disease.

Some individuals accept the popular stereotype that they are a potential health
risk to others even if they are not in a situation in which they are exchanging
bodily fluids with others (e.g., drug use, sexual behavior, or breast feeding). For instance, one woman stated that she could not reveal her status to others because
she feared infecting them. Thus, people with HIV struggle with identity issues.
For some, HIV becomes core to their identity: "It's the biggest thing in my life" or
"My whole life revolves around my HIV, the medication, treatments." Issues with
self-blame or self-concept may inhibit disclosure.

Fear of Rejection or Being Misunderstood.   The third self-focused motivation
for nondisclosure is fear of rejection or being misunderstood. People are also motivated to restrict privacy boundaries due to concerns about being rejected, stigmatized, misunderstood, ostracized, or discriminated against. People with HIV may
fear losing their jobs, insurance, housing, or child custody, and so forth. In today's
society, these fears are well placed despite legislation and other efforts to protect
civil rights (cf. Burris, 1999). The worries that people with HIV have (not only about
losing jobs but also about being rejected by family, friends, or intimate partners, or
even being physically assaulted; see Brown, Melchior, Reback, & Huba, 1994;
Gielen, O'Campo, Faden, & Eke, 1997; Kimerling, Armistead, & Forehand, 1999;
Rothenberg & Paskey, 1995; van der Straten, King, et al., 1998) may influence decisions not to disclose. Fear of rejection was the most common reason cited not to disclose an HIV diagnosis in Klitzman's (1999) study. In Agne et al.'s (2000) study of 107
people with HIV (predominantly MSM), 33% reported fear (e.g., "I was afraid of
her response," p. 249) as the reason for not disclosing HIV diagnosis to their health
care provider. People with HIV have specific concerns about tangible things such as

violence, housing, or insurance. These tangible fears influence decisions to maintain privacy. The possibility of relational rejection or disappointment is psychological, but it can also motivate nondisclosure. A man with HIV described how he would not tell some family members about the diagnosis because of concerns about their negative reactions:

> As for my uncles and aunts, I have the basic, old-fashioned, country family that are set in their ways. And so it's better that they don't know [about the diagnosis] because they are the type that I know would turn their back on me instead of be[ing] there for me.

Not only do people fear rejection from their family members, but this anxiety may partly explain why some might not disclose to sexual and intimate partners. Participants in Green's (1994) study reported fear of rejection was common, but reported few actual reactions that included rejection (see also chap. 5). The incidence of post-HIV disclosure divorce is unknown (see chap. 5 for more detailed actual reactions to HIV disclosure). A man with HIV refused to tell his girlfriend about his diagnosis because he felt certain that she would abandon him. He said, "I thought she liked me. I believed it would affect our relationship if I did tell her. I wouldn't want to lose her in that way." Although the decision not to reveal this health condition denies the girlfriend needed information about her relationship with this man, calculating the decision is complicated. As we see from the man just described, he did not want to disturb the relationship, yet he also wanted to protect his girlfriend from the disease. Thus, he mentioned using a condom when having sex with this partner "just to be safe." In this way, the decision in favor of concealment is justified (in the man's thinking) by also enacting behaviors that tried to protect the unsuspecting other.

Wishing to keep the relationship at its current level or not tamper with the relationship may motivate not disclosing the HIV status. Disruption to the relationship is a possible expectation when a partner finds out that he or she has been sexually intimate with someone with HIV. The burden of telling may be more stressful than the burden of concealing the information. Ignoring the situation gives the person with HIV some time to come to grips with the knowledge. Unfortunately, those who choose to conceal from their partners eventually add another layer of issues to their dilemma. One woman with HIV explained her reasoning to withhold her status in the interest of preserving some sense of enacting a "normal" relationship. However, her account also illustrates the risk individuals take in making this decision:

> I finally did tell him about two months into the relationship. Everybody else around me knows that I have it, but I had "me–him" away from all the AIDS-related stuff. He was full of anger when he first found out, and I said that I just wanted to be normal one last time. I don't want to be fucked with AIDS. I wanted to be fucked. He understood it after we talked about it for a while. But I felt like I was leading a double life

because here I've got AIDS stuff all over my house. I have t-shirts, my car [stickers], everything's got it. He'd ask me, and I'd say I do AIDS education. I do a lot of guest speaking because of my nursing background. He had accepted that, but I just wanted to be fucked one last time. He was the one person that didn't know, and I wanted to keep it from him. I didn't want to get treated any different or to scare him away.

For this woman, the choice to not disclose was based on the concern that it would change the relationship.

Motivations for developing rules to restrict disclosure also stem from both psychological threats as well as potential threats to health and safety of the infected individual (e.g., Herek, 1999a; Herek & Capitanio, 1993; Kimerling et al., 1999; Leary & Schreindorfer, 1998; Rose, 1998; Rothenberg & Paskey, 1995). The risk of physical assault among people with HIV needs to be examined further. For instance, there is evidence from surveys that a male partner's knowledge of a woman's HIV positive status is associated with sexual coercion—such as insistence on having sex or the man getting angry if the woman refuses to have sexual intercourse (see van der Straten, King, et al., 1998)—but not necessarily with physical violence (see Vlahov et al., 1998). One woman with HIV who had recently stopped dating altogether described her decision to withhold her HIV status from her sexual partners, fearing physical abuse:

> The last relationship I had lasted 2 years. Then something separated us. I never told him. We kept in touch through letters, and I just never told him. I know some people that, if they tell a guy, the guy might beat them up. I know a girl that told a guy and he beat her up badly. That's what happens when you get in a relationship and don't tell first. I wasn't good at that so I decided to stop altogether [having intimate relationships].

Reports of HIV disclosers being physically assaulted are not isolated. Greene and Faulkner (2002) in a similar vein reported adolescents with HIV did not personally fear being assaulted but were concerned that others (their brothers or uncles) would beat up the supposed source of infection (the boyfriend or ex-boyfriend). This has not been reported elsewhere in the HIV or disclosure literature—situations in which a family member or friend would be violent toward a third party out of concern for the infected person—and it should be explored further. Fear of negative reactions are processed in decisions to disclose or maintain privacy. These fears range from tangible issues such as assault to relational and psychological issues.

Decisions Leading to Nondisclosure for Other-Gain

Some decisions to not disclose are based on other-gain or protecting the other person. Although many of the motivations to withhold information about one's HIV positive status are centered on protecting the individual with HIV, there are also reasons that concern the protection of others.

Protecting Others.   Many people with HIV are worried about other people's ability to cope with the knowledge of their HIV status. They do not want to upset or worry others and cite this as a reason for not disclosing about their diagnosis (e.g., Armistead, Klein, Forehand, & Wierson, 1997; Derlega, Lovejoy, et al., 1998; Diaz, 1998; Greene & Faulkner, 2002; Hays et al., 1993; Klitzman, 1999; Mason et al., 1995; Simoni et al., 1995; Winstead et al., 2002).

There are many explanations of why people with HIV weigh others' needs in deciding whether or not to disclose about the HIV diagnosis. For example, individuals who place a high priority on family loyalty may withhold the information about their HIV status from family members to save them from embarrassment, shame, or other negative consequences. In one case, a woman told us she did not disclose about the diagnosis to her mother because she had numerous problems of her own. She said about her mother, "she's emotionally unstable and an alcoholic. I'm afraid the news would send her back up in a hospital. She's also pre-Alzheimer's and she's suffering from dementia, and there's just too many problems with it." This consideration is similar to findings with sexually abused children (Petronio et al., 1996) in which children did not reveal the abuse to their grandmothers, sisters, brothers, or other family members when they (the others) were perceived to be unable to handle the disclosure. These findings suggest that although consideration for the other is apparent, an additional motivation may be to select confidants who are able to handle the responsibility of knowing the high-stress information. Once a disclosure is made, the recipient implicitly or explicitly is asked to be accountable for taking care of the information and for coping with the shared knowledge. In both cases—learning a child has been abused and that someone has HIV— the burden on the confidant is potentially great. Thus, projecting how the confidant or recipient might respond is justified both in terms of the outcome for the recipient and for the person who is HIV positive.

At times, people balance self and other concerns in disclosure decisions. As one man stated, his decision not to tell his daughter was based on considerations for both her and for himself:

> I feel like it would hurt her and confuse her more than it would help by telling. I would say that the health I am in right now that I've got a pretty good while to go. So, I just put that [telling her about the diagnosis] on the back burner for now. I don't know if I'll ever tell her.

There are also attempts to limit interfamilial disclosure. Even if some family members are informed about the diagnosis, others might not be told to protect them. For example, most of a family knows but they do not tell one sister because of her situation. In addition, family members who know the diagnosis might see the dissemination to outside sources as a reflection on them. Robinson, Walters, and Skeen (1989) reported in a sample recruited through a network for parents and friends of lesbians and gays (PFLAG), most parents wanted no one outside the family to know of their child's hypothetical HIV infection. As another example, a mother with HIV was asked by a television station to participate in a program about AIDS to be broadcast locally. When this woman asked her daughter whether it was okay to be on the television show, the daughter said, "Mommy, please don't do that to me." The mother then declined to appear on the program.

These examples illustrate the ramifications of jointly sharing the information and highlight how some family members view others knowing. In a sense, the nature of the mother–daughter relationship (in the preceding example) made the daughter perceive a kind of contagion in which her mother's HIV status was thought to affect her reputation (see courtesy stigma discussion in chap. 5). On the other hand, the mother sharing the information gave the daughter the ability to voice her objection to further widening the privacy boundary.

Decisions Leading to Nondisclosure for Interpersonal-Gain

Some decisions to not disclose are based on interpersonal factors. Although many of the motivations to withhold information about one's HIV positive status are centered on protecting the individual with HIV or the other (recipient), there are also reasons that concern the relationship. We explore the superficial relationship next.

Superficial Relationship.   Many people with HIV are worried about their relationship with the potential receiver of disclosure. If people with HIV do not feel the relationship is good, they may choose not to disclose. For example, one woman with HIV responded to a question about why she had not shared her diagnosis with a friend. "Why would I tell her? We used to be close, but not now." Another man had disclosed to some members of his family but did not want to tell his sister (and asked others specifically not to tell her):

> We just don't have that kind of relationship. I send her a card for her birthday, we exchange gifts at Christmas, but that's about it. I haven't seen her outside of a family gathering in maybe 5 years, and we live an hour apart.

For these people with HIV, poor relationships resulted in tightening of privacy boundaries. They could not conceive of reasons or situations in which they might share their diagnosis with these particular people.

Someone would be unlikely to disclose information as sensitive as an HIV diagnosis to someone with whom they had a poor relationship, even if the role was close. Serovich et al. (1998) reported negative reactions to women's disclosure of HIV infection occurred mostly in the context of poor relationships. Similarly, Petronio et al. (1996) reported concerns over loss of control and major trust problems (such as what happens to information once it is disclosed) as critical in disclosure decisions about sexual abuse. Limandri (1989) described prerequisites for HIV disclosure: compassion, understanding, trust, and rapport with the respondent. We cover additional features of relationship context in a section later in this chapter on relational quality, including illustrations and citations.

Summary of Decisions Leading to Nondisclosure

As this discussion has verified, people are motivated in numerous ways to conceal their HIV status. The particular needs of individuals influence the ways they disclose about their health condition. Both the level of risk and issues that motivate individuals are important in the way they develop rules that regulate revealing and concealing. However, these are not the only factors that contribute to managing private information. In addition, relationship ties are critical to decisions about disclosure to others because once the revelation is made, the recipients jointly share the information (Derlega et al., 1993). As those who share the responsibility for the information, all parties need to coordinate how they mutually manage the privacy boundary around HIV status. The reasons for nondisclosure reviewed were third-party leakage, self-blame, fear of rejection, protecting others, and superficial relationship. Thus far, the chapter has reviewed stigma and reasons for HIV disclosure and nondisclosure. In the next section we examine specific relational contributions to managing disclosure and privacy decisions.

RELATIONAL CONTEXTS FOR DISCLOSURE DECISIONS

In this chapter we have discussed stigma and motivations influencing disclosure decisions. In motivations for disclosure and nondisclosure we examined self, other, and interpersonal aspects of disclosure decision making. We explore further here the interpersonal or relational influences on HIV disclosure decisions. The scheme of relational contexts presented here contrasts with the earlier discussion in this chapter of motives or reasons for disclosure and nondisclosure.

One potentially useful view of contexts was proposed by Ickovics, Thayaparan, and Ethier (2001) to understand HIV transmission and progression for women from an ecological perspective, with an emphasis on "a reciprocal and bidirectional association between individuals and the social contexts in which they live" (p. 818). Four social contexts are described: sociocultural, interpersonal, temporal, and situational contexts. This contextual framework has utility for incorporating work on the relationships of people with HIV (see also Greene et al., 2002). Persons with HIV and those with whom they interact in relationships are embedded within these four contexts.

Features of relationships influence how people make decisions to reveal or conceal their HIV infection (e.g., Agne et al., 2000; Greene & Serovich, 1995). If disclosure does occur, a level of coordination is necessary so that consistent rules for disclosure may be used. However, coordination is not always attained, and we also see instances in which the members of the relationship are unable to reach a functional level of coordination. As a result, lack of coordination (or CPM discordance) takes place, and this can be especially troubling given the stigma associated with HIV. Although uncomfortable for the participants, this disagreement can help to develop a better sense of coordination once the members work through the discord.

The relational aspects of disclosure decisions are significant. Intimate relationships carry an implicit expectation to share aspects of self (Millar & Rogers, 1987). Self-disclosure is a component in this development of intimacy, and intimacy is crucial for the development of close relationships (e.g., Chelune, Robinson, & Kommor, 1984; Dindia, 1997, 2002; Prager, 1995; Reis & Shaver, 1988; Simmel, 1964/1950). The amount and intimacy of self-disclosure is related to stage of relationship (Taylor & Altman, 1987) and friendships (Miell & Duck, 1986).

For individuals with HIV, several critical issues mark potential relational effects on disclosure decisions. First, anticipated responses to revelations about HIV status may increase or decrease the likelihood that someone will be selected as a disclosure target. In addition, the individual with HIV may also measure the extent to which another person is able or willing to negotiate mutually held rules for how to manage this information. The nature of the relationship between the confidant (i.e., the disclosure recipient) and the person with HIV can also influence disclosure choices. In other words, the strength of ties between and among the potential recipients identifies possible disclosure choices. Another relational feature is past discussion of HIV. People may use discussion of HIV-related issues with the recipient to explore disclosure decisions. Finally, the relational quality also affects not only if someone tells about their health condition but also how much he or she tells. We examine each of these relational aspects in this section: anticipated response to disclosure, strength of relational ties, past discussion of HIV, perceived relational quality, discloser's past experience, and ethnicity and gender.

Anticipated Response to Disclosure

Because the nature of a relationship with someone selected to be a confidant is often critical, one way in which people make decisions about disclosing or not telling HIV status is through anticipating responses to disclosure (Petronio, 2002; Petronio & Martin, 1986). There is great uncertainty if someone does not know how the other will respond in a situation (Albrecht & Adelman, 1984; Berger, 1987) or to disclosure (e.g., Greene & Serovich, 1995; Kelly & McKillop, 1996; Petronio, Martin, & Littlefield, 1984; Vangelisti, Caughlin, & Timmerman, 2001).[1]

---

[1]There has been an upswing of research using uncertainty reduction theory, particularly in health settings. We should be cautious with the assumption that uncertainty generally does and will produce anxiety (e.g., Afifi & Weiner, 2002; Brashers, 2001). For example, some people are not tested for HIV (e.g., "I don't want to know"), preferring to remain unaware of their HIV status even if they practice risky behaviors. Sometimes uncertainty is not only tolerable but is even preferable (and this may differ between and within cultures; Hines, 2001).

Afifi and Weiner (2002) explored the notion that individuals are motivated to seek information to reduce uncertainty. For example, many people seek health information on the internet (Cline & Haynes, 2001). Managing information about many medical conditions is challenging, perhaps even more so with HIV because of the complexity of medications and relatively short research time (e.g., Brashers, Goldsmith, & Hsieh, 2002). People can use information to manipulate uncertainty (increase or decrease it) and thus may actually seek to either confirm or contradict present information. The information seeking may be more or less direct, and people may avoid information (because it can be overwhelming or they are distressed). For example, one person with HIV stated, "I just stopped listening, even going to meetings or the doctor. There was so much to read and learn, I just couldn't handle it." Information seeking about these issues can be passive, not just active, information gathering (see Berger, 2002).

In considering whether someone is likely to receive HIV disclosure, anticipating his or her reaction is often used as a rule (Greene & Faulkner, 2002; Greene & Serovich, 1995). People with HIV seek to anticipate the recipient's reaction before they are willing to disclose (Limandri, 1989) and often seek to explore the other's reaction (Dindia, 1998). For example, Kimberly et al. (1995) reported that women with HIV cite that the expected response from the target determines whether they will tell someone about their infection. Greene and Serovich (1995) found that only if someone anticipates a positive reaction (not a neutral or a negative one) are they willing to disclose an HIV diagnosis. It may be necessary, given topics as sensitive as HIV and AIDS, for people to be relatively certain of a positive response before they disclose about the HIV positive diagnosis.

One woman described why she waited to tell her boyfriend: "No way, uh-huh, no way would I take a chance on telling unless I was really sure what he'd do." This woman wanted to be clear about how the person might respond before sharing (which she eventually did), similar to a man in his 20s who was uncertain about telling his sister (which he had not yet done):

It's not worth it to guess on what she might say. She's my only sister, I can't mess that up. I'll wait 'til I'm pretty sure where she is, then I can decide if I want to tell her. It'd just kill me if my baby sister didn't talk to me, so I can't risk that right now.

Another woman described how she did not disclose to her father about the diagnosis because:

My father is very naive when it comes to life in general. My father is not educated into AIDS or HIV. So I feel that if I did tell my father he would treat me as though I was a disease.

Thus, if people expect a negative response they are less likely to disclose about the HIV diagnosis (Greene & Faulkner, 2002; Limandri, 1989; Moneyham et al., 1996; Simoni et al., 1997).

People are sometimes surprised by unanticipated responses to HIV disclosure, that is, they are more positive or negative than expected (Greene & Faulkner, 2002). On a more upbeat note, sometimes people respond much better than expected, but alternately people can be surprised by a negative reaction. For instance, Mansergh, Marks, and Simoni (1995) reported HIV disclosers had very positive reactions when they disclosed, which were different from the anticipated negative reactions of the nondisclosers. Thus, people may incorrectly expect the worst in terms of others' reactions to HIV disclosure, but given the risks discussed previously, nondisclosure may still be a prudent decision.

With each disclosure statement there is an implicit demand characteristic within the message that signals expectations for a certain kind of response (Petronio, 1991). Disclosure messages about HIV status are no different (explicit messages are explored in chap. 4). Adam and Sears (1994) noted that the process of HIV disclosure contains an implicit expectation for the type of response from the listener: "The revelation of a potentially discreditable aspect of self [such as HIV infection] carries with it at least an implicit appeal for trust and compassion by the other" (p. 72). Thus, people have clear ideas about how they would like the other to react or respond.

People with HIV often have an idea of what response to disclosure they want and make estimates of a person's likelihood of responding in the desired way (Greene & Serovich, 1995; Petronio, 1991). The disclosure process works smoothly when the expectations are met. For example, one individual commented, "I knew he [cousin] would be supportive too. He hugged me." Not all expectations, however, are positive. In another case, this person expected a negative response: "Well, I was always wondering if they were going to, you know, treat me differently or treat me the same way they been treatin' me." Finally, one girl shared her fears about poor reactions: "I think what really hurt me the most is if, I don't want them to act scared of me, you know." What people want to get out of a disclosure about their HIV status may affect the anticipated responses in the way they communicate the message and the implicit demands for certain responses to their message. Clearly, unanticipated reactions can lead to stress and discordance, and we explore these actual reactions to disclosure in chapter 5.

The ability of the discloser to accurately perceive and predict how the recipient copes with the information is also a factor in the disclosure process. In the decision to disclose, accurately perceiving the receiver's skills to handle the information is crucial. If the discloser makes a mistake and discloses to someone who cannot handle the information, the reaction will likely have a negative effect on both parties. Likewise, misreading the need to protect someone from the information also has potentially negative outcomes (see Greene & Faulkner, 2002, for a discussion of relational violations).

There are certainly times when the discloser feels that the receiver needs to be protected from difficult news like an HIV diagnosis (Hays, Chauncey, & Tobey, 1990; Yep, Reece, & Negrón, 2003). One man with HIV described why he could not tell his father: "He can't handle it; he'd lose it and not be OK." In Greene and Faulkner's (2002) interviews with adolescent girls with HIV, participants systematically would not disclose to someone who was considered too old, not physically healthy (or had an ill family member), or if the recipient did not have adequate social support (also see Greene & Serovich, 1995; Kimberly et al., 1995). For instance, an adolescent with AIDS reported, "she's [grandmother] too old, in bad health, got heart problems. I can't tell her, she'd fall out and die." Because a judgment is based on perceptions rather than actual reactions, there is always room for dealing with misjudgments about how a person might react to learning about an HIV diagnosis. The anticipated response of the recipient to the disclosure can affect decisions. We turn next to how strength of relational ties can influence this privacy management.

Relational Ties

In the United States, an average of 6 to 8 affected relatives or intimates (e.g., parent, sibling, partner, friend, etc.) exist for every person diagnosed with HIV (see Cowles & Rodgers, 1997), but not all these people are chosen to receive disclosure or function in a support role. The relational ties that people have with one another influence the decision to disclose and ultimately the level of control given over the information (Petronio, 2002). When there is a weak relational tie, recipients may be less willing to keep the information confidential. Strong relational ties with a recipient evoke a wholly different set of assumptions. This idea of relational ties is different from relational quality. Throughout the literature, we see many examples of the differences in judgment people make because of the strength of relational ties. Not only does it influence the initial disclosure decisions but also the level of disclosure and interaction thereafter (see Stokes, Fuehrer, & Childs, 1980; Tardy, Hosman, & Bradac, 1981). As Dindia (1998) argued, one chooses disclosure targets to manage risk, perhaps based on relational ties.

The factors influencing decisions to disclose to one recipient (e.g., a mother) are different from factors influencing decisions to disclose to another (e.g., a partner; see Derlega et al., 2002; Greene, 2000, 2001; Greene & Serovich, 1996; Marks et al., 1992; Simoni et al., 1995). Marital or significant relationships and even those previously holding strong ties (lovers, spouses, ex-spouses, friends) are often viewed as the most appropriate recipients of disclosure of HIV infection. In an extensive study, Wolitski, Rietmeijer, Goldbaum, and Wilson (1998) followed 701 MSM in four cities, and 6 months later 97% had disclosed to at least one other person (often a friend or partner). Of course, this does not suggest that ties within the nuclear family (e.g., parents, siblings, children) are unimportant. Indeed, research suggests that close family members are viewed the next highest (after partners) as potential recipients of disclosure of HIV status (Greene & Serovich, 1996; Marks et al., 1992; Serovich, Greene, & Parrott, 1992; Simoni et al., 1995). In comparison, a group that is less likely to receive the disclosure about HIV status is that of extended family (e.g., grandparents or in-laws), and the least likely is the general public.

Serovich et al. (1992) looked at the potential recipient of HIV-testing information. Individuals overall reported the most desire to restrict access to HIV-testing information to the general public, less to the community, and least to the marital subsystem. Serovich and Greene (1993) expanded this work by looking at potential family recipients of release of HIV-testing information. Overall, participants reported the most support for access to HIV-testing information to the marital system (e.g., lovers, spouses), moderate to the nuclear family (e.g., mother, son), and least to the extended family (e.g., aunt, mother-in-law). One drawback to these studies is they are based on perceptions of people who were not infected with HIV, but at present very little data area available on attitudes toward privacy of individuals with HIV.

Greene and Serovich (1996) replicated these studies and reported that persons with HIV also have clear distinctions in perceptions of appropriate recipients of information about HIV infection. In addition, persons with HIV reported less desire (compared with non HIV infected) for HIV disclosure to all subsystems. Marks et al. (1992) similarly reported individuals with HIV were highly selective in choosing recipients of disclosure and tended to inform significant others (parents, friends, and lovers) more than nonsignificant others (employers, landlords, and religious leaders). Thus, the strength of relational ties matters for people who are disclosing about their HIV status.

Disclosure to people one knows well enough to anticipate reactions seems to matter. In addition, it may be that a certain assumption about loyalty can be made with intimates and family members that cannot be made with strangers. Unlike other situations in which weak relational ties might be seen as preferable, someone with HIV needs to feel confident that they select people who have a vested interest in keeping the information confidential. However, the way that choices are made for disclosure may differ depending on with whom the person with HIV has strong relational ties. We explore disclosure to targets varying in relational tie strength next: partners, parents, siblings, children, family, friends, coworkers, and health care workers.

Disclosure to Partner. Decisions to disclose about an HIV diagnosis to a relational partner (lover or spouse) are complex. Besides possibly attaining social support, there is an added dimension of the need for safer sex or other potential risk-avoidance practices. The partner of a person with HIV is in a different position from others in that this person may be at substantial risk for exposure to the virus. Concealment could not only affect the relationship but the health of both the person with HIV and the partner. Infected persons are at risk for reinfection with another strain of HIV; additionally, they may be at risk for other sexually transmitted diseases (STDs) that are dangerous to persons with HIV (see, e.g., Kalichman, 2000). Not only is the person with HIV at risk, but the partner could be at risk as well. Therefore, decisions to disclose to partners are defined by different senses of obligation, both moral and legal. For example, Klitzman's (1999) participants reported disclosure was an important issue, "a moral one," and most felt main partners should be told.

One initial difficulty is that some individuals with HIV are reluctant to disclose to partners. Rates of reported disclosure to sexual partners have varied and range from 31% of a sample of homosexual and bisexual men with HIV (Stempel, Moulton, Bachetti, & Moss, 1989) to 89% of an HIV positive sample (Mansergh et al., 1995), with many studies reporting rates somewhere in between. Mason et al. (1995) described a range of disclosure to partners of 69% to 96% among Latino and White individuals with HIV. Marks, Richardson, and Maldonado (1991) reported that of men who were sexually active (other than kissing) post HIV diagnosis, 52% had not disclosed to one or more sexual partners. Marks et al. (1992) reported 24% had not disclosed to an intimate lover and 17% had not to a spouse (respectively, 76% and 83% disclosure). In contrast, Simoni et al. (1995) reported

87% disclosed to lovers, and Hays et al. (1993) found 98% of gay men disclosed to lovers. These differences in rates of disclosure to partners need to be better understood, perhaps as a feature of ethnicity, gender, or sexual orientation discussed later in this chapter.

It may be that the type of partner relationship predicts disclosure. Marks et al. (1992) reported that for Hispanic gay men with HIV, disclosure decreased with the number of sexual partners (see also Stein et al., 1998). Wolitski et al. (1998) reported 66% had not disclosed their infection to nonprimary partner versus 11% who had not to a primary partner. As Vázquez-Pacheco (2000) stated, "It seems the common social practice, however, is that if your sex partner is a stranger, then you don't tell him anything, not your serostatus, not your marital status, not even your real name" (p. 24). Stempel, Moulton, and Moss (1995) described 82% disclosure to a primary sexual partner compared with 56% to new sexual partner. Cranson and Caron (1998) reported that 90% of men and 86% of women had disclosed to primary partners and not as many disclosed to past partners (see Greene & Faulkner, 2002; Klitzman, 1999). In new relationships, significantly more women disclosed than men, indicating gender should be considered. Moneyham et al. (1996) reported women did not necessarily tell long-term partners out of concern that HIV disclosure would end the relationship. Finally, Marks et al. (1994) reported a disclosure rate of 86% to partners with HIV but 50% to partners who did not have HIV. Thus, it is important to distinguish type of relationship, casual or new, and whether or not the sexual partner is also HIV positive (see also Adam & Sears, 1994; Fisher, Kimble Willcutts, Misovich, & Weinstein, 1998; Klitzman, 1999; Markova, Wilkie, Naji, & Forbes, 1990; Norman et al., 1998).

Some people who know they are infected with HIV fail to tell their sexual partners. The good news is that reported disclosure to partners is increasing in recent years, and it may be higher for women (e.g., Greene & Faulkner, 2002). Even though the percentage of people revealing their status to partners may be on the rise, this is one of the most compelling reasons for exploring decision making about HIV disclosure. Men and women with HIV may choose to conceal their health status from the very people who are most affected (also see chap. 5 in which we discuss consequences of HIV disclosure). There are many reasons why a partner is not selected for disclosure. Disclosure decisions to partners are complicated, as they may fear losing the relationship, worry about violence, or not see the relationship as long term. The patterns of disclosure to partners vary widely, and these differences may be accounted for by year of diagnosis, length of time diagnosis has been known, symptoms, use of condoms, HIV status of partners, and relational status (one night vs. steady dating; e.g., Crosby, 2000; Green, 1994; Klitzman, 1999; Stein et al., 1998). We turn next to disclosure decisions to parents.

Disclosure to Parent(s). Choosing whether to disclose the diagnosis to parents is a stressful decision (see Kimberly et al., 1995), as disclosure to a parent can be important for social support of a person with HIV (Hays et al., 1993). People with HIV may fear parents' rejection and perhaps withdrawal of financial or emotional support (Gard, 1990). Individuals with HIV cite parents' health, age, and lack of education or sophistication as reasons for not disclosing to them (e.g., Gard, 1990; Greene & Faulkner, 2002; Kimberly et al., 1995).

Aside from the possible embarrassment, shame, or humiliation that comes with having to tell parents about one's HIV status, people also may have to engage in related disclosure. People with HIV sometimes feel a need to provide background information to go along with the disclosure of the HIV diagnosis. As described by some individuals with HIV, the first question asked is often, "How could this happen?" or "How did you get it?" To answer that, many people also have to describe their sexual behavior, drug habits, or other circumstances that frame the way in which they contracted the disease. This situation is relatively unique to HIV as a health condition. Consider for a moment the plausibility of someone asking a person with Lupus or colon cancer, "How did you get it?" People with HIV are asked this very question about source or mode of infection regularly. This is often the first question asked after HIV disclosure and may be prerequisite knowledge for disclosure, especially to parents. In fact, virtually no one in Marks et al.'s (1992) study revealed their HIV infection to parents if the parents did not already know about their gay or bisexual orientation.

When people do disclose to parents, they are more likely to tell their mother than father (e.g., Greene & Faulkner, 2002; Stempel et al., 1995), but this difference is not always large. Marks et al. (1992) reported 23.8% of their HIV positive sample had disclosed to their mothers, compared with 8.1% to fathers, but Simoni et al. (1995) reported moderate disclosure with 59% to mothers and 31% to fathers. Mason et al. (1995) reported a range of disclosure to mothers 39% to 61% and lower to fathers, 22% to 40%. Reports from Hays et al. (1993) are more similar, with mothers 48% and fathers 40%. These are in sharp contrast to a sample in which 82% of mothers and 78% of fathers had knowledge of a child's HIV infection (Greene & Serovich, 1996). Studies are clear that mothers are more often told than fathers, but this may also reflect an overall increase in disclosure over time.

Although the father may be unlikely to be told directly by the person with HIV (Greene & Faulkner, 2002), the mother or another family member may share the diagnosis with him. For the father, this may be a problem because he was not told directly and may not be able to acknowledge the information. In this case, his role may be restricted to receiving information through another person (such as the mother). This is a specific case of the phenomenon of third-party disclosure discussed in depth in chapter 4. Thus, the father knows but may have to pretend that he does not know to the child and others in the family. The father may be placed in a difficult situation if he wants to provide social support. This summary indicates people with HIV more often choose to disclose to mothers than to fathers, but they do disclose their diagnoses to parents. We also note the absence of research including stepparents. We turn next to disclosing an HIV diagnosis to siblings.

Disclosure to Siblings.   Decisions to disclose to siblings are not well under-stood in the literature. Some information helps direct further research in this area. For example, Mansergh et al. (1995) reported moderate disclosure to brothers (49%) and slightly higher levels to sisters (53%) (cf. Marks et al., 1992). Simoni et al. (1995) reported disclosure to sisters of 54% and brothers 49%, similar to Hays et al.'s (1993) report of disclosure to sisters 53% and brothers 43%. Mason et al. (1995) found similar disclosure patterns with sisters (37% to 60%) and brothers (36% to 54%). Some researchers have reported more disclosure to sisters than to brothers (e.g., Greene & Faulkner, 2002; Stempel et al., 1995). Thus, although the gender of the sibling matters in terms of how often information is disclosed, both sisters and brothers are disclosed to. This research should be interpreted with cau-tion based on the absence of other potential factors such as disclosure of sexual orientation or drug use.

Perhaps adult siblings receive more disclosure about the nature of their brother or sister's HIV status because they are more in-tune with generational life choices and may have been privy to intimate information in the past. In addition, the sibling may not respond by passing judgment in the same way that the parents might. Disclosure to a parent, on the other hand, may mean the risk of causing hurt or an angry response. A parent may also feel the child's choices or behavior reflects poorly on them, but a sibling is less likely to feel this way. It is also possible that relational quality with the sibling (discussed later in the chapter) is higher than with the parent, explaining the disclosure decision. We turn next to disclo-sure to children.

Disclosure to Children.   One consequence of the AIDS epidemic is the increas-ing number of AIDS orphans (Pequegnat & Szapocznik, 2000). Probably one of the most difficult situations is deciding about disclosing HIV diagnoses to children (both a parent's infection and the child's infection). By doing so, the child is drawn into an adult world with all of the associated responsibilities of privacy and the stigma of HIV and AIDS. Not only does the telling become problematic, but the aftermath can be especially difficult for children. It is difficult to know how to make the decision to reveal or conceal HIV status to children. For example, moth-ers may have limited resources for making decisions about disclosure to children (e.g., Chung & Magraw, 1992; Kimberly et al., 1995). Thus, it is especially difficult to process this disclosure decision. Schrimshaw and Siegel (2002) described that among mothers with HIV, two thirds had disclosed to one or more of their chil-dren (see also Greene & Faulkner, 2002; Winstead et al., 2002). There was a greater likelihood of disclosure to children if the child lived in the home. Pliskin, Farrell, Crandles, and DeHovitz (1993) reported slightly lower disclosure, in which 55% of mothers disclosed the diagnosis to their seronegative children. In-terestingly, many studies related to disclosure of HIV—some focusing on gay men—have failed to explore children as recipients of disclosure (e.g., Hays et al., 1993; Mansergh et al., 1995; Marks et al., 1992; Simoni et al., 1995). Many people with HIV, including gay men, are parents, and this topic deserves further research attention.

For parents, disclosure to children is a difficult decision. Parents report thinking about this matter weekly, with an enormous emotional toll from concealing this information (Wiener, Battles, & Heilman, 1998). Researchers studying when to inform a child of any parent's serious illness focus on to what extent the child can perceive the seriousness of the disease and impending death (see Wiener, Septimus, & Grady, 1998). Bauman, Draimin, Levine, and Hudis (2000) focused on what children understand of death; nondisclosure may deny the child the opportunity to mourn with support, and disclosure could help the child manage grief, fear, and stigma. Parents must also consider plans for the future, including issues related to the care and custody of children (Bauman et al., 2000; Wiener, Septimus, et al., 1998). Age ("Are they ready?") and ability to keep the secret (Gewirtz & Gossart-Walker, 2000; Greene & Faulkner, 2002; Moneyham et al., 1996; Winstead et al., 2002) are also issues parents must consider in deciding whether or not to disclose to children.

For the parent, making the decision to reveal HIV status can be especially difficult when it is one's own child (e.g., Wiener, Battles, et al., 1998). The disclosure decision not only concerns one's own mortality, but the life and death of the parent matters greatly to the child (Wiener & Figueroa, 1998). Although disclosure allows the child to prepare for the death as well as coping with health problems and the medical management of HIV (Armistead et al., 1997; Gewirtz & Gossart-Walker, 2000; Rotheram-Borus & Lightfoot, 2000; Siegel & Gorey, 1994; Winstead et al., 2002), the parent must select ways of telling that are helpful rather than detrimental. It may also be important to prepare the child for the parent's ordeal, possibly changing living circumstances (if the parent becomes incapacitated due to illness). On the other hand, if the information is concealed and the child is protected, ultimately this choice may have more negative ramifications than positive ones (Bauman et al., 2000). The child may witness symptoms and become frightened because he or she does not understand the problem. As the illness progresses, depending on the age of the child, he or she may want to discuss the future with the parent. By not disclosing to the child, the parent does not allow a line of communication that is necessary to cope with the radical changes in the child's life. We turn next to disclosure to family.

Disclosure to Family.   *Family* is a broad term, varying in specificity by culture. We previously covered several specific family relations, parents, siblings, and children, but some studies collapse all family members in to the category of family compared with employer or general public, and so forth. Family has an important role in disease prevention and health promotion (Pequegnat & Szapocznik, 2000). HIV as a chronic disease creates a strain on the family system

(Gewirtz & Gossart-Walker, 2000; Pequegnat & Szapocznik, 2000), and relatives are often caretakers (Pequegnat & Bray, 1997; Wiener, Septimus, et al., 1998). Other research shows that it is important to separate family members in terms of the different roles they have in the life of someone with HIV (see Greene & Serovich, 1996; Serovich & Greene, 1993). For example, differences in disclosure to mothers and fathers such as those reviewed previously suggest that disclosure to family varies by specific relationship. Families often have secrets they do not talk about outside the family unit (Vangelisti et al., 2001), but the number of family secrets is inversely related to people's level of satisfaction with their family (Vangelisti, 1994).

Reports of disclosure to family overall are relatively low, but higher for some specific family members reviewed previously. Stempel et al. (1995) reported 37% disclosure to family 1 year post diagnosis. Wolitski et al. (1998) reported 35% to family, but Lester, Partridge, Chesney, and Cooke (1995) reported that 75% of women with HIV had disclosed to family. Perry, Ryan, Fogel, Fishman, and Jacobsberg (1990) reported only 35% of gay men with HIV had disclosed to any family member. Additionally, we know little about disclosure to family members such as in-laws, grandparents, cousins, aunts, and uncles (for exceptions, see Greene & Faulkner, 2002; Greene & Serovich, 1996; Simoni et al., 1995), but disclosure to extended family is lower (Simoni et al., 1995; e.g., grandparents 24%, cousin 28%, and aunt or uncle 22%). There is a need for continued work to explored disclosure decisions to extended family, especially with increased life expectancy for people with HIV and some families where multiple members are infected.

Disclosure to Friends. The decision to disclose about the HIV diagnosis to friends is another complex yet different issue. Reports that individuals disclose most to friends are not surprising, as friends are freely chosen and distinguished by mutual trust and similarity (see discussion of relational quality found later in this chapter). For example, if people experience problems in romantic relationships, they most often turn to friends of the same age and sex for assistance (Goldsmith & Parks, 1990). Several studies have reported relatively high disclosure to at least some friends: Perry et al. (1990) reported 68%, Marks et al. (1992) reported 58% disclosure to a male friend and 43% to female friend, Simoni et al. (1995) reported 78%, Mason et al. (1995) reported 74% to 87%, and Stempel et al. (1995) reported 92% to a gay friend 1 year post diagnosis. This is in contrast to Hays et al. (1993) in which 95% had disclosed to a gay friend but only 77% to a heterosexual friend (cf. Lester et al., 1995, in which 65% women reported no disclosure to any friend, but this sample is composed of pregnant, disadvantaged mothers who were especially stressed with the health care system, and even seronegative controls were distressed). These estimates are difficult to interpret because they may be based on disclosing to one or several friends but not take into account the three or perhaps dozen friends not disclosed to. It is also uncertain if there are gender effects here (cf. Dindia, 2002), whether people are more or less willing to disclose to male or female friends, or if HIV disclosure is affected by some combination of the discloser's and recipient's gender and/or sexual orientation.

Social networks also complicate HIV disclosure to friends. If friends know each other, it may be difficult to tell one person and not another. Also the partner of a friend may influence disclosure choices. For example, one man stated:

> I wanted to tell a high school buddy of mine, we'd always been close. But his new wife, she's real religious and always making comments. I don't want to put him in a bad spot with her, where he'd have to lie about my HIV. No way would I want her to know.

Thus, common sense would lead us to believe people disclose to friends, and studies show there is a high level of disclosure. However, these decisions are not automatic and have unique complexities. Some of these differences can be explained by differences in the term *friend* (vs. *acquaintance*), as the term *friend* is used loosely by some and more strictly by others (see Argyle & Henderson, 1984, for discussion of "lapsed friends" or former friends people were once closer to and how rules change in these friendships). We turn next to disclosure to coworkers.

Disclosure to Coworkers.   Some people with HIV struggle with decisions to disclose (or not) to coworkers. Much of the employee HIV literature focuses on transmission risks (e.g., health care workers, food service), legal issues, or attitudes of noninfected workers (Simoni et al., 1997). With changes in the epidemic, many people with HIV remain in or never leave the workforce. Thus, a person may spend a significant portion of time (perhaps one third) in a work setting with others, some of whom will become friends. These decisions to share a diagnosis are also complicated with risk of reprisal, as people have reported termination, harassment, or hostile work environments following HIV disclosure. If illness affects attendance, the person with HIV may need an explanation for missing work and choose to tell a supervisor with the hope it is not shared further. People in specific types of jobs (e.g., day care, hospitals, food preparation) may also process information about fears of contagion in their disclosure decisions. The most extensive study to date on disclosure of HIV infection in the workplace is Simoni et al. (1997). In this study of MSM with HIV, there was increased disclosure if the person with HIV was European American, diagnosed more than 4 years previously, employer was gay or bisexual, "out" at work (had disclosed his sexual orientation), and symptomatic.

One possible explanation for differences in HIV disclosure for some people is how "out" someone is about their sexual orientation. Disclosing sexual orientation may have preceded discussion of HIV diagnosis (Marks et al., 1992; Mason et al., 1995). Research indicates if a person with HIV has disclosed at work that they are gay, lesbian, or bisexual, they are more likely to disclose an HIV diagnosis. For example, Simoni et al. (1997) found that being out about one's sexual orientation increased the likelihood of HIV disclosure at work. These findings may be helpful for some people with HIV who are gay or bisexual, but it will not apply directly to others, for example, heterosexuals.

There may be different issues in disclosing to a boss and a coworker. Many people form relationships with coworkers that are similar to friendships, and these may be different from boss–employee relationships. Alternately, a boss might be told rather than a coworker if there is any question about transmission risk or to assist with coordinating appointments, and so forth. For example, Hays et al. (1993) reported 47% disclosed to a boss and 60% to coworkers. Similarly, Stempel et al. (1995) reported 31% of employers and 46% of coworkers were told by 1 year post diagnosis. Thus, current evidence indicates people disclose more to coworkers than employers.

Many people are adamant about not disclosing in a work setting. A man with HIV said:

> I didn't tell anybody at work because I was a professional at work. I never discussed anything personal. Work is work. I have no interaction with those people after work. I came here to do a job, and let's get the job done and go home.

For this man, the information is not relevant for others. Another woman expressed more ambiguity about her decision. She had been retired for nearly a decade; however, she remembered her concerns about possibly exposing others to the infection:

> I decided not to tell the girls that I'm close to at work, because we did a lot of things together there. We had cooking parties at work and we had picnics together. We were like a close family. When one girl's parents died, the whole office went. So I was close to those girls. But I definitely didn't want to tell them because I would think they would have thought about all the food that I cooked and if [they became infected with HIV] they got it from me. I was really afraid. I said, "Maybe I did. Maybe I gave them something." I wasn't even aware of being educated at the time about it [HIV transmission]. So I was pretty scared.

This woman did not want to disclose even to coworkers, and this created much distress. The research on disclosure in the workplace indicates it occurs more to coworkers than employers and is higher if someone is out and diagnosed longer. Disclosing HIV in the workplace continues to be an area for future study.

Disclosure to Health Care Workers.   Common wisdom indicates people with HIV should disclose to medical providers to obtain the best medical care possible. Another reason for disclosure is to avoid endangering the health care worker. The probability of a patient infecting a health care worker is much greater than a health care worker infecting a patient (Clark, 1999; Limandri, 1989; Marks, Mason, &

Simoni, 1995; Oddi, 1994). This finding does contradict entrenched public perceptions of the Kimberly Bergalis case (Singleton, 1993). In 1991, Bergalis was supposedly exposed to HIV through David Acer, her dentist. Acer was HIV positive and may have infected six of his patients (including Bergalis) through contaminated instruments, and the case received extensive publicity.

This disclosure decision to health care providers, however, is confusing because not all medical professionals necessarily need to know. For example, a nurse who draws blood is at some risk of contracting HIV (although it is minimal if precautions are taken). However, this situation is different from a case in which a person is taking blood pressure, height, and weight, or deciding which medications might interact (and must know what the person is taking). More complex decisions would occur in situations related to dentists or dental hygienists in which there is some risk of accidental transmission of HIV (see Charbonneau, Maheux, & Beland, 1999; Cline & McKenzie, 2000).

People generally expect medical professionals to have more accurate knowledge about transmission and to be less prejudiced in their attitudes about someone with HIV. Unfortunately, some health personnel also stigmatize people with HIV (Crawford, Humfleet, Ribordy, Ho, & Vickers, 1991; Gerbert, Maguire, Bleeker, Coates, & McPhee, 1991; Kelly et al., 1987a, 1987b). Patients may be concerned that some health care workers will not treat them, and refusal of care has been reported (e.g., Derse, 1995). This type of stigma will lessen willingness to disclose to health care workers, even when disclosure has clear benefits (Agne et al., 2000; Doll et al., 1994, found the type of medical screening by health personnel had a significant effect on HIV disclosure). Consider the Greg Louganis episode. The Olympic diver split open his head and needed stitches but had not told the team physician about his HIV positive status (see Clark, 1999; Louganis, 1996). The incident created a great deal of controversy, from the blood in the pool to the physician who stitched Louganis and failed to take universal precautions of putting on gloves. In this case, the balance of privacy led Louganis to disclose several years after the incident but not before.

Reported rates of HIV disclosure to health care professionals have varied but are higher if a patient feels comfortable with the provider (Agne et al., 2000). For example, Perry et al. (1993) reported 88% disclosure to physicians. In contrast, Stempel et al. (1995) reported 71% disclosure to physicians, 57% to psychotherapists, but 37% to dentists 1 year post HIV diagnosis. These results are similar to Wolitski et al. (1998) findings of 17% disclosure to health care workers and 59% to physicians. Marks et al. (1995) reported 21% had not disclosed their infection to any health provider. Moneyham et al. (1996) reported women with HIV had not always disclosed to health care workers out of concern regarding discrimination and their name being recorded in a database. In one study of a specialized health facility (Barnes, Gerbert, McMaster, & Greenblatt, 1996), patients disclosed to 70% of dentists but often in response to a direct inquiry (only one half volunteered the diagnosis). Finally, a study by Agne et al. (2000) found that individuals with HIV typically do disclose their diagnosis to health care workers for better coordination of health care but are still cautious about possible risks. The study also noted that HIV disclosure increases dramatically in response to a direct question from the health care provider. Disclosure to health care workers should be studied further, and at present does not include a wide range of mental health providers, for example therapists or religious figures.

Summary of Relational Ties.   We have reviewed in this section the unique features of relational roles (e.g., partner, sibling, coworker) that contribute to decisions to open or close the privacy boundary around an HIV diagnosis. We explored this in the context of relational ties. We turn now to how people use past discussion of HIV to assist in making HIV disclosure decisions.

Past Discussion of HIV

Relational quality and relational ties previously discussed are entwined with past discussion of various topics, including HIV. It is reasonable to expect more previous discussion of most topics with those you are closer to. People with HIV or AIDS often report discussing AIDS, health issues, or homosexuality before they share an HIV diagnosis (Dindia, 1998; Greene, 2001). In part, they may do this to test the reactions of others and to gain information before they decide (or not) to disclose. Dindia (1998) described how people can "test the waters" or check the environment by slowly approaching a topic of disclosure to check the reaction. In this case, an individual with HIV might first talk about a sick friend, describe the illness, and finally reveal he or she has HIV or AIDS (also see Powell-Cope & Brown, 1992). One woman reported, "When I start thinking about telling someone, I try to talk about related things to kind of feel it out first." For some, the disclosure decision is tentative and very slow. Another man described similarly, "First I talked to my sister about a mutual friend who had AIDS. She was very supportive of him, so that made it easier to decide to tell her." At the time of the interview, this man had not told his sister but intended to do so, and the AIDS discussions were important in his decisions. One study reported that past discussion of AIDS predicted perceived willingness to disclose HIV infection, but that was not in an HIV positive sample (Greene & Serovich, 1995). In this study, the more people had discussed HIV with the target person (e.g., mother, friend), the more willing they would be to disclose if they had an HIV infection.

People use discussion of AIDS or other issues to explore others' reactions or to prepare them before they decide to disclose. In these instances the decisions to disclose are based on how the potential recipient handles related discussions. Individuals with HIV evaluate and anticipate possible reactions through these discussions and choose disclosure recipients carefully (Holt et al., 1998). We look next at the effect of relational quality on disclosure decisions.

Perceived Relational Quality

Perceived relational quality is a part of the relational context that influences disclosure decisions. Perception of a relationship is a significant determinant of willingness to disclose HIV infection as well, beyond past discussion of AIDS-related issues. People choose disclosure targets they feel closer to (Collins & Miller, 1994; Dindia, 1998, 2002; Dindia & Tieu, 1996; Greene, 2001; Marks et al., 1992; Spencer & Derlega, 1995; Vangelisti & Caughlin, 1997; Wheeless, 1976) and trust (Cozby, 1973; Pearce & Sharp, 1973; Wheeless & Grotz, 1977). Vangelisti et al. (2001) noted that the quality of relationship with the target (psychologically close) is part of the criteria used for disclosure beyond the relationship role. Thus, in addition to the role a relationship plays (e.g., sister), the quality of that relationship is likely to differentiate relationships. For example, a person can have varying degrees of relational quality with a sister such as very close, frequent contact or more distant and conflictual. This perception of the relationship may be a deciding factor in disclosure decisions. A woman with an AIDS diagnosis told her mother because "We've never kept secrets, and I wanted her to know why I was sick. I didn't want her to be scared because I was getting sick all the time. At least now she knows why." For this woman, the relationship was significant in the disclosure decision.

Individuals may also not disclose about the HIV diagnosis to someone because they do not feel close to them. The other person may be a neighbor, a casual acquaintance, or a coworker who is not known well enough, who "doesn't need to know," or someone with whom there is no ongoing relationship. Even relationships with family members who are not seen very often or who are not close (for instance, in-laws, cousins) may be perceived as too superficial to justify disclosure of the diagnosis (Greene & Faulkner, 2002; Greene & Serovich, 1996). A man in his 40s described how he did not tell his adult siblings about his HIV diagnosis because:

> I guess my brothers and sisters and I are not really close anyway. You know, I never really shared anything else with them. I am so much older than my brothers and sisters. I was never around for them anyway. I was the big brother who was gone.

This man sees his family relationships as distant so he chooses to disclose to other people, mostly his friends. A woman about 30 mentioned how she did not disclose to relatives about her diagnosis because she did not feel close to them:

> I clearly decided that the only time I need to tell someone is when I feel very close to them and I want them to know about all of the important issues in my life. And, you have cousins, you have distant cousins, who you see once a year or whatever. I don't have the desire to tell them. They don't need to know. I don't want to start to have a close relationship because I am sick because that's not a genuine relationship.

This woman also brought up that relational quality must be positive before disclosing a diagnosis. She did not want an illness to be the reason she became close to extended family members.

Some individuals do not tell sexual partners about the HIV diagnosis because they do not feel close to them or are no longer together in a relationship. Past sexual partners are less likely to be told about the HIV diagnosis, compared to current or potential partners (Marks et al., 1992). Stein et al. (1998) reported that people with HIV who had high spousal support were more likely to disclose their diagnosis. Greene and Faulkner (2002), however, reported African American adolescents with HIV disclosed to many past sexual partners but all current partners. Less research is available tracking disclosure to past sexual or needle-sharing partners. Someone with HIV is also more likely to disclose about their HIV status to a primary sexual partner than to someone with whom they had a one-time, occasional, or brief relationship (e.g., Norman et al., 1998; Stempel et al., 1995), as discussed previously in our section on partners. A study conducted by Fisher et al. (1998) illustrates the relationship between perceptions of closeness and self-disclosure to sexual partners among MSM with HIV. Sixty percent of the participants in the study had talked about their HIV status with primary sexual partners, but only 34% talked about their HIV status with anonymous partners (whom they met for a "cruise" or one-night stand).

Some people even choose short-term relationships and refuse to date anyone very long to specifically avoid dealing with disclosure decisions (e.g., "If I don't go out with him for long then I don't have to tell him."). There is also research suggesting that some individuals with HIV may find sexual partners for short-term relationships because they feel less responsible for having to disclose their HIV status in superficial relationships (Fisher et al., 1998; Markova et al., 1990). One man described this:

> I'd rather date around, just pick up men when I want to. I always use condoms, but why would I tell someone I picked up at a truck stop? I don't want to see him again or date, it's too much to deal with if you talk about HIV. It gets too intense.

Thus, relational quality explains some decisions to conceal or reveal an HIV diagnosis. Also remember that for disclosure purposes relational quality is perceived from the discloser's (not receiver's) perspective. An aunt may see a relationship as very close (or not), yet this view may not be shared by her nephew. This perception of how close a relationship is will affect disclosure decisions from the point of view of the discloser. We turn next to discloser's past experience.

Discloser's Past Experience

Past experience refers to history with the process of disclosure itself (disclosure experience) and the outcomes and degrees of satisfaction associated with past HIV disclosure (past experience). Taken together, the discloser's experience can affect current and future disclosures (Moneyham et al., 1996; Squire, 1999) and conversations (Kellerman, 1987). Disclosure experience is affected by affective, cognitive, and behavioral factors. Affective factors include self-confidence, personal attitudes toward one's own HIV infection, and emotional state, among others. Cognitive components include one's beliefs about HIV, knowledge about one's own disease progression, and so forth. Behavioral factors refer to skills related to the process of revealing personal information about the self, including past HIV disclosure experiences.

For a number of gay men with HIV, coming out as gay in many ways served as practice for disclosing seropositivity (Squire, 1999). Although such experiences do not necessarily mitigate the emotional challenges associated with HIV disclosure, they provide some people with a potential repertoire of disclosure skills and psychological readiness that individuals who lack such experiences may not have (Mansergh et al., 1995). It is also important to remember that coming out as practice for disclosing HIV is not applicable for many people with HIV; some homosexuals (and bisexuals) have never come out, and the process is certainly not the same for heterosexuals. One man with AIDS stated, "I just didn't know what to say. I mean, how do you tell your mother something like that? Do you just walk up and say, 'Hey, I'm dying but I love you?'" He did not see himself as having the ability to share his diagnosis. Another woman described her efforts to disclose: "I started to tell him [boyfriend] lots of times, once last week I picked a time, but then I'd lose my words. I just couldn't think of anything to say." This woman wanted and intended to share but was unable to put the desire to disclose into action. The last (or first) disclosure may be especially crucial in a person's with HIV's experience with the disease. If a person had a bad experience the first (or most recent) time they shared the diagnosis, disclosure may be even more difficult. Disclosing may become easier over time (see chap. 4); however, negative disclosure experiences are likely to reduce future disclosures.

Past experience with disclosure influences the process of revealing one's HIV status to others. As one gay man with AIDS reported, "After my sister, what my sister did, telling me God gave me AIDS to punish my sins, why would I want to tell anyone?" In spite of the stigma attached to being HIV positive, past research (e.g., Adam & Sears, 1994, 1996; Mansergh et al., 1995; Schnell et al., 1992) suggests that reactions to HIV disclosure are generally more positive than negative (see chap. 5). However, a negative past experience can have a traumatic impact on the discloser as one woman recalled:

I was pretty open about my HIV diagnosis at the beginning. I'm healthy and my mother and friends are very supportive. Then I met this man … we really liked each other … and we seemed to understand each other. We had this chemistry. I knew that I had to tell him before we did anything [sexual] … and when I told him, he was very angry at first because I did not tell him right away. I mean, what am I supposed to do? Say "Hi, my name is X and I'm HIV positive?" But I did not wait that long … I told him after 3 weeks of dating. It wasn't easy for me, and he seemed to forget that fact. Then he told me that he was falling in love with me and that HIV did not matter. Like a fool, I believed him and continued to go out until one day I heard his message on my answering machine telling me that he cannot see me anymore ... and not to ever call him again. I was devastated, and I felt ugly and contaminated. It took me over a year to start dating again ... and telling my dates about my diagnosis reminds me of the message on my answering machine.

Although this woman met more accepting and supportive men, including her current boyfriend of 18 months, her past experience made her anticipate HIV disclosure with more anxiety and trepidation. As this discussion indicated, disclosure decisions are set within a context of individual and relational past history. This past experience can also be linked to ethnicity and gender, which is discussed next.

Ethnicity and Gender

Ethnicity and gender are important social factors and identity categories that affect how individuals experience and disclose about an HIV diagnosis, manage and cope with stigma, seek and receive social support, and perceive and gain access to health care services (see, e.g., Flaskerud & Nyamathi, 2000; Jackson et al., 1998–1999; Roth & Fuller, 1998; Yep, Merrigan, Martin, Lovaas, & Cetron, 2002). In short, ethnic and gender identities are intimately tied to every facet of experience related to HIV. In terms of HIV disclosure, ethnic and gender differences can further exacerbate the difficulties associated with such revelations (Gramling et al., 1996; Marks et al., 1992; Mason et al., 1995; Moneyham et al., 1996; Serovich et al., 1998; Simoni et al., 1995).

Ethnicity.   HIV has disproportionately affected ethnic communities, particularly African Americans and Latinos (see, e.g., Centers for Disease Control and Prevention, 2001). In addition, ethnic membership appears to be related to different patterns of coping with HIV. For instance, HIV stigma in ethnic minority communities might be different than in Euro-American, gay male communities (Yep et al., 2003). Additionally, perceptions of HIV and AIDS support services such as ASOs are often seen as uninterested in non-White, non-middle class clients (Siegel & Raveis, 1997). Ethnic minorities with HIV may be even further isolated if they have limited access to health services (Yep, Merrigan, et al., 2002). Others have emphasized the role of homophobia in certain cultures, for example African American churches (see Fullilove & Fullilove, 1999; Rose, 1998). Clearly there is a need for more research in this area, as studies are limited. However, some research exists. Examples include Yep et al.'s (Yep, Merrigan, et al., 2002; Yep et al., 2003) work with Asian Americans; Siegel and Raveis' (1997) research with African Americans and Puerto Ricans; Mason et al.'s (1995) and Diaz's (1998) work with Latinos who were and were not Spanish speaking; Simoni et al.'s (1995) research with Latinas who were and were not Spanish speaking; Stein et al.'s (1998) work with European American, Latino, and African American participants; and Greene and Faulkner's (2002) research with African American women.

Several studies have suggested that European Americans may disclose more than ethnic minority groups, although much more work is needed to explore why and when these differences occur. For example, European Americans disclose more to employers (Simoni et al., 1997) than Latinos or African Americans. Euro-American men with hemophilia disclose more to their children (Armistead et al., 1997) compared with African American fathers. Mason et al. (1995) reported Spanish speaking Latino men are especially unlikely to disclose HIV infection or homosexuality to significant others. Stein et al. (1998) reported European Americans and Latinos disclosed more to partners than African Americans.

Gender.   Women and HIV is an emerging area of research (see Greene et al., 2002; Roth & Fuller, 1998). Similar to ethnic minorities, women have been less visible in the epidemic, and this may affect stigma and disclosure decisions.

There is some question as to whether women are more likely to disclose their HIV diagnoses than men and additionally if women are more likely to be chosen as HIV disclosure recipients than men. At present little data exist to directly tap either question with HIV, but studies of self-disclosure generally may provide some insight. There are more studies of gender differences than any other issue in self-disclosure (Dindia, 2002); therefore, use of review articles is especially important. Dindia (2002) reported a small effect in a meta-analysis of gender and disclosure such that women were disclosed to slightly more often (a *meta-analysis* is a study that uses a statistical technique to summarize patterns of results from numerous studies). Specifically, there was greater disclosure to women and same-sex targets (see Dindia & Allen, 1992), findings moderated by self-disclosure measure and target sex (but not year published; therefore, the gender differences have not decreased). Dindia's (2002) review would lead to the conclusion that the gender effect is interactive with more disclosure to women overall (higher same-gender than cross-gender disclosure), but studies to this point with HIV have not tested this specific idea.

Gender and ethnicity may also interact to produce different disclosure patterns. For example, in a study of African American adolescent heterosexual women with HIV, Greene and Faulkner (2002) found different disclosure rates than those reported for Euro-American gay men. Women in Greene and Faulkner's study disclosed more readily to mothers, aunts, grandmothers, and sisters than reported in other studies for gay men. In addition, African American women were more likely to disclose directly to other women than to men (except their boyfriends) in their social networks. Disclosure to male targets other than their boyfriends tended to be told via a third party. These African American young women also reported having difficulties dealing with gossip after their disclosure. In short, gender and ethnic differences seem to produce different patterns of disclosure (e.g., African American HIV positive adolescent women disclosing more about their HIV infection to sexual partners than MSM) and their associated challenges (e.g., gossip). Further research utilizing combinations of gender and ethnicity would be helpful.

CONCLUSIONS

This chapter illustrates how HIV stigma, reasons for and against HIV disclosure, and relational factors influence whether someone is told about the HIV diagnosis. Persons living with HIV weigh stigma, relational features, and reasons for and against disclosure in deciding whether to disclose based on their own, their partner's, and their relationship's needs. CPM argues that individuals develop self-protection strategies, and decisions about disclosure may become routinized. A person may develop a set way of telling a new sexual partner or a friend.

By not disclosing one's HIV status, someone with HIV can maintain normal social relations with others in the face of negative public attitudes toward the disease. However, these concerns about protecting social relations may be greater for someone who recently found out about the diagnosis than for those who have been living with the diagnosis for a long time. Individuals who live with HIV for an extended period may develop self-protective strategies that assist in undermining the impact of HIV-related stigma. People with HIV may participate in self-help, support, and community groups to empower themselves and to challenge the HIV stigma (e.g., Crocker & Major, 1989; Siegel et al., 1998). In later stages of AIDS, the person lives with the increased risk of serious illness, hospitalization, and death. It may be difficult to "pass" as a person who is not infected when physical signs of illness and decline are visible (Alonzo & Reynolds, 1995). Also, in the later stages the impact of HIV stigma on disclosure decision making diminishes if needs for physical and emotional support outweigh concerns about disrupting relationships with significant others. These changes are factored in when making disclosure decisions.

This chapter focused on HIV decision making from the perspective of the individual with HIV. However, the decision about who to tell about the diagnosis does not occur in social isolation (Monette, 1990; Powell-Cope, 1995; van der Straten, Vernon, et al., 1998; Van Devanter et al., 1999). Significant others (including family members, friends, intimate partners) who already know about someone's status frequently give (and attempt to impose) their opinion about who should be told about the diagnosis. We also discuss third-party disclosure (indirect disclosure) in chapter 4. Hence, weighing the reasons for and against HIV disclosure in many cases is a joint process that takes into account the needs of the individual with HIV, others who already know about the diagnosis, as well as the needs of those who have not yet been told.

Features of HIV Disclosure Messages

Chapter 3 explored the HIV disclosure decision-making process. We focused on the criteria people use to develop rules to manage their privacy boundaries concerning revealing and concealing the HIV diagnosis. Once someone makes a disclosure about their HIV status, CPM (see chap. 2) argues that a personal privacy boundary becomes a collective boundary as the discloser and the disclosure recipient are linked together. Boundary linkages may result from the verbal and alternative message strategies people use to disclose. This chapter explores how people disclose their HIV seropositive status through an exploration of specific message strategies.

For someone with HIV, disclosure can be an ongoing process of linking people into privacy boundaries around their HIV status. The disclosure might only reveal partial aspects of information concerning HIV status or a full disclosure might take many different interactions to become known (Petronio, 2002). Thus, one particular disclosure event may be short or long in duration, while there are also new people who may be linked into this privacy boundary. Because there is a need to talk about HIV, also given that it is risky to do so, disclosure often takes into account the nature of the message, how the message is articulated, and the way messages are used.

Accounting for the delicate nature of the disclosure event, those diagnosed with HIV not only use verbal messages, they also use alternative messages to let people know their status. The self-disclosure literature usually focuses on verbal statements such as "I feel," "I think" (see also Derlega & Grzelak's, 1979, definition of self-disclosure emphasizing verbal aspects of disclosure, as well as Derlega et al., 1993). In this chapter we focus on the verbal disclosure messages and include alternative message strategies. These other message strategies may be labeled in a variety of ways (e.g., nonverbal, environmental, symbolic, behavioral, indirect, nonvocal); however, we choose the terminology *alternative message strategies* to adopt the widest and most inclusive approach. Using alternative messages allows the examination of options such as avoiding directly stating the

HIV diagnosis. For example, some MSM do not feel that they can talk about their serostatus with new sex partners; consequently, they may prefer to use indirect ways to disclose (e.g., wearing an AIDS t-shirt or leaving medication out). The majority of research conceptualizes disclosure generally to reflect verbal messages. Although we do discuss verbal ways of defining disclosure, we also include alternate messages that are not verbal, as the previous example illustrates. Clearly these are not mutually exclusive, as verbal and alternative message forms can occur simultaneously (and may reinforce or contradict each other). We describe message features associated with verbal messages first, then turn to alternative messages later in the chapter.

The most frequent message choice to disclose is verbally. Although there is a growing body of research on HIV disclosure in recent years (e.g., Derlega, Lovejoy, et al., 1998; Derlega et al., 2002; Greene & Faulkner, 2002; Greene & Serovich, 1996; Hays et al., 1993; Mansergh et al., 1995; Marks et al., 1992; Mason et al., 1995; Moneyham et al., 1996; Petronio & Magni, 1996; Serovich et al., 1998; Simoni et al., 1995), considerably less work has focused on the actual message used to disclose and link others into a privacy boundary around HIV status. Studying verbal messages is helpful because doing so provides insights not only into the choices people make in how to disclose, but message choices also frame how the confidant is able to respond (Petronio, 1991). As a consequence, knowing the mode of communication people with HIV select (such as face-to-face or third-party routes), knowing the context in which people with HIV link others into their privacy boundary, and knowing the particular message features such as the explicitness, length, and content of the message all affect the disclosure process. In these ways, people link others to their privacy boundaries around their HIV status. We organize the discussion of verbal messages according to these three factors (mode, context, and message features).

MODE OF COMMUNICATION

When people decide to disclose about their HIV infection, they have a range of communication modes or channels from which to select. Individuals living with HIV might choose to reveal their health status in a face-to-face encounter (e.g., a conversation in person), in a non-face-to-face encounter (e.g., a letter, phone call, or e-mail message), or by using a third party to deliver the news (e.g., a designated person such as a sibling, friend, or health care provider). The mode is important because it influences the way others become co-owners of the information about HIV status. We compare non-face-to-face and face-to-face disclosure first.

Face-to-Face Versus Non-Face-to-Face Disclosure

There is considerable debate about how the personal news of HIV diagnosis should be delivered (Yep, Merrigan, et al., 2002). Choices include disclosing in person, face-to-face, or in a non-face-to-face encounter like a letter, card, telephone call, or e-mail. Each mode of communication has its pros and cons, functioning differently for individuals. There may also be a history of particular message usage in the relationship (e.g., many e-mails or phone calls if long distance).

Non-Face-to-Face Disclosure. Non-face-to-face revelations tend to be either more implied or communicated in a situation that may limit lengthy conversations and how much the confidant knows about the illness. The most rapidly expanding mode in this area of non-face-to-face is computer mediated communication (CMC) such as the Internet. The health care industry and Internet are related in important ways (Rice & Katz, 2001). Research has explored how people tailor their Internet use to suit individual health needs, such as use of interactive health software packages (e.g., Smaglik et al., 1998; see also chap. 5). As one participant described, "When I was diagnosed I spent a lot of time in HIV chat rooms, mostly looking at what others wrote. I learned a lot and eventually started participating, talking with people about meds, how to tell." Use of Internet to disclose and receive social support is an emerging area for research.

In these non-face-to-face situations, visual (and most nonverbal) cues are unavailable to both parties in the interaction (Schegloff, 1986). Thus, the non-face-to-face form seems to control the conditions of knowing about the HIV status and how the person is linked into the privacy boundary around the HIV status. For example, an adolescent girl with HIV wrote a note to an ex-boyfriend revealing her infection after she chose not to have sex with a new partner: "It was because I was keeping these issues in ... and we [the ex] had sex and that's when I wrote him this note. Because I did not have sex with the boy because I had HIV." The girl later revealed she wrote to her ex-partner because she "could not look him in the face" given she was so angry that he had not told her about his infection. Choosing to send a note also allowed this girl to organize the information in the way she wanted and control her emotions. Thus, non-face-to-face disclosure such as this one can be a strategy to prepare a message and anticipate potential responses, such as keeping the interaction brief. Through this message process, a person may be able to constrain potential responses to the disclosure.

It is also possible with non-face-to-face disclosure to have interactions specific to the mode. For example, the recipient might never acknowledge receiving the e-mail, letter, or phone call, further increasing uncertainty and perhaps hurt. This is less likely to happen in a face-to-face mode, although a person could leave or refuse to discuss the issue. One man sent an e-mail to an ex-lover, disclosing the infection and encouraging him to get tested. "I waited for weeks, and he checks his e-mail all the time, he's obsessive. And he never said a word. To this day I have not heard from him. That's 2 years and counting." In this case, the person was relatively certain the disclosure message was received because there was a change in pattern of interaction. Similarly, a person could leave a phone message and not have it returned, with some uncertainty as to if it was ever received (or who received it).

Separate from the difficulties possible with non-face-to-face disclosure, some people report lengthy exchanges through non-face-to-face communication. For example, one woman wrote back and forth with her brother for weeks after disclosing her diagnosis to him before the family was to gather for the holidays:

> I wanted to tell him, but I knew looking at him I'd just sit and cry and have to watch him cry, so writing was much better. We wrote maybe 15, maybe 20 messages back and forth about this before we talked on the phone. We had time to be upset and respond to the other one when we were ready.

For this woman, the non-face-to-face mode served the purpose of helping her control and process emotions. She also took the additional step of telling her brother's wife (again, disclosing to her through e-mail) to ensure that he had support.

Another non-face-to-face option is writing a letter or card. A woman in her late 30s, who was separated from her husband and has children, had gone out dancing a few times with girlfriends. This woman met a man at a club. She said, "We got to talking. We stayed at the club longer than I thought we were going to stay there and [I] never mentioned anything about HIV." She described what happened afterward:

> And all of a sudden he said, "Can I have your number?" And I said, "Sure." And I gave him my number. And I am thinking to myself, "Why did I give him my number? Why did I give him my number?"
>
> He gave me his number. We started talking [on the phone]. We talked for a couple of weeks. He called me every day, two, three, four times a day. [He said], "Why don't you meet me up here [at the Naval Base]. I am on my break. Why don't you meet me here? We can eat in the mess hall." I would say, "Well, no." I found myself getting close to him. I knew he was attracted to me. I was attracted to him. I found that we enjoyed the conversations that we had and that this could be a real possibility for a relationship. So, I said, "I've got to tell him, I've got to tell him." So I wrote him a letter. And I said, "There is a whole lot about me that you don't know. We've gotten to know each other and obviously we're attracted to each other."
>
> Anyway, he had called me and expected me to meet him. I did not meet him. I called my girlfriend who was with me when we went out and I said, "Can you please meet him at this place and give him this letter because I can't let this keep going on." And we [he and I] had done nothing. There was nothing intimate, nothing had happened. So, anyway, I gave her the letter.
>
> He read the letter. And in the letter I told him that if he did not want to call me or talk to me again, I would truly understand. Because some people just cannot deal with HIV and don't want to deal with it, period. "But I want you to know you're the first person who has made me feel normal. You've made me feel just being [HIV] positive doesn't mean that you don't have the same desires, the attractions, the

needs, whatever. All that's still there. I like you. You have the right to know. You can make a decision, a choice, from this."

He called and he told me that reading that letter was just like talking to me. And he said, "Just in the time frame I've known you, I feel like I can trust you, probably more than some people in my family or somebody I have grown up with. You're very open. You're very honest." And he said, "This doesn't matter to me. But I don't know a whole lot about it." But his whole personality changed. Where he was very quick to give me flattering comments and things like that, it was like this shock, scare, and he didn't say anything like that. He did say, "You're a beautiful woman. I never would have guessed. Looking at you, I can tell you work out. You look very physically fit and I never would have known."

I told him that you can't tell by looking at people. So I kind of educated him a little bit. We had this conversation. After this conversation, I never heard from him again. It kind of hurt me but at this point it didn't hurt so bad because I kind of set myself up. I said, "Well, if it can be anything then it will. If it won't, then I've got to take this chance. I've got to be honest. I've got to tell him." But I found that he was afraid and he never called me.

This use of a letter opened the possibility for other conversations. The ultimate outcome was difficult for the woman who disclosed because she felt rejected, yet she also felt she "did the right thing" in sharing her diagnosis.

More frequent than e-mail or letters is use of the telephone in non-face-to-face disclosure (Greene & Faulkner, 2002). One adolescent girl telephoned her aunt to disclose her HIV positive diagnosis because she lived too far away and wanted to tell her aunt before she heard it somewhere else. "Well at first she didn't believe me, she didn't believe me, 'cause she thought I was joking." People with HIV may choose non-face-to-face disclosure in cases of great distance, awkward work schedules (e.g., working opposite shifts), or if they are worried about extreme reactions such as hysteria or violence.

For example, a woman described how difficult it was disclosing over the phone, especially when she needed assistance:

I told her [over the phone]. I heard mother cry and I heard her hang the phone up. So I tried to call her back and she wouldn't answer. So I called my middle sister. She is the only one of the rest of my family that I would ever talk to. So, I told her, and she just broke down and started crying right then. I said "I need your love and support. I don't need tears, and I don't need your sorrow." And she said, "Okay, okay." And she called my mother. Then I finally got back in contact with my mother and she said, "Okay, you know everything will be all right. I'll pray for you."

This example demonstrates several difficulties of non-face-to-face, particularly nonresponse. In this case, the person was creative and utilized a third party, also via non-face-to-face disclosure. Selecting a mode that takes place in person occurs more frequently than non-face-to-face options to link others into a privacy boundary. Nevertheless, as these examples illustrate, doing so increases the control over how much information one discloses at a time.

Face-to-Face Disclosure. Using a face-to-face mode of communication by the person disclosing sometimes affects the control the person has over the amount of information that is revealed during the course of the interaction. One woman wanted to tell her partner even though they were breaking up; she wanted to disclose the information but not discuss it with him:

> I went to tell him, he had to know, we're having sex but also having problems. I just wanted to tell him so he'd get tested, but he kept asking more and more questions, so many questions. What a fucking mess.

In this situation, the face-to-face mode encouraged more discussion than the woman felt comfortable with, but she was glad she told him.

Face-to-face disclosure sometimes occurs spontaneously, especially if people are talking to others with whom they have significant relationships or family members (e.g., someone is upset and "it just comes out"). Some people also describe that not disclosing face-to-face would both harm the relationship with the person and show a lack of respect for the other person (Greene & Faulkner, 2002). One woman described how she dreaded the disclosure and put it off for months. "There's no way I couldn't go there, look her in the face and tell her for myself. But damn, I didn't want to." In this situation there was a clear image in the woman's mind about the appropriate mode to use for this particular person, even if it was difficult. Another man lived across country from a sibling, and he wanted to tell her but only in person:

> My sister, she's great. We always had fun, could talk about anything. I'd never hurt her by calling to tell her or letting my mother do it. I didn't have the money right then, but I figured out how to fly to see her for the weekend [and told her].

He made a special trip to see her to disclose face-to-face, which was expensive and physically draining for him but he reported was "well worth it."

Talking face-to-face is less predictable and more difficult in managing the type of boundary linkages with others. Although a person may wish to only tell some of the details about their HIV status, talking face-to-face may mean that they end up revealing much more information because the other person is right there asking lots of questions. One heterosexual man told his parents, and they asked many questions that were hurtful to him:

> All they wanted to know was if I was gay, were my male friends "boyfriends." I just wanted to leave, it was so hard to tell them, and then they want to know more and more stuff that's not even relevant.

In this case the man disclosed in person but the event itself grew, and he ended up answering many unwanted questions. This extended the disclosive episode, it became very heated, and he grew defensive.

These examples have demonstrated both face-to-face and non-face-to-face disclosure, one issue to consider when disclosing. The selection of the mode is an important one. This choice may be conscious or may just happen (planning is discussed later in this chapter). One final aspect of communication mode is the use of third parties.

Third-Party Disclosure

Not all disclosure messages involve only two people. Direct disclosure (face-to-face or not) is too threatening for some. Disclosure can also occur through third parties either via face-to-face or non-face-to-face modes. There has been research on using an indirect mode of information acquisition labeled *third parties* (Berger, 1987) to seek information (for example to ask common friends to "check out" a potential date). Hewes, Graham, Doelger, and Pavitt (1985) estimated 30% of people's information is from third-party sources, but this has not been studied in the context of HIV disclosure. For this third-party communication mode, individuals with HIV deliberately use another person to make a third-party disclosure to link others implicitly in their privacy boundary around HIV status (see Greene & Faulkner, 2002; Petronio, 2002; Petronio et al., 1996; Yep et al., 2003). This route to inform others of HIV status is useful because someone else makes an initial disclosure of the information about HIV status to pave the way for the person with HIV to talk (or not) about their illness. For some individuals disclosure by a designated third party (e.g., a family member, friend, partner, or health care provider) is preferred in a given situation. For example, a man in California depended on his sister to spread the information by disclosing to her first so that she would in turn tell his parents. He described the following:

> My sister and I are very close. We talk every week on the phone. She lives in San Francisco with her husband and two children. She was the first person I told when I was diagnosed with AIDS. She was very understanding and came to visit me at the hospital when I had pneumonia. I am okay now ... my parents also live in San Francisco and they don't know that I'm gay or have AIDS. I know that it'll be difficult for them ... I'm their only son ... although my health is better now, I asked my sister to talk to my parents before they come down to visit and see all the [AIDS] medications I'm taking.

This man had a clear plan to use a third party (his sister) to facilitate disclosure with his parents (and prepare them). At the time of the interview he had not yet seen his parents but anticipated his sister would be a invaluable support.

Third-party disclosures such as this may also function to save energy for the person with HIV (crucial for some to maintain healthy immune functioning). Although the act of revealing helps the person with HIV, it also takes emotional strength to go through the revealing process each time (these consequences are described more fully in chap. 5). As one heterosexual man described:

> It takes so damn much to tell. I feel worn out for days, and I can't do that any more. My health has to come before relationships at this point, and sharing takes too much. My friends tell other friends I meet, so they take care of it. If they don't understand down the road, I'll deal with it.

In this instance this person, because of the emotional drain, did not generally consider direct disclosure. He utilized third-party disclosure for any new people he chose to inform. In this way, he had a clear rule for how he was going to link others into a privacy boundary around his HIV status by using a third-party source. By doing this he preserved what emotional strength he had, and he also shared responsibility with others to manage disclosure about his HIV status.

Besides conserving emotional strength, an additional benefit may be that the third party or support person already "in the know" may be closer to the disclosure recipient than the person with HIV, perhaps easing the process. Greene and Faulkner (2002) reported over one fourth of the HIV disclosure in their sample of adolescent African American females with HIV occurred via a third party. This third-party disclosure was, in fact, the only means of sharing the news with in-laws, uncles, and grandfathers, and it was the main mechanism of disclosure to grandmothers, aunts, and cousins. They did not report which third person was used for which specific disclosure, so it is possible that the third party chosen for a particular disclosure may be closer to the recipient (e.g., a mother telling her sister, the aunt). Who acts as the third party is an area for further research.

Third Party as Support. Although a somewhat different dynamic than the use of third parties in the previous example, there are times when people with HIV bring a third person who already knows about their diagnosis when they plan to disclose to a new person. A man with HIV took his partner along, who was told six months previously, when he disclosed. "My partner … went with me when I told my sister. I waited until he was off from work to go over there. I asked him to go, so we'd all be OK." This person wanted assistance with the process and asked for help from a third party that he trusted. In this way, he had the emotional support from his partner who helped manage the disclosure about his HIV status with his sister. Alternately, a woman in her 30s revealed, "I took [my sister] with me to tell my aunt, so she'd [the sister] be there for her [aunt]. [My sister] is the one who told my aunt; I just couldn't look at her." In this case, the third party, who was there not to tell but to support the recipient and the discloser, ended up disclosing when the woman could not. The sister with HIV gave permission to reveal the HIV status, linking the aunt into the privacy boundary around the information. By having the sister tell the aunt, the person with HIV gave the responsibility to disclose the situation to her sister as an attempt to reduce difficulties. In fact, this is a different aspect of third party than when a third person discloses; in this case the third person (or more) is invited to join the disclosive event.

An additional feature of third-party support involves receiving the HIV diagnosis. Many people report taking a third party (often a friend, partner, or family member) with them to learn about the HIV test results, a slightly different issue. One woman asked a friend to go with her to get test results:

> I took [my best friend] to the health department to get the test back. I asked her, and she said, "You know I will" and she did. She was great, I was numb and couldn't listen to anything the woman [social worker] said.

This woman wanted a close friend present when she received the diagnosis. She was overwhelmed and brought another person to be sure to get the needed information. This practice is commonly reported, taking a friend or parent when getting tested or results of tests, and couples are frequently tested together.

Third-Party Intention.   As these examples illustrate, some third-party disclosure tends to be intentional and deliberate. These descriptions emphasized asking a third party to disclose the HIV diagnosis or choosing to bring along another person when disclosing (or receiving test results). These message choices are generally intentional and preplanned. For other third-party situations, family members or friends find out about a person's HIV status without the person with HIV intending to disclose. When the inclusion of a third party is unintentional, such as if the person with HIV receives emergency medical care and has to inform family members, the difference is a level of control over who is in the privacy boundary. Boundary leakage that is accidental, inadvertent, and unplanned can wreak havoc for the person with HIV (Petronio, 2002; Petronio et al., 2003). One key difference here is the intent of the person with HIV versus the intent of a third party.

Obviously, if not intentional, the individual with HIV had little control over how his or her private information was disclosed, yet must live with the consequences. Participants in Klitzman's (1999) study were troubled at how they lost control of information with a third party, especially in families. Sometimes this type of situation leads to privacy dilemmas in which there is no easy way to cope with the ramifications of the disclosure (Petronio et al., 2003). In one case of leakage, a man described how a neighbor had overheard his girlfriend talking to a friend:

> It was really hot one night, and they [girlfriend and a friend] were outside on the porch. They thought no one was around, we do that all the time, talk out there. I'd been having trouble with my meds, throwing up a lot, and they wanted to get me to

the doctor. The next week, my neighbor comes around, asking all these questions like she knew something. So we figured out she'd overheard, and shit, that woman talks.

In this example the information was overheard, not intended by any of the parties, yet they must deal with the outcomes.

A slightly different situation exists when a third party chooses to tell others without the infected person's knowledge. This phenomenon occurs when the discloser and recipient use different rules to manage the information and is markedly different from privacy. Greene and Faulkner (2002) reported negative perceptions of a similar phenomenon labeled gossip (also see chap. 3 motivations for nondisclosure) in which adolescents with HIV would not tell another person if they thought the person would violate privacy boundaries. In that study there were very negative reactions to unplanned third-party disclosures such as several family members no longer being on speaking terms. One adolescent's brother told many community members, and now she "won't talk to him" because "he had no right to do that [share her diagnosis with others]." These third-party rules are important because breaking them can lead to difficulties in the relationship (like CPM turbulence). In fact, Argyle and Henderson (1984) demonstrated how friends breaking rules for a third party (such as keeping confidences) can dissolve relationships. This illustrates one of the difficulties with third-party disclosures. CPM (see chap. 2) argues that as the information moves away from the original owner and the ties of loyalties to that person weaken, the commitment to negotiate mutually held rules for how the private information is managed also weakens (Petronio, 2002). Consequently, although the third parties are "in the know," they come by the information in a way that precludes negotiating co-ownership rules and feel less responsibility to abide by any rules except the ones they want to use for further disclosure.

One man had not told any family members about his HIV positive diagnosis for several years. When he told his mother, she criticized him and also told others in the family about the diagnosis against his wishes:

> Two years ago, I finally told my mother that I was HIV positive. She started chewing me out, but then she wanted to act like she loves me. I didn't want her to really talk to the rest of the family yet. I wanted to tell them, but she went on and ran her mouth. She told a couple of her sisters and everybody had me on a deathbed. One of my aunts went to South Carolina and told everybody I was laid up in the hospital near death's door. My twin sister found out through word of mouth, and I never wanted her to know that way. Technically, I never wanted my twin sister or my nephew to ever know. For some reason, I thought I could hide it from them.

For this man the third party (mother) intentionally shared with many others, in this case family members. From her point of view it was family information subject to different rules, but the person with HIV still wanted to make choices about who knew (and what, as the misinformation about his illness was distressing).

One way to deal with this third-party sharing problem may be to address specifically further disclosure in the initial disclosure message. Individuals with HIV have described asking others to keep the information confidential. "I asked him not to tell anyone." Petronio and Bantz (1991) described the use of "prior restraint phrases" (PRPs). An example might be, "Please don't tell anyone, but I tested HIV positive." These PRPs could occur before the disclosure ("I want to tell you something but you have to keep quiet about it") or after the disclosure (one woman described how, after talking with her sister—and disclosing the diagnosis—for 2 hours she said, "Now you know you cannot tell anyone, especially X, X, X [names of family members]"). The question remains, however, does this request for confidentiality function as intended? Petronio and Bantz's (1991) research indicates that people who receive these requests do not necessarily keep the information completely secret (see also Petronio, 2002). In fact, disclosers using these PRPs expect the information to be passed along but selectively, not just telling anyone and everyone. In this case the phrase may function to warn another to share with fewer others (rather than not share with all others). Unfortunately, this could create difficulty if the expectations are unclear, particularly in the case of HIV.

We have discussed communication mode, face-to-face, non-face-to-face, and third-party disclosure. These choices of mode affect the disclosure message. We turn next to the effect of context on disclosure messages.

CONTEXTUAL CONSIDERATIONS

To this point, we have discussed the mode of disclosure messages (face-to-face, non-face-to-face, and third-party), yet these disclosure message choices are also set within contexts (Pearce & Sharp, 1973). In chapter 3 we described the use of context (with four types), and we expand on some of these ideas of context here. Similarly, Altman, Brown, Staples, and Werner (1992) argued for research that connects cultural and social contexts of relationships with the physical environments in which those relationships are embedded. CPM theory also argues that one of the criteria used to develop privacy rules that manage boundaries is the definition of the context (Petronio, 2002). The contextual considerations may be the physical elements or social environmental aspects of the communication process that include setting and timing of disclosure. They must be considered, along with communication mode, in disclosure decisions to determine the privacy rules.

Setting

Close relationships are intertwined with physical environments such that people and place are inherently connected (Altman et al., 1992). The physical environment where disclosure takes place results from rules people have for telling the private information (Petronio, 2002), and that physical environment constrains conversations (Kellerman, 1987). McCall and Simmons (1978) argued activities are limited to locales, and locales provide social and cultural boundaries with consequent imposed rules and constraints. Thus, settings influence perceptions of privacy (Petronio et al., 1996), and settings range along a continuum from more public to more private (Altman et al., 1992). For example, private settings (where individuals may have considerable control over information management) such as an individual's home, office, or automobile can facilitate disclosure by enhancing the potential discloser's sense of privacy (Altman, 1975; Altman & Werner, 1985; Werner, Altman, & Brown, 1992). Alternately, public settings (where individuals have reduced control over information management) such as a park, café, or restaurant can constrain the disclosure process, as the potential discloser might feel reluctant to reveal highly personal and sensitive information in these environments (Petronio & Martin, 1986). Klitzman (1999) reported men were unlikely to disclose HIV in a bar because they believe the setting was inappropriate.

The choice of setting may be deliberate and preplanned if a person thinks through where to share news of an HIV diagnosis. Conversely, the setting may simply reflect where an opportune moment arose or a related question was asked. People do not always choose or plan private settings for disclosure. As one study of child sexual abuse illustrates (Petronio et al., 1996), there are also instances in which a person might deliberately choose a public setting to disclose highly stressful information like their HIV infection. For example, one woman with HIV reported how she decided about where to tell her husband her HIV diagnosis, stating that, "I took him to a nice restaurant to tell him so he couldn't go off and had to talk about it." As this example illustrates, sometimes a setting is chosen because it limits the ability of others to overreact to the information.

As such, settings can function as control devices as observed in the next example. In this situation the man recalled that he took his partner to the physician's office:

> He knew I was sick, but I wanted to tell him where there were people who knew a lot about it [HIV]. We live in a small town, and that way he could ask all the questions he wanted, which he did.

In this situation and the previous example the individuals with HIV controlled the linkage and flow of information through the selection of certain kinds of settings to manage how much is known and who tells the information.

Aside from choosing settings that control others' reactions, the level of access others might have to overhear the information is also controlled with selection of setting (Petronio, 2002). Individuals with HIV may select a more restricted setting for disclosing to maintain control over their privacy boundaries through regulating the setting. It is important to remember, however, that in generally viewed private spaces (e.g., an office or an apartment) one can also be overheard. One woman with AIDS was talking with a friend in a cafeteria about changing her medications and realized a coworker had overheard. Thus, these choices manage the potential for others hearing the information unintentionally. For instance, one adolescent described how she told her best friend:

We were going to school together, and I had missed a couple days, so she had called and she wanted to know what's wrong with me. So, I went out there to see her at school, and I told her mom to get her out of school early so I can talk to her. And her mom did, and we went to her house, and I told her there.

As this example shows, rather than talking on the phone or at school, the girl with HIV orchestrated a meeting that precluded anyone else's involvement in the disclosure. By doing this, she restricted access to information about her status and maintained her desired level of control over the information to unwanted others.

In another situation, a gay man reported waiting until after leaving some friends to tell a potential new partner:

We'd been out a few times, were enjoying each other and getting to know each other. It hadn't gotten physical yet. That night I wanted to introduce him to some of my friends, good friends who have been there for me through all this [illness]. My friends made some comments related to it [HIV] but I wanted to wait to tell him when we could talk, so I steered the conversation another way. After we left, I was driving him home and I pulled over near this park. And I told him that I had HIV, that I wanted him to know. He asked some questions, so I was glad I waited until we were alone.

This person intentionally chose a more private physical setting for disclosure, in addition to avoiding disclosing in a group. In this and the other examples, the main issue for individuals with HIV is the maintenance of control over disclosure of their HIV status. Thus, the setting functions to retain control over unwanted others being linked into a privacy boundary surrounding the HIV status of a person.

According to CPM, however, it is not always possible to control the setting for disclosure, especially when someone asks a direct question soliciting private information (Petronio, 1991, 2002). When someone asks explicitly if a person is HIV positive, the message strategy gives the discloser few options about how to reply. In a face-to-face situation when a person is asked directly, an explicit demand is imposed because of the message and the situation that calls for an immediate reply, even if the setting is not optimal (Petronio, 1991). For instance, people might be asked if they have HIV in front of others who they do not know. The adolescent in the next example was pressed for information by her boyfriend:

Well, I started some kind of conversation and he just said "go ahead and tell me what the doctor said." And I wanted to go home and tell him, but he was at work at the time. And I just came right out and told him.

In this situation, even though linking the person into the privacy boundary is not what the person with HIV desired, social pressure and the publicness of the request forced a level of linkage. Socially, ignoring a direct question or request even if it asks for HIV disclosure, particularly in front of others, is difficult and threatening. Consequently, when a woman's partner repeatedly asked her things about her recent visit to the doctor, even though the woman never really replied, it resulted in feelings of frustration. The woman yelled that she was HIV positive to her partner in the midst of a group of their friends. She stated, "It just came out, right there in front of God and everybody. Loud and blunt [she laughs]." In this situation, the requests for information were repeated but the ultimate disclosive act occurred in front of others, not as desired. The woman was upset about the way it was handled. The actions of others can, at times, be viewed as leaving little room to protect personal privacy. Yielding to such demands may result in feeling violated even though the disclosure about HIV status may actually be made by the person with HIV despite the reservations and negative feelings. The direct demand to know, consequently, leaves little opportunity to negotiate the privacy rules on the person with HIV's own terms. As this discussion illustrates, the nature of disclosure settings vary from more private to public spaces and are important in developing and changing privacy rules.

Timing

We have described the influence of setting on message choices, exploring why people choose more private or public spaces to disclose. Also critical to development of privacy rules is the extent to which timing of disclosure plays a part in choices about revealing (Petronio, 2002). Ickovics et al. (2001) noted the temporal context including epidemiological stage, disease stage, and life stage (see also Greene et al., 2002) can affect relationships of people with HIV, even disclosing. There is some variability in timing of general disclosure, but premature or inappropriate disclosure is costly (e.g., Chelune, Sultan, & Williams, 1980; Taylor & Altman, 1987) because inappropriate timing violates social norms (see Gilbert, 1976; Kiesler, Kiesler, & Pallak, 1967). Kellerman (1987) indicated timing is a crucial issue for politeness in initial interactions, specifically that the social appropriateness of self-disclosure regulates information flow (Chaikin & Derlega, 1974). As Derlega et al. (1993) argued, timing plays an important role in disclosure episodes generally and appears to be significant in HIV disclosure specifically. For the research on HIV, timing refers to three potential questions: (a) When should one disclose after learning an HIV diagnosis, (b) should disclosure be spontaneous or preplanned, and (c) when within a conversation should disclosure occur? All three questions revolve around the extent to which a person gauges when a disclosure about HIV status is made to others. Timing influences the extent to which a person is linked into a privacy boundary around the HIV status and when others know about an individual's HIV status.

When to Disclose After Learning Diagnosis

Research results are mixed concerning when to disclose an HIV diagnosis. In general, research suggests that individuals with HIV believe that telling sooner is better than waiting to disclose (Adam & Sears, 1994, 1996). However, many people wait to disclose the diagnosis (see Greene & Faulkner, 2002; Kimberly et al., 1995). Gielen et al. (1997) reported that many women with HIV disclosed right away, but some delayed any disclosure. In this study, 18% of the women had disclosed to zero or one person by 1 year post diagnosis. For women who delayed disclosure (26%), the time delay ranged from a few days to many months. The women who delayed cited reasons such as being in denial and worry about the impact on others.

Getting the information out earlier appears to relieve the burden or stress of the diagnosis, but Pryor, Reeder, and Landau's (1999) model of AIDS stigma indicates people process the HIV diagnosis over a period of time and adjust (see also Klitzman, 1999). People may conceal the diagnosis for a while and then disclose through an unlayering process (Limandri, 1989), perhaps similar to studies of disclosure of sexual abuse (e.g., MacFarlane & Krebs, 1986; Petronio et al., 1996), although the recipient selection is done carefully. Often people need time alone with the knowledge of the disease to simply come to grips with the implication of the diagnosis (e.g., Klitzman, 1999; Stevens & Tighe Doerr, 1997). Holt et al. (1998) described most nondisclosure occurring immediately after learning about the diagnosis (when dealing with the acute trauma). People may need an opportunity to adjust to the diagnosis before dealing with others' reactions. For example, in one study (Kimberly et al., 1995) all women with HIV did not disclose to anyone for a period of 6 months following the diagnosis. Waiting, as these women did to disclose, gave them time to digest the consequences of learning the diagnosis and possibly estimate how others would handle the information. Disclosure increases with time diagnosed (e.g., Greene & Faulkner, 2002; Simoni et al. 1997) in part because it is an additive process, including new people disclosed to rather than simply new people met but also choosing more confidants.

Because of the significant changes that occur after learning the HIV diagnosis and because of the social stigma of the disease, those with HIV tend to become selective after the initial need to talk has passed (Derlega, Lovejoy, et al., 1998; Greene & Serovich, 1996). Greene and Faulkner (2002) reported in their sample of African American adolescent females with HIV that on the first day they were diagnosed many told mothers and some told boyfriends. Metts and Manns (1996) explored who was told the diagnosis first: close friend (57%) and mother (46%), and some told both. Thus, selectivity is played out in the timing or when those people close to the person with HIV are told and when those with weaker ties learn about the diagnosis, possibly later.

As CPM suggest, the timing for disclosure often depends on selecting confidants who can be trusted. Another study by Serovich and Greene (1993) reported that willingness to disclose HIV testing information was most likely in the marital subsystem (e.g., partners, spouses) and least likely in the extended family (e.g., aunt, mother-in-law). Hence, it seems plausible that recently diagnosed individuals are more likely to disclose to members of their marital subsystem right after receiving news about their diagnosis. The logic of the decision to turn to close family members is illustrated in the following example. One man in his 30s described why he told his mother almost immediately: "We've always been close, and I wanted to tell her sooner. I knew we could talk it through." In a second example, a woman, although apprehensive, told her boyfriend with whom she felt a close tie the day she was diagnosed. "He was going to be mad at me, upset I think, mad at it. I told him cause we're together and that I felt that he needed to know, to what was going on." Thus, the choice of timing may involve telling those closest first (e.g., friends, partner, parents) and selective others later.

Disclosure as Inevitable. Although these examples underscore a choice about revealing the HIV positive status, there are situations in which the decision to disclose seems more an inevitability than an option. Members of an immediate family are often already joined in a larger family privacy boundary that carries explicit expectations for some level of disclosure within the family on matters significant to a family member (Petronio, 2002; Vangelisti, 1994). Because the family is a system, one family member's problem often affects other individuals in the immediate family (e.g., Vangelisti, 1994; Vangelisti et al., 2001). Consequently, many consider the inevitable nature of having to disclose to family members. For example, one adolescent girl described why she told her aunt. "She was going to find out sooner or later, and once I started going to the doctor over here then she was gonna start asking questions. Right after, I started going to the doctors in [city], so I told her." This girl saw the disclosure not as much a choice but as an evolving process, one that would eventually happen. Similarly, one man said the following:

> I'd wanted to wait until I was sick to be normal for as long as possible, but with my family, it was like a rock rolling downhill and picking up speed, with no way to stop it once I told my brother. Everyone knew, it just kept growing, I couldn't keep track.

In this case, the person waited a long time to disclose, but when he did he accepted that the whole family would know.

This theme of disclosure eventually occurring also raises the question of the association between disclosure and illness progression. Individuals with HIV have concerns about the future progress of the disease and the need to adhere to strict guidelines in taking HIV medications, and some have reported they will wait to disclose until they are more ill (e.g., Greene & Faulkner, 2002; Klitzman, 1999). Several studies have found that HIV disclosure is more likely when people report more physical symptoms associated with the illness (e.g., Armistead, Morse, Forehand, Morse, & Clark, 1999; Crosby, 2000; Fisher, Goldschmidt, Hays, & Catania,

1993; Hays et al., 1993; Marks et al., 1992; Schrimshaw & Siegel, 2002; Simoni et al., 1997). Thus, evidence indicates that disease progression affects disclosure, and Marks et al. (1992) argue that this is independent of time since diagnosis. After someone contracts HIV, they may live for years without any manifest symptoms associated with HIV (the asymptomatic phase of the disease; Bartlett & Gallant, 2001). Following this asymptomatic phase, the individual may develop various physical symptoms including night sweats, fever, weight loss, herpes, shingles, and thrush (the symptomatic phase). In the advanced stage of HIV associated with AIDS severe and life-threatening physical problems, including *Pneumocystis carinii* pneumonia, pulmonary tuberculosis, and invasive cervical cancer, may occur. Effects during the symptomatic phase may be much easier for others to notice, and it is at this symptomatic (or advanced) stage that increased disclosure is more common.

Incremental Disclosure. Even though there might be some sense of inevitability, participants in the Greene and Faulkner (2002) study reported progressive disclosure (disclosure in stages) that maintained a level of control over how much information was told and when it was revealed. These respondents tended to indicate intentions to disclose, yet these statements were vaguely represented as sometime "in the future" or "sometime soon." For example, people might first disclose that their health has not been very good and later discuss their weakened immune system before disclosing they are HIV positive. The notion of progressive or incremental disclosure was initially discussed in a study on child sexual abuse (Petronio et al., 1996) and is found in a variety of situations in which someone is managing highly sensitive personal information. In child sexual abuse cases, children told only some of the information or hinted at other aspects of the abuse before they were willing to make a full disclosure (Petronio et al., 1997; Petronio et al., 1996). Only when they felt confident about the recipient's likely reactions to disclosure were children willing to make a full disclosure. Consequently, people experiencing high stress situations such as HIV may need to test out the reactions of others by beginning with a partial linkage through hinting and then moving to a full disclosure.

Incremental disclosure may be particularly significant for boundary linkage with HIV diagnosis. Opening the boundary a little allows one to decide whether to create a more complete linkage without precluding the option of maintaining a relatively closed boundary if the potential confidant does not respond as desired. This can be seen as a way of gathering vital information regarding the risks and potential benefits involved with disclosure. For example, research indicates that following an initial period of adjustment after diagnosis many individuals living with HIV infection begin to make sense of their condition (Crossley, 1999; Ezzy, 1998, 2000; Kimberly et al., 1995; Rose, 1998; Stevens & Tighe Doerr, 1997). Because this is a highly stressful situation, people typically need time to digest what has happen to them before they can even talk about it to others. People with HIV may change their definition of self as they come to see themselves as a person living with HIV, and this affects the disclosive messages shared. To do this they need to reconstruct their identities and change many ways they have come to view who they are as people (Hassin, 1994; Roth & Nelson, 1997), experience emotional growth and transcendence (Boerum, 1998), find community (Bloom, 1997; King, 1995; Remien & Rabkin, 1995; Squire, 1999), and resume, continue, or find new intimate relationships (Adam & Sears, 1994, 1996). These issues are explored further in chapter 5, but they are raised here to note that how a person is dealing with the disease can affect how he or she discloses the diagnosis.

People with HIV also describe disclosing incrementally in which they share sexual orientation or drug use first and later reveal about the HIV diagnosis. If the reaction to the first disclosure is poor, they may choose not to disclose further. One woman stated

> My mother, she thought I'd stopped using in college, years ago … and I wanted to tell her about the HIV, but I knew she'd want to know why, how, and everything. And I didn't want to half-tell, so I told about the drugs first [sharing needles with her boyfriend who is also positive]. A few months later I told her the rest, but I wouldn't have if she'd judged me about the drugs.

This woman wanted to be certain before she was ready to disclose further and started by disclosing drug history. Similarly, one bisexual man described telling his sister:

> [My sister] knows I had an encounter [with a man] when I was 18, but she thought it was just the one time. I've been seeing men ever since, bringing ladies home to family events. But dating men is a part of who I am, part of my HIV now, too, so I told her about my current boyfriend … then I came clean about the HIV. I didn't know what to expect, but she was great. I guess I thought she'd not handle the gay thing and then I wouldn't tell my family about my HIV.

This person also chose to disclose in stages with his bisexuality first. Similar to the previous example, it was important for the recipient to accept the stigmatized piece of information first as a precondition to disclosing the HIV diagnosis.

This incremental disclosure pattern is not linear, as people go back, modify, and withdraw information (Dindia, 1997). The most relevant data here concern sexual abuse in which people "test the waters" (Miell, 1984) before disclosure proceeds (Petronio et al., 1996). When disclosing sexual abuse, people reverse their story or retract or recant their disclosures (e.g., Sorensen & Snow, 1991; Summit, 1983). In Sorensen and Snow's (1991) study, 22% of participants recanted their disclosure of sexual abuse, but 92% of these later reaffirmed their original disclosure. The incremental disclosure pattern is important to study for HIV because similar patterns may emerge; for example, people who disclose they are gay may later say they are bisexual or had a one-time sexual encounter with a person of the same sex.

Relational Development.   Timing can also be conceptualized in the context of development of a person or a relationship, and that can affect disclosure timing (Petronio, 2002). There is general agreement that we tell first those who are closer to us. There are, however, exceptions to this finding, specifically children and dating partners.

When the targets of disclosure are children, there seems to be general agreement to wait until the children are "ready" (e.g., Moneyham et al., 1996). Thus, children form a special case of close family relationships because they are close but disclosure is often delayed. Andrews, Williams, and Neil (1993) reported most mothers had not disclosed to young children. Rotheram (1995), however, indicated 75% disclosed to at least one of their children, and this may create problems if one child knows but not others. One man reported his family did not want him to tell his nephews, ages 7 and 8, "Basically, I was like do you think I should tell because by them being little kids, you know, they might not deal." One lesbian with AIDS reported she would tell her son, "When I think he can understand." She was uncertain when this might be and worried about planning for her death and the care of her son. Another adolescent had not told a sibling. "X [My brother] he's 4 years old. I'm close with him, but I can't talk to him yet because he don't get it."

The child's age is the best predictor of disclosure (Rotheram, 1995); that is, disclosure increases with the child's age (e.g., Bauman et al., 2000; Schrimshaw & Siegel, 2002). Bauman et al. (2000) additionally included a child's developmental stage, which also predicts disclosure from parents. We know that mothers are not likely to tell children (and nieces or nephews) under the age of 11 years old (see Greene & Faulkner, 2002; Kimberly et al., 1995). If a child is not developed enough to understand the illness, often he or she is not told, and it is difficult to know when anyone, especially a child, is ready. For example, one woman in her early 20s described how her daughter "won't get it" and decided to delay disclosure. Alternately, the child may be able to comprehend the illness but not yet fully grasp the concept of privacy and boundaries. The family may fear the child will gossip or not keep the secret (Armistead et al., 1997), albeit unintentionally. A woman was afraid her son would tell his playmates and thus the neighborhood, putting her housing at risk:

> How can I tell [my son]? I want to, to help him understand why I don't feel well, but what happens when he goes to the playground with his friends? He doesn't understand what to say or not say yet. I'll tell him when he gets older.

For this woman, the potential risk or further disclosure or expanding boundaries resulted in her decision not to tell her son (at that point).

Besides children, timing may also be unique in decisions to disclose to potential sexual partners (or needle-sharing partners). For some, disclosing right away is the best choice. From this point of view, the dating partner has the information before he or she can become emotionally attached (or any physical intimacy occurs). For others, disclosing this soon is too threatening and they prefer to disclose the diagnosis only if they become intimate (e.g., Klitzman, 1999). The link between disclosure and physical intimacy is crucial. "It gets harder to disclose *after* you fuck, especially if you are HIV positive" because it violates trust if you have not disclosed (Vázquez-Pacheco, 2000, p. 26). One man told his boyfriend. "When he [the partner] wanted to have sex I had to tell him then." This situation does, however, become more complicated if people with HIV feel they should disclose after they really know the person but before they are intimate. The most difficult situation occurs when a person with HIV is sexually active with another and has not told but feels "it's the right thing to do." In this case, the perception is that the timing is too late. Thus, the timing for disclosure to sexual partners is related to how people perceive intimacy and responsibility (discussed further in chap. 5).

Disclosing about HIV early in a relationship, if rejection is the outcome, may still cause emotional pain. A woman gave the following account of attempting to get close to a man with whom she wanted to start a relationship:

> Well, I would like to get into a relationship. I need a man in my life right now. I got a lot of time on my hands. I need the affection. I need the attention. I go to a [support] group on Monday. In fact, I go to group tonight and there's this young guy there. ... I had to tell him about my problem, that I was HIV positive. I liked him. I figured we could have a relationship. I wrote to him and told him [and] I haven't heard anything from him. I'm kind of messed up over that, too.

This woman disclosed earlier in a potential relationship, with a difficult outcome for her. She wanted to share early to avoid problems and was hurt by the lack of response to what she viewed as very responsible behavior. Timing of disclosure in a dating relationship is complex, to balance knowing someone with the responsibility of sharing possible risk.

Thus far we have covered the effects of overall timing on disclosure message choices, and we turn next to the level of planning involved in this message timing.

Preplanned Versus Unplanned Disclosure

Another aspect of timing is disclosure message planning. Although some people living with HIV have reported unplanned disclosure of their diagnosis when it comes up rather than thinking out the details of disclosing, Yep et al. (2003) found that participants preferred preplanned and deliberate disclosure. Because people are more likely to want control over who is linked into their privacy boundary around HIV status, the unplanned disclosures often tend to be seen as mistakes or instances they regret. More likely, those infected consider who they want to know, how they will link that person into their privacy boundary, and when (and where) it might take place because they understand the risks and consequences of disclosing this information.

There are very little data available to address this planning question, with the most extensive being Stempel et al.'s (1995) study. Stempel et al. (1995) asked people at HIV testing (2 weeks prenotification) about their willingness to disclose to various targets. One year later (post notification) they were asked about actual HIV disclosure, which was much higher than people with HIV anticipated at testing. Specifically, Stempel et al. (1995) reported unanticipated disclosure most often to lovers (41% intended vs. 83% actual), to gay friends (51% intended vs. 94% actual) and nongay friends (30% intended vs. 76% actual), coworkers (13% intended vs. 47% actual), employers (11% intended vs. 31% actual), and psychologists (33% intended vs. 57% actual). Also note all actual disclosure was equal to or higher than intended disclosure (not lower in any case). Participants in Stempel et al.'s (1995) study were relatively accurate in anticipating disclosure to physicians and dentists. These findings of unplanned disclosure contradict Holt et al.'s (1998) study in which MSM reported no instances of unplanned disclosure (only third-party unplanned in which X told another person), yet there may be differences in time frame (1 year vs. immediate future plans). Additionally, Greene (2001) described over 90% of her participants reported they would tell a sexual partner ("absolutely") if they tested HIV positive (see also Greene, 2000; Greene & Serovich, 1995), clearly overestimating HIV disclosure to partners based on other studies reviewed in chapter 3, but this was with a general population sample (not people with HIV or people tested for HIV). Thus, the frequency of unplanned disclosure in the HIV context is an area for further exploration.

Given that the need for control over privacy boundaries around HIV status is so important, many people with HIV can recall instances when they did not plan to disclose their diagnosis and link someone into the boundary (although there is some evidence that self-disclosure decision making may occur at an unconscious and automatic level; see Bargh & Chartrand, 1999; Langer, 1978; Omarzu, 2000). A man who had been diagnosed 9 months previously was spending time with a group of his friends. He recalled how he was preoccupied that night and while helping with dishes after dinner, one of his friends asked "what was wrong?":

> I told her, right there in the kitchen. I'd never meant to, I really didn't want these friends to know, but I was upset and in that moment it was OK. Now most of the group knows and I'll have to deal with that.

For this man, he clearly did not plan to disclose but did anyway. In this case, friends were supportive and maintained privacy. However, unplanned disclosure can still create distress, as one participant in a study by Moneyham et al. (1996) reported:

I think sometimes it just comes out, and you don't plan it. I've slipped a couple of times when I wasn't planning ... I [told a friend] I had just met in the neighborhood, and I am still scared to death of what will happen ... I was sitting there for days afterward, shaking. Oh, my God! What if she tells someone? (p. 214)

This spontaneous disclosure caused stress for the woman, who regretted her impulsivity.

Another example of the less planned disclosure is disclosing in response to disclosure, or reciprocity. If someone discloses their HIV positive status (or AIDS diagnosis), someone might simply respond "I do [have it], too," in an unplanned way. People can also disclose to get disclosure (also called reciprocity; see Gouldner, 1960); however, in this case it is more likely to happen in very specific situations. One similar event is portrayed in a scene in the Broadway show *Rent* (Larson, 1996, Act I, Scene 5) in which Tom Collins meets a man named Angel, and Angel is going to an HIV support group meeting. Angel says, "This body provides a comfortable home for the acquired immune deficiency syndrome." Tom replies, "As does mine." The disclosure would not have been planned; it occurred at that moment in response to another person bringing it up. One gay man went out with a group of friends, and one of them also was HIV positive:

So we were out having a good time, and John's friend ... was joking about the food, and he says "Well it's nice they finally adjusted the damn meds so I can eat decent food." He looks at me and says, "Oh, sorry, I have AIDS and was having trouble with side effects from my cocktail." I don't know what came over me, but I said, "So do I." I'm not sure who was more surprised, me or my friends. They know how cautious I am about telling, now I share in the first hour of meeting someone [shaking his head]. But I guess it was OK, he's dealing with the same things.

These instances have provided specific cases when disclosure can be reciprocated by disclosure in an unplanned manner. This is not necessarily unique to HIV, as a person who had a specific surgery might mention it and another person reciprocate they had that surgery as well.

We have described how most people plan disclosures and provided examples of the less frequent unplanned events. The unplanned disclosure might be the result of stress, a direct question, or reciprocity. The timing for these various plans is different, and we explore next the timing associated with HIV disclosure within a conversation.

When to Disclose in a Conversation

When considering timing, the sequencing of the conversation and how it unfolds is also critical (Derlega et al., 1993; Petronio, 2002). Once a decision is made to disclose (planned), a person must choose how and where in a conversation to share the diagnosis. Often those with HIV consider whether telling should be the first thing mentioned in a conversation, whether the person with HIV should lead up to the disclosure, or whether a full disclosure should be the last issue mentioned before ending the conversation. Unlike incremental disclosures, this issue concerns where in the sequence of the conversation the disclosure should occur, not which parts to share in increments or stages. Certain conversational acts create openings (e.g., reciprocity) or invitations in which disclosure may be more comfortable.

Conversations have particular norms and regularities (Cappella, 1994) dominated by politeness forms (Brown & Levinson, 1987). Initial messages often contain more demographic, polite information (Berger, 1973; Sunnafrank, 1986), with some superficial talk early in relationships and conversations. Kellerman and Lim (1990) developed a model of conversation termed *memory organization packet* that focuses on routines established in conversations to achieve goals. The beginning or opening of a conversation is an important area in which participants establish what will be talked about in the interaction (Schegloff, 1986). This includes not just content (what) but priority placement (where or in what order; Schegloff, 1986). The parties mutually agree on content (Tracy, 1985), but often one has to bring a subject up (it may not be known to both, as in the case of HIV disclosure). Who initiates the topic is important (Wilson et al., 1998), saying you have HIV or being asked, "How are you feeling, you've lost weight?" More urgent topics are discussed earlier, which are also labeled "newsworthy" (Button & Casey, 1984); HIV disclosure would be considered both urgent and newsworthy.

One possible critique of research on timing of self-disclosure is that it mainly utilizes conversations with strangers (Derlega et al., 1987), and most HIV disclosure is not to strangers. Researchers generally report people who disclose early in a conversation are seen as disclosing everything (not selective), with later disclosure in a conversation perceived more favorably (Wortman, Adesman, Herman, & Greenberg, 1976). Research shows that when negative information is to be revealed, the most favorable time from the perspective of the recipient tends to be early in the conversation (Archer & Burleson, 1980; Derlega et al., 1993; Jones & Gordon, 1972). From the perspective of the receiver, the most constructive option for individuals wishing to talk about their HIV status tends to be earlier in the interaction rather than later. Thus, research on conversations and timing of negative disclosure appears contradictory. We explore three options for disclosing an HIV diagnosis within a conversation: immediate, intermediate, and late.

Immediate Disclosure in Conversation.   One choice is to tell very early in the conversation, even preview the information (e.g., "I have something to tell you after dinner"). This kind of communicative strategy is not only used in incremental disclosure to initiate the conversational sequence, it also functions as a way to prepare the recipient for being linked into a privacy boundary (Petronio, 1991, 2002). However, one issue is this preannouncement can be blocked or the potential confidant can discourage disclosure. Reports from some people with HIV indicate, at times, they disclose immediately so that their status is revealed in the first few words of a conversation. They describe doing so because they have built up tension surrounding the disclosure, and for some they are afraid they will "chicken out" if they do not share immediately. This idea is similar to Stiles' (1987) fever model of disclosure. Stiles (Stiles, 1995; Stiles, Shuster, & Harrigan, 1992) argued that when people are distressed, they experience a need to relieve their anxiety, stress, and strain by telling someone about their problems; he drew the analogy to having a physical fever that needs to be reduced to return to a normal body temperature. So too can be the case when a person is diagnosed with HIV. The individual often experiences a great need to unburden himself or herself of the knowledge. In this way, the person with HIV is almost propelled to link others into the privacy boundary around the information to share the weight and responsibility of dealing with the disease.

Whether someone diagnosed with HIV feels compelled to disclose in the manner suggested by Stiles (1987, 1995) may depend, in part, on how long they may have suspected they had the illness, how often they see the person, how much time they have, or the quality of the relationship. People who have been diagnosed longer may feel more comfortable integrating the disclosure into a conversation, perhaps in the middle. If considering disclosing to someone they do not see often, they might want to reconnect a bit before disclosing. If there is limited time, a person might choose to tell someone immediately so they have time to talk about it afterwards. Finally, if the parties are very close, they might share earlier in the conversation, whereas if they are not as close the person might share later in the conversation, waiting for an opportune moment.

In one specific case there may be a need to disclose immediately, in the first part of a conversation, such as with a health care worker (see Cline & McKenzie, 2000). The situational constraints still affect conversational timing, but the direction of a health-related conversation might change dramatically if that information is disclosed immediately. Health decisions may be shifted rapidly based on knowledge of HIV status. Also recall the situation in 1988 in which Olympic diver Greg Louganis did not disclose his HIV diagnosis to a team physician (we first mentioned this incident in chap. 3). During competition in the Olympic Games in Seoul, South Korea, Louganis struck his head on the diving board, he required stitches but completed the competition, and the physician did not utilize the universal precaution of wearing gloves when treating a patient. In 1995, Louganis disclosed that he was HIV positive at the time of the accident (see Clark, 1999). Some press reporters argued vehemently against this disclosure choice to retain privacy, proposing that he (or his coach) should have told the physician immediately so he would protect himself (there were other related arguments about blood in the pool and on the pool deck and whether he should have told the Olympic committee to warn other divers, but experts acknowledge the chlorine and minute portion of blood was a very small risk to others; see Clark, 1999; Louganis, 1996).

Although not the case in this well-known situation, generally there is considerable benefit to the patient to disclose to health care workers immediately (Bartlett & Gallant, 2001; Cline & McKenzie, 2000).

It is also possible to indicate a topic for discussion vaguely early in an interaction to set up a later discussion. People may foreshadow early in a conversation what may come later (Schegloff, 1986), for example, "Remind me to tell you something before I leave." Someone may even forewarn the person before the conversation. "I have to talk to you about something really important when we have dinner." In these instances, people may use the introduction or early interaction to preview a later significant conversational topic such as HIV disclosure.

Disclosure Intermediate in Conversation.   Rather than jumping into a full disclosure immediately, others report they are more comfortable first leading into the topic, catching up with a friend or family member before disclosing. One woman wanted to disclose to a friend but was extremely upset. "We went out to dinner. She knew I was preoccupied but waited until I was ready. So after a while I was able to tell her, it just took a long time, and we sat there and she was great." For this woman, her friend allowing her time was very important and they were both pleased with how it went (although they stayed in the restaurant long enough for it to close and be asked to leave, which they found amusing). A man who had disclosed many times described the following:

> Yeah, I have a plan I guess. I like to go on walks, take a bit of time to be sure the other person has no immediate crisis, then tell. By that point, we're usually halfway through the park and can go back together. [laughs] I've not been walked out on yet, so maybe it's working.

This person uses physical constraints of setting and timing to reinforce his desire for others to talk through their reactions to his disclosure.

In addition to assessing the discloser's needs, there are situations in which the person with HIV takes into account who is the confidant or target of the disclosure. After deciding to disclose, when to reveal is one of the things that marks the conversational plan of action (Petronio, 2002). Though not the same topic of information, children who had been sexually abused did consider the recipient and whether the timing was beneficial for the discloser (Petronio et al., 1996). If they focus on the recipient, the person with HIV may assess how the potential recipient is doing—if they are ill, having a tough time—and choose to disclose at another point. This requires a plan to disclose after seeing how the person is doing; as such it cannot be immediate disclosure. One woman spent the weekend with a friend she does not see much, but the friend was going through a breakup: "I'd planned to tell her that weekend, but we were so wrapped up in the X [boyfriend] mess, I didn't feel it was right to add that on top of things she already had." This woman planned to disclose but decided to wait based on her friend's needs (more relational timing than conversation timing in this case). Intermediate disclosure has some benefits and it is utilized by people to disclose their HIV diagnosis.

Disclosure Late in Conversation. In general, waiting until the last moment, for example, right before a person has to go to work or their bus is leaving, makes follow-up conversation difficult and contradicts a desire to receive the negative information early rather than later in the conversation. From the perspective of the confidant, it makes sense that recipients would not want this type of explosive information made available right before they were leaving for work or unable to get all of the details. Obviously, disclosure without the benefit of following up would no doubt upset the recipient(s) and make it difficult for them to resolve and discuss the issues. For example, the brother of a woman with HIV reported the following:

> I remember when she told me, at Thanksgiving, the morning I was leaving. My plane left in two hours and she tells me then. Don't get me wrong, I was glad she told me, but why not before, when I could find out more, be there with her?

He has visited his sister since this disclosure event, and the difficulty of the initial timing is past, but it was awkward when it occurred.

One possible explanation for late disclosure is that people may be aware of how difficult it is to continue a conversation after such a revelation. There is great difficulty moving away from troubles talk in conversation (Atkinson & Heritage, 1984; Jefferson, 1984); people have to deliberately get off the topic by disengaging and moving to a new topic. For example, one man commented, "What are you supposed to say after? First, it's 'I have AIDS,' and then 'How 'bout that Yankees game?' Like that's going to work well." This flow is awkward and may be intimidating for people considering disclosing HIV infection. If they think about how to talk about other things after disclosing, individuals with HIV may choose to disclose late, despite the awkwardness for the recipient. In fact, participants in Klitzman's (1999) study reported dates often ended after HIV disclosure. Thus, HIV disclosure may actually signal the end of a conversation (recall the earlier example where the mother hung up).

On the other hand, perhaps disclosing late in a conversation is a deliberate strategy by the discloser to limit conversational options. One woman wanted her boyfriend to know but did not want to have a discussion with him. She chose to tell him right before he had to leave for work. "I knew he had to leave, that's why I told him then." He was upset about how she shared, yet she was pleased with the outcome. "That [delay before they could talk] forced him to think before he opened his mouth." Telling late in a conversation could also function to set up a future conversation, perhaps let the person process and talk about it later. One man decided to tell a friend from childhood. They do not talk or visit often but still remain close. He called the friend, talked for about an hour, and then as the conversation was winding down shared his diagnosis:

I didn't want to talk about AIDS for an hour, I wanted to talk to my friend. But he should also know. I didn't know how it would go, he doesn't like parts of my life. So he called back a few days later and wanted to talk some more.

This example of late disclosure was planned, but it could also simply happen if a person cannot find the motivation to share for a while: "I didn't have the courage [to disclose] until the waiter brought the check."

The placement of HIV disclosure at the end of a conversation may be problematic and violates norms, as the closing is not normally a place for new conversational material (Schegloff & Sacks, 1973). Recipients like earlier disclosure better, and these late examples are not appreciated by receivers but may suit the needs of the discloser. This may be a case in which two views (discloser and recipient) of appropriateness are different, a question to answer in the future.

We discussed three different aspects of timing in this section: when to disclose, planning, and timing in a conversation. All of these are important choices in a message strategy, and we turn next to discussion of specific message features.

MESSAGE FEATURES

Besides modes of communication and contextual considerations, it is important to consider message features as ways that people disclose HIV status. Message features are the characteristics of the actual disclosive messages. Messages can vary in terms of explicitness along the directness–equivocality continuum. In addition, the content of disclosure messages can vary in length (e.g., concise, gradual, lengthy) and associated information included (e.g., mode of infection, current health status, sexual orientation, drug history). Finally, messages vary in content or what specific information is shared.

Directness–Equivocality

When individuals decide to reveal their HIV status to others in a planned manner, they are careful about selecting the message strategy that can best produce expected outcomes. People can discuss the same topics repeatedly, disclosing in more detail or more explicitly over time (Spencer, 1994). The directness–equivocality continuum refers to the degree of explicitness in the disclosure message. This topic was addressed previously, but it is presented here in depth with examples of message characteristics.

At one end of the continuum, we have what Petronio (1991) referred to as *explicit message strategies*. These are communication tactics that contain high certainty demand characteristics. Such messages contain clear intentions, obvious demands, low ambiguity, and low uncertainty. With these messages, control is given to receivers and therefore they are placed in a more threatening position in which protection from vulnerabilities is more difficult to attain. Because less autonomy is given to recipients of the disclosure message, they have fewer options available as a response to the information delivered. For example, if a person tells a date, "I have AIDS," the message is explicit and the person would be expected to respond in some manner (like an acknowledgment or an affirming statement). In Klitzman's (1999) study, participants reported important differences in disclosing that they were HIV positive versus they had AIDS, with the latter much more difficult to disclose.

At the other end of the continuum, we have equivocal or *implicit message strategies*. These are communication tactics that are characterized by low certainty demand features (Petronio, 1991). Agne et al. (2000) described indirect messages such as "I can't find a physician who understands this HIV" reported by a small (8%) portion of their sample, but this is only for disclosure to health care providers. These HIV disclosure messages contain much ambiguity and uncertainty and can be potentially interpreted in numerous ways, therefore allowing the partner more autonomy to respond to the implicit demand in the communication. Implicit message tactics protect the communication boundaries for both the discloser and the recipient of the disclosure. The receiving partner has the freedom to probe for clarification, continue exploring the subject, or simply acknowledge the original message. For example, if a person living with HIV tells a date about a new antiretroviral drug or protease inhibitor to fight HIV reported on the evening news, the message is implicit and equivocal and the date can respond in a number of ways (like making it more personal, changing the topic, or treating the topic impersonally). Examples of less specifically direct disclosures from Klitzman (1999) include "hint my lover died of AIDS" or "mention my T-cells are fluctuating."

People living with HIV use a variety of message strategies for disclosure of their condition ranging from extremely direct (e.g., "I have AIDS" vs. "I'm HIV positive") to extremely indirect (e.g., "I know someone who volunteers for an AIDS organization"), and most have developed their repertoire of tactics by trial and error (Adam & Sears, 1994, 1996). People likely vary, choosing a level of directness appropriate for a given disclosure episode. Gradual disclosure, starting with implicit and equivocal messages and moving to ones that are more explicit when reactions are favorable (this also combines timing previously discussed in this chapter), appears to be common (Adam & Sears, 1996; Greene & Faulkner, 2002; Siegel et al., 1998; Spencer & Derlega, 1995). Spencer and Derlega (1995, p. 9) reported on the message strategies used by a gay man with HIV who was interviewed in their study:

> I was dating someone not too long ago, went out, was asked out. I didn't tell [about his HIV diagnosis] right at that point. The way I handled it on the first date, I steered the conversation around to AIDS-related topics; because of my volunteer work, I was able to do that—start talking about them and seeing what their reaction was. Were they going to try to change the subject, were they uncomfortable, or were

they comfortable and compassionate with the whole thing? That was it for the first time, and the second time I brought it up again. I brought up that a former lover of mine had recently tested positive, which he had. Which sort of puts it into their mind that I probably would be, too, and if they were horrified, well that was it and I wouldn't see them again. If that [went] fine, then the next time it was, "Yes, I have tested positive myself." But until I told them, nothing physical had gone on; I had not put anyone in danger. But that's the way I do it; just sort of a gradual thing, test the waters a bit, not just jump right in it, telling them and scaring them to death.

This example illustrates deliberate and gradual disclosure to a potential relationship partner. A man also described how he would talk about HIV related movies and news with a member of his family before disclosing: "You know, to lead up to telling I was sick, I'd talk around it, before I finally said the word AIDS."

In contrast to the gradual examples, some disclosures are abrupt and explicit. One woman reported blurting it out when she broke off a relationship because her partner wanted to become more physical and she was uncomfortable. A teen also illustrated the direct approach when his friend kept asking "over and over again, what was wrong. He wouldn't let up, so I got in his face and said 'I got HIV. Are you happy now?' And he backed off a bit." These examples illustrate differences in directness and length of HIV disclosure narratives. Others may try an indirect approach before becoming more explicit. Agne et al. (2000) described how a person with HIV "told a nurse in the ER to 'put on gloves' three times. Finally, I said, 'look, I'm HIV+, put on gloves (p. 242).'" In this case, when the other did not respond, the initial choice of indirect message to not have to disclose but protect the other was not effective, and this person felt forced to become explicit.

Responses to Questions.   One aspect of directness is being specifically asked for information. Agne et al. (2000) reported that 7% of patients' disclosures to health care providers were in response to a direct question (e.g., "They asked me if I had any medical issues that they should know about in assisting me medically. I said 'yes.' They asked me and I told them I was HIV positive."). In Klitzman's (1999) study, many men with HIV disclosed only when or if asked their status. In some cases, if asked directly about HIV status, some replied "don't know my own status but it's probably positive." Thus, even when some people know, they may not directly admit it.

Although not specifically related to HIV, Berger and Kellerman (1989) examined evasive tactics or strategies people use when asked direct questions. For example, a person could ask, "Are you sick?" and that is a very different type of direct question compared with "I heard you have AIDS." Once such a direct question is posed, it creates a dilemma. This response to a question is not voluntary disclosure but it still requires action or a response. There are three main groupings of possible responses to such a direct question about HIV status. First, the person could use the opportunity to disclose by confirming, "Yes, I do have AIDS." This would allow the person an opportunity to expand on the topic in many ways. Second, the person could either deny or redirect the question. A denial could be "No, I do not have AIDS," and individuals with HIV do report times when they directly misrepresent their HIV status. This direct denial is different from redirecting, for example, "AIDS? I have a type of bone cancer." This redirecting response may invite many more questions. Both denial and redirecting strategies can be considered deception but in different ways. In Klitzman's (1999) study, one date asked, "Are you healthy?" and he replied "Yes" even though he knew the person was asking if he was HIV positive (deliberate misinterpretation). Finally, the third possible way to respond to a direct question is to avoid. For example, "Why is X always talking about other people?" and proceed to discuss the person who spread the information. Another variation would simply be to change the topic. If the other is very persistent, the avoiding strategy may be difficult. This is an example of how responses to disclosure can either encourage or discourage elaboration on the topic (Maynard, 1997). Responding to direct questions about HIV status may be difficult, but there are options (we presented 3 here).

We described how disclosure can vary in level of directness and how people can respond to direct questions. We turn next to length of disclosure messages.

Length of Message

Disclosure of HIV status can vary in length within a given episode (not like directness discussed previously, which can be across conversations). Agne et al. (2000) reported 45% of disclosure messages to health care providers were limited to indicating HIV status and thus were brief (e.g., "I recently found out that I'm HIV positive"). As seen previously, some disclosures may be gradual or concise. Some might be concise, whereas others are lengthy and expository. The following is an illustration of concise disclosure:

> I had told her earlier, I had said I have something to tell you. Anyway, I said I'm gonna wait and then I told her. Well, I was still gonna wait for a little bit. Once my momma got off the phone, I was trying to wait until my momma got off the phone but L. was like, "What are they arguing, what is she arguing with him for?" ... so I went ahead and told her. That's why she was like this is a dream, un-uh, you [are] lying, it's a dream. I said "I'm HIV positive."

Here is another example in which the message was more lengthy and expository when a woman disclosed on the phone to her boyfriend:

> "Was I, what did they actually say? What did they actually say?" That's what, that's what he was saying, "What did they say, what did they ask you?," That's all he could ask me. How did they say it? ... I won't, I can't say how he really was 'cause I couldn't see him, so I don't know. He said, "What'd they say?" ... I said, you know what, you

know what it is. I said, something like, I was saying something like, "You know what it is, you already know what it is. Remember when you said I was going to die anyway, you know what it is." Something I kept saying. He was like, "What did they say?" Positive or something he said ... so I said "yeah." He said what, did, they say what did they say, he was saying, said, "Did I have AIDS or did I, or was I HIV positive." That was what he was meaning. I just said I was HIV positive and I just said it blunt, just like that and left it alone. I was like now what? And that was when he said like, who did I tell? Who have I told, that's what he asked me, and the conversation went on from there.

In this situation, the needs of the discloser and receiver are not the same in terms of message (and interaction) length. She clearly wanted a short event, simply to tell him. He, however, wanted an in-depth conversation about the details. Thus, different needs can affect the outcome of message length (and it may not go as planned).

The preceding discussion focused on the directness and length of the HIV disclosure episodes. We turn next to message content.

Message Content

Disclosers, after assessing their own expectations and message strategies, must make a decision about what precisely to tell (Petronio, 1991, 2002). In other words, as CPM proposes, as part of developing privacy rules the individual with HIV needs to formulate the actual content of the disclosive message. They may actually rehearse what they plan to say, much like people rehearse proposing marriage or asking for a raise (in the appendix we present examples to assist with this HIV disclosure rehearsal process). Content considerations include the type of information disclosed, beyond using terms *HIV* or *AIDS*. Many people with HIV may simply state, "I am HIV positive" without additional information (e.g., Agne et al., 2000, disclosure to heath care providers).

The individual with HIV also needs to consider telling (or being asked) other issues potentially associated with the condition, like mode of infection, sexual orientation, drug use, and current health status, among others. Revealing one's HIV diagnosis for some includes the process of telling about one's health status and sexual orientation at the same time (Adam & Sears, 1996; Gard, 1990; Hays et al., 1993) or the process of telling about their health and drug use history simultaneously (Hassin, 1994). One woman recalled how she was afraid of this link between HIV, sex, and drug use. "I thought everybody would be, God ... at first I thought people was gonna think I was sleeping around a lot, you know. Might think I'm on drugs or something." She was reluctant to disclose her diagnosis, and when she did she made it very clear she got it from her ex-husband. This example is also reminiscent of Arthur Ashe's (see chap. 1) disclosing his HIV status and how often and vehemently he repeated he had gotten the HIV infection during surgery in the 1980s. An adolescent reported how she was worried about disclosing:

I wouldn't tell [grandmother] 'cause, I don't know, she would be too shocked. Because see I know with my grandfather he kind of had an idea before I told him because the way my life style is. I mean it's like I ain't never had sex but one, two, three, four, four maybe five times if it's somebody I forgot.... The only bad habit I got, right, is smoking and sex. And I'm not gonna stop that, I care, but I ain't gonna stop it.

In this case, the grandfather was more prepared because the grandmother was not aware the girl was sexually active. This created a bind in disclosing to them, specifically about what to say (she had not resolved what to disclose at the time of the interview but wanted to tell them).

The disclosure of HIV infection, even if separate in minds of the person with HIV, is linked with mode of transmission in the minds of many people. One gay man described his dilemma:

My parents, I was raised Catholic, and I can't see them understanding. I want to tell them about the HIV, but I've never been able to face them about being gay. And they will want to know how I got it.

A man in his 30s described telling the woman he was dating for 8 years:

My girlfriend thought I was clean, she knew I'd done crack years ago, but I'm still using. I must'of got it that way, 'cause we've been tested together. So when I told her I had AIDS, I had to tell her about the drugs. She was really hurt.

This person felt obligated to share the associated information (drug use) in addition to the HIV diagnosis. This linkage of HIV with mode of infection is not exclusive to HIV, but it is unusual (see stigma discussions in chaps 3 and 5). It can be seen in descriptions of disclosure messages, what people actually say when they disclose about their diagnosis.

How HIV was contracted motivates some decisions to conceal a diagnosis (e.g., Kalichman, Roffman, Picciano, & Bolan, 1998; Marks et al., 1992). For example, a man with HIV described the following conversation with his grandmother about why he delayed telling her or other family members about his diagnosis:

Not only did I have to tell her [grandmother] about the HIV, I had to tell her I was a gay man, too. Then she wants to know why it took all these years [to disclose about the HIV]. I said, "Because I didn't think you would understand." Instead of taking these people [family] through that [being homosexual], I just never told anybody.

This example illustrates the potential need for a double disclosure when the information was high risk for both issues. Often to know about the HIV infection means that a person must consider the rules he or she wants to use for two high-risk sources of private information. The individual may have difficulty separating one from the other. Sometimes people may be willing to talk about the infection but be less willing to disclose how they contracted it because they must reveal more about their lives than they feel comfortable doing. The disclosure about HIV status may mean therefore that the individual is left coping with not one difficult situation but two powerful revelations in need of further explanation. Consequently, the decision to conceal or reveal increases in complexity because of the way a person becomes infected. This is true for those using injection drugs, having extrarelational affairs, or any other source of infection that has a potential to place an added burden when the reason for contracting the disease is not easily revealed.

In this section, we discussed a number of factors associated with verbal disclosure of HIV infection: mode, context, and message features. For mode or channel considerations we examined face-to-face, non-face-to-face, and third-party disclosure. For context considerations we examined setting and timing. Finally, for message features we discussed directness, length, and content of what information was shared. All of these discussions focused on verbal or written disclosure messages. We now turn to alternative messages used to disclose about an HIV diagnosis.

ALTERNATIVE DISCLOSURE MESSAGE STRATEGIES

To this point in the chapter, we have focused on verbal HIV disclosure messages. There are, however, alternate forms of HIV disclosure that might be described by terms such as *symbolic, environmental,* or *nonverbal.* None of these terms adequately captures the range of alternative messages. As discussed in chapter 3, disclosure of HIV status is a difficult and challenging relational event for the discloser and the disclosure target. Because of the potential social stigma, rejection, and personal vulnerability involved, some people living with HIV and/or AIDS choose to disclose in other ways, avoiding the verbal option. Klitzman (1999) reported disclosure often occurred using subtle cues in codes and through indirect hints. Crosby's (2000) study, conducted with a sample of 92 MSM with HIV in San Francisco, found that most of these men had difficulties revealing their diagnosis to new sexual partners. One individual captured well the overall sentiment regarding HIV disclosure:

> Gay men [in San Francisco] do not feel like they can talk about their serostatus with new sex partners, period. Consequently, many of us are using symbolic ways of disclosing our status that are not particularly direct and could very easily be misunderstood. (Julian, 1997, p. 13)

These symbolic ways of disclosure are often indirect and emblematic. It is also possible to use direct disclosure that is not verbal in form. In this way, people are able to send a nonambiguous message without using a verbal strategy:

I didn't tell her. I gave her a pamphlet. Well, she asked me what was wrong with me. She said "what did they say was wrong with you?," and I gave her the pamphlet, and I was crying and she just read it and she was like "What?, for real?, Are you serious?" You know, like that kind of shock.

In this instance, sharing the pamphlet was a replacement for a verbal disclosure. Many attempts are not directly verbal but take other forms. Although using this pamphlet strategy is not verbal, it is still very direct.

An additional direct, yet not verbal, disclosure strategy, is the use of a tattoo. One man interviewed for this book had "HIV+" tattooed on his bicep about a year after he was diagnosed. As he described:

I was still going out, picking up guys, and I got tired of all the mess with talking about it, being safe. It was so awkward. I always wear a muscle shirt to the club to show off my body, so a friend jokingly suggested I get this [points to tattoo], and I thought it was a perfect solution. This way, there is no way he [a potential date] wouldn't know but we don't have to talk about it.

For this person, disclosure was important. Yet he saw verbal disclosure as requiring too much time and energy, and he wanted an efficient strategy. Other people we interviewed were aware of this tattoo strategy (had seen or heard of it), but it appears to be relatively infrequent.

Physical appearance, at times, precludes both the necessity and choice of disclosing. In some cases, physical effects of the disease and treatments are an almost certain indication of HIV infection. One man described the following:

I've been on [HIV] combination therapy since late 1995. It saved my life. I am 6'2" and was down to about 130 pounds before I started [HAART]. Now, with my anti-HIV and growth hormone therapy [to combat HIV wasting], I've gained all my weight back and more. I guess some people call me a G. O. D. [gay on steroids]. I am very muscular now. But the HIV medications have side effects, and I show signs of lipodistrophy. I don't have a "Crix belly" [an accumulation of fat around the stomach attributed to Crixivan and other protease inhibitors] but I have sunken cheeks and skinny limbs with a big chest and huge arms. So, I have an "HIV body" and I assume that people I date will know by just looking at me. I don't usually tell them that I am HIV positive unless they ask. But, from my experience, most of the men I dated could tell just by looking at my body.

For this man, others could generally tell his HIV diagnosis by looking at his body. Using a visual indicator, however, is not the same for all people with HIV and may become problematic if people assume those who look healthy are not HIV positive (see, e.g., Markova & Power, 1992; Metts & Fitzpatrick, 1992). Although disclosure strategies that are not verbal may be less effective than verbal disclosures, individuals with HIV use them to some extent to let others know about their health. People with unknown or seronegative status may also use them to discover whether their potential partner has HIV (Brouwer, 2000).

Crosby (2000) described nonverbal attempts by individuals with HIV or AIDS to disclose their serostatus to potential sexual partners. Limandri (1989) described "invitational disclosure" in which a person provides cues and sees if the other follows up with questions. Although it is worth emphasizing that these disclosure and discovery tactics may be ineffective and extremely unreliable, a number of individuals with HIV reported using them (Julian, 1997; Klitzman, 1999). Some of these strategies include leaving out copies of *POZ* magazine (a publication about living with HIV infection; see Appendix), leaving out HIV- or AIDS-related medications (like AZT; generic name is *zidovudine*), leaving medical reports or receipts in view for visitors, and attending AIDS-related events (e.g., AIDS fundraisers, HIV medical updates in the community). Other gay men report a similar strategy of displaying safer sex posters in their apartments (Crosby, 2000). One gay man reported, "I always leave my medication on my dining room table, so it'd almost be impossible to miss. If he wants to ask about it, I'm willing to discuss it." For this man, he feels he provides enough information and others can ask if they have questions.

Alternative message choices may be deliberate, conscious decisions to share information in a way that may be less threatening and provide potential topics for conversations such as "I went to the AIDS walk on Saturday." One heterosexual woman said, "I want anyone I'm dating to know [my diagnosis]. So I have all these t-shirts and AIDS stuff all over my house, my car." This woman self-describes as "out" concerning her HIV infection, but she also recognizes that not directly stating that she has HIV might be misconstrued. Another alternative strategy is the "sushi test," which refers to an individual's refusal to eat sushi, to protect the compromised immune system of an individual with HIV against uncooked foods for fear of parasites (Brouwer, 2000). Some gay men report asking a date if he wants to get sushi for dinner as a way of judging his HIV status (this could be considered a "secret test," see Baxter & Wilmot, 1984). Needless to say, these alternative strategies can be extremely indirect and potentially misunderstood by the target of the disclosure.

Vernacular Tactics

Brouwer (2000) examined vernacular tactics of HIV discovery among gay men. Vernacular tactics are "those behaviors, practices, gestures, and discourses that individuals and groups perform in the course of their everyday lives … [through] the local methods that individuals use to make meaning of their own" (Brouwer, 2000, p. 98). The nonverbal aspects of such tactics become critical in the absence of explicit verbal communication about HIV status. For example, a person's sudden weight change (e.g., drastic weight loss) or lesions might be read as indicative of seropositive status. Family, friends, coworkers, and others may notice these cues. Vernacular tactics also can be seen as information seeking strategies or means to discover if a partner is "safe" and may function as ways of reducing uncertainty. Metts and Fitzpatrick (1992) mentioned that people's preferred method of safer sex is their belief in their ability to "select a safe partner" (p. 2). In fact, people often seek information to confirm the suitability of a prospective sexual partner. They devise strategies to confirm the partner is not at risk, to reduce their uncertainty. Kitzinger (1991) reported people clearly believe they can tell by looking at a person if they are HIV positive (see also Metts & Fitzpatrick, 1992; Markova & Power, 1992). Use of alcohol or other drugs may also inhibit accurate perceptions. In a study by Murphy, Monahan, and Miller (1998) the more intoxicated women thought they became the more confident they were that they could tell the risk status just by looking at another person (picture of a hypothetical date).

Two vernacular tactics were identified in Brouwer's (2000) study: "trick examinations" and "trick intuitions." People use them to seek information about another's HIV status without specifically asking. Trick examinations are strategies used by a person in a sexual encounter to discern the HIV status of the partner. Such strategies may consist of touching and feeling the partner's lymph nodes under the disguise of erotic play. Although potentially inaccurate and ineffective, swollen lymph nodes may be read as signs of HIV infection in a dating situation (and implicitly the absence of swelling is taken as an indication of noninfection).

As opposed to actively using touch to decide on the HIV status of a sexual partner, trick intuitions refer to the perceived ability "to accurately read nonverbal signs of HIV infection" (Brouwer, 2000, p. 107). People also make inferences based on cues (e.g., hygiene, apartment cleanliness; Crosby, 2000). Although dreadfully inaccurate and potentially hazardous to one's health, some men regard nonverbal cues like "emotional tenor" (e.g., degree of calmness during unprotected sexual intercourse) and facial expressions and characteristics as indicators of their partner's HIV status. Both of these tactics—trick examinations and trick intuitions—are actually not about HIV disclosure per se; they can be better characterized as one communicator's attempt to discern and read their partner's serostatus. In Klitzman's (1999, p. 46) study, one participant reported he "picks those [partners] I can trust" similar to knowing by looking if a person is seropositive (Markova & Power, 1992; Metts & Fitzpatrick, 1992). People are also more confident that someone they know (is a part of their social network) is HIV negative.

Clearly not as much research examines aspects of disclosure (or information seeking) that are not verbal, although it has been reported sporadically. Further research would be useful to understand how alternative HIV disclosure messages (and detection) function.

CONCLUSIONS

In this chapter we have discussed the message features associated with disclosure of HIV status. Specifically, we examined the verbal disclosure process and alternative attempts to discern someone else's status as well as strategies to reveal one's HIV diagnosis. We examined the verbal disclosure process by identifying communication mode (e.g., face-to-face, non-face-to-face, third-party disclosure), contextual (e.g., setting, timing), and message factors (e.g., directness– equivocality, message length, and content). Each of these factors must be dealt with in every disclosure event. Finally, we discussed alternative forms of HIV disclosure by examining tactics used by persons with HIV to disclose their diagnosis and vernacular strategies used by individuals to discern the HIV status of their potential sexual partners.

As we demonstrated in this chapter, there are a wide range of disclosure messages people use to share their HIV diagnoses. There is agreement about how some message features work, but for other message features people make decisions that vary from situation to situation. Most people with HIV agree that the disclosure messages become somewhat easier to share with time and practice. However, the disclosive episodes require investment and energy and do not always turn out as planned. In the next chapter we examine the consequences or outcomes of HIV disclosure.

CHAPTER FIVE

Consequences of HIV Disclosure and Nondisclosure Decision Making

In this chapter we examine the consequences of HIV disclosure and the choices to maintain privacy for persons with HIV and for others to whom they might or might not disclose the diagnosis. A person deciding if or when to disclose takes into account how benefits weigh against drawbacks (described in chap. 3); included in this process is uncertainty about how the others will react and possible unforeseen consequences. This balance is crucial because of the potential outcomes: specifically, disclosure can provide opportunities for social support but also opens a person to risks. Many of these consequences occur only after disclosure, that is, the consequences are not apparent when the person has not disclosed. However, as CPM argues, given that people manage their privacy, some anticipate consequences and make judgments about revealing or concealing based on reactions they expect (Petronio, 2002).

To fully grasp the consequences of HIV disclosure, it may be necessary for the person with HIV and others to wait for some period of time. There may also be differences between immediate (what happens literally during or right after the disclosure) and longer term consequences (the next day, week, or month) of someone knowing the HIV diagnosis. Additionally, there may be differences associated with direct and indirect disclosure, for instance when a person simply states, "I am HIV positive" or hints around without fully disclosing. Yet much research focuses only on a person knowing the HIV diagnosis (not necessarily how he or she found out) and not on the disclosure recipient (Petronio, 2002). Because the recipient is so critical in maintaining the level of protection or dissemination of a discloser's health status and because that person is necessary for valuable support during the illness, it is imperative to consider how recipients co-manage knowing about a person's HIV status.

In this chapter we first describe reported responses to HIV disclosure based on personal accounts. Then we examine outcomes of social support. Next, we look at the effects of disclosure on psychological health and identity, as disclosure can influence how people cope with HIV. Another outcome of disclosure is being stigmatized, and these reports are widespread and influence further HIV disclosure

121

decisions. The last outcome discussed is the effect of HIV disclosure on close relationships because relational contexts are important areas for how people with HIV
manage their lives; specifically, we examine relationship closeness, significant others as caregivers, effects on children, and impact on safer sex and other risk behaviors. Finally, the chapter examines the effect of nondisclosure of an HIV diagnosis.

CONSEQUENCES OF HIV DISCLOSURE

To set the stage, consider the following three cases of Marie, Philip, and Revelle
that illustrate possible consequences of trying to coordinate rules for when to
open the privacy boundary and give access to information about HIV status.

Marie.   Marie learned about her HIV diagnosis in late 1992. She reported that
at first she was "in denial" about the diagnosis. She told no one but her twin sister
who lived across the country. Marie at the time had a daughter who was 6 years
old, but she did not want to tell her child about the diagnosis because she was too
young. After a couple of years, Marie joined an HIV support group. Gradually she
"got more bold" in dealing with HIV and chose to tell the rest of her family. One
day Marie went to her parents' house to tell her family about the HIV diagnosis:

> When I decided to tell everybody, my brother was home working on a car and my
> mom was in the house. I told him that I needed to tell him something about my
> health. He said, "What are you talking about? I think I already know what you are
> going to tell me." I said, "How would you know?" Then I told him about the diagno-
> sis. What I did not know is that my sister had already told him about my diagnosis
> when he went out to California to visit her. He had behaved over the last 2 years as if
> he didn't know. It is funny, though. I have had a lot of problems with my car and he
> has been coming over to my house and helping me out. All of us in the family have
> never been close. I thought it was weird that he was being so helpful.

Marie continued:

> When I went into the house, I told my mother that I had donated blood and found
> out that way about the HIV diagnosis. She asked me if I was certain about the diag-
> nosis. I said, "Yeah." I also told her that my daughter had been tested and that she
> was negative. My mother didn't say anything. We have never been close.

We asked Marie if she and her family were able to talk about the diagnosis in the
months and years that followed. She said the following:

> Ever since I told them [the family] about the diagnosis, nobody will talk to me about
> it. They choose to ignore it. They won't address it. I think they are afraid that I am, or
> that I could be, dying. I explained to them about all the medicines for HIV that are
> out now, that the disease is manageable and people are living longer and that I might

not be dying. I might be able to live a normal life span. But you can't just sweep it [their fear of my death] under the rug. It's there.

This description of Marie's disclosure experiences illustrates both direct (to sister) and unplanned or unrequested third-party (sister to brother) disclosure and choices not to disclose (to child). Marie's story reveals careful selection in disclosure choices and the effect of relational quality discussed in chapter 3. We explore further in this chapter the consequences of HIV disclosure, which may be positive or negative. In the case of Marie, the consequences for her were disappointment and lack of social support.

Philip.   Another person living with HIV, Philip, has told very few people about his diagnosis, including his lover, a cousin, and a few friends. He has never told his father because "My father would treat me as though I was a disease." He has not told other family members. Philip said he wanted to maintain the closeness he has traditionally enjoyed with other family members—even if it means that they do not know about his HIV diagnosis. He said the following:

You look at people who are real close and real dear to you and you say, "Well, I wonder how they would react if I were to tell them." And you want to tell them but then you say, "Well, this closeness that we have, I want to keep it. So, I better keep it to myself."

Philip had been concerned about his lover's reaction, whether he would get up and walk out and never come back when he learned about the diagnosis. Philip did tell his lover, adding, "If you leave, I will understand it." Philip's lover did not leave him; indeed, he said "Telling him about the diagnosis brought us closer together."

Philip, like Marie, illustrates careful choices in disclosure and nondisclosure. His story reveals some positive consequences, specifically that his lover felt closer to him. It also illustrates the concept of anticipated response (both anticipated and actual) we described in chapter 3 and how concerns about HIV stigma may inhibit disclosure. We explore stigma consequences of disclosure later in this chapter.

Revelle.   Revelle is a woman in her 30s who reported becoming infected via a boyfriend who did not tell her about his HIV infection. She has only disclosed to her immediate family and one friend. Revelle was diagnosed in 1988 and told her parents shortly after she found out:

I told my mother that the test results came back and that I was HIV positive. She was pretty much in shock. She was scared I was going to die the next day. I was scared to tell my mother. I felt guilty that I brought this news to my family. I didn't want to hurt my parents and I felt that they would react to HIV as a behavior problem, as if I had done something wrong. I also told my sister at that time. My sister is a very loving person. When I told her that I have this disease, she cried. I think it was the first time that I saw my sister cry. She told me she didn't want to lose me. I was the only sister she had. It was very emotional.

Revelle noted that her mother and sister have grown with her in coping with the disease:

They are learning themselves about how to deal with a member of the family who is infected with HIV. They are learning a lot of medical stuff. They are learning about medicines. They are learning about T-cells. Pretty much through all these years, my sister and mother ask me, especially when we talk on the phone, how are you doing, have you been to the doctor, how are your T-cells. They have learned all this terminology that we never talked about before.

Revelle's story illustrates predominantly direct verbal disclosure. The consequences she experienced were initially difficult, but over time Revelle received more support and acceptance.

These anecdotes involving Marie, Philip, and Revelle indicate some consequences associated with HIV disclosure. As CPM theory proposes, individuals with HIV weigh the pros and cons of disclosing to others about the diagnosis (see chap. 3). Yet they also live with expected and unexpected consequences of disclosing or not disclosing to others about the diagnosis. The way they are able to coordinate their privacy boundaries with others and determine collective rules for maintaining the privacy frequently rests on the level of benefits or costs assessed by the participants (see chap. 2). There may be beneficial outcomes to disclosure, including the opportunity to express thoughts and feelings about the diagnosis that may have been pent up for days, months, or even years (see Derlega & Grzelak, 1979). There may be the satisfaction of being open and honest with loved ones. There is the opportunity to obtain emotional and tangible support in coping with a life-threatening disease. However, HIV disclosure may also incur a price with significant negative outcomes for all involved. Significant others may experience their own shock, discomfort, and denial about the diagnosis. Those who know about the diagnosis may worry about becoming infected themselves, they may have misgivings about the personal life of the individual with HIV, or they may have difficulty interacting with a loved one who has a chronic or life-threatening disease. Being the confidant means taking responsibility for the information with the discloser (Petronio, 2002). Sometimes recipients want to help, but when they find out the diagnosis they are often unable to get past the emotional trauma of knowing. Yet, in some situations, disclosure of the diagnosis may not necessarily change relationships—for better or for worse—compared to how they were before.

We examine the effects of coordinating rules for HIV disclosure and maintenance of privacy boundaries for individuals with HIV and their significant others in several areas including social support, stigma, and close relationships. Because the consequences of HIV disclosure and nondisclosure contain risks and benefits not only for the person infected but also for the confidants selected, it is necessary to consider the way that all people are linked into the privacy boundary around the HIV status of an individual. Although we mainly focus on the consequences of HIV disclosure when the person with HIV tells others about the diagnosis, we also consider what happens when others may find out via a third party (recall chap. 4), as with the example of Marie at the beginning of this chapter. We begin by summarizing reports of responses to HIV disclosure.

Actual Responses to HIV Disclosure

In chapter 3 we discussed the role of anticipated response in HIV disclosure decisions. This chapter summarizes research on some of the actual responses to HIV disclosure reported, similar to yet different from anticipated responses about how people think others will respond. Some researchers conceive of responses to disclosure as positive, negative, or neutral. Schegloff (1986) suggested that in general conversations, a neutral response shuts down a topic, whereas a positive or negative verbal response (even nonverbal signifiers) prompts expansion of the conversation. In both positive or negative response situations it is possible to continue the discussion, even by asking for clarification (e.g., one mother followed up by asking, "What does that mean, are you really sick, are you going to die?," allowing the conversation to continue). This may be the case as well for HIV disclosure if a positive or negative response continues discussion of the issue (even a negative response could lead to an argument or further discussion of the disagreement). Kimberly et al. (1995), however, argued that someone must anticipate a positive (not neutral or negative) response before they are willing to disclose an issue as important as an HIV diagnosis (see also Petronio & Martin, 1986). One study (Limandri, 1989) found that individuals with HIV report many more negative responses to disclosure than positive responses, but these negative responses may simply be more vivid and memorable (especially compared with neutral ones). Greene and Faulkner (2002), however, reported fewer negative responses to HIV disclosure overall than people anticipated yet some specific negative responses (e.g., violence and treated differently) not expected by people with HIV.

The different results found by Limandri (1989) compared with Greene and Faulkner (2002) may be accounted for by the time in the epidemic (late 1980s vs. late 1990s, respectively) or samples. The fact that people with HIV might be expecting negative responses, however, may be more crucial than whether or not people actually respond negatively. If people are estimating costs of disclosure to be high, they will develop rules that limit the amount and frequency of revealing (Petronio, 2002). Likewise, when they do disclose, they will want to enter into a discussion that limits further revelations about their HIV status. Thus, it is useful to consider both the expected and actual responses to knowing someone's HIV status to understand the way people might navigate this tricky terrain.

Research suggests there are different kinds of reactions people diagnosed with HIV actually experience when others learn about the diagnosis. Simoni et al. (1995) asked women with HIV to place their families' reactions to the HIV disclosure into three categories: provided emotional support, became angry, and withdrew. Participants reported that mother, father, and friends all generally provided support and were rarely angry. Lovers provided support but were more likely to withdraw or become angry (20% left the relationship). Mansergh et al. (1995) used the same three-category reaction system as Simoni et al. (1995) with a sample of men with HIV and reported very similar reactions. These two studies provide initial evidence for reactions to disclosure, yet they are constrained by the use of only three apriori categories for responses.

Serovich et al. (1998) examined reactions experienced by women who disclose their HIV status from a constant comparison approach (Glaser & Strauss, 1967). This method allows categories to emerge from the data (interviews) through close and repeated reading of the text. They interviewed 12 women with HIV and developed a 31-response typology based on the women's descriptions of reactions to HIV disclosure. The six broader categories of responses included intellectual, physical, spiritual, relational, instrumental, and emotional. The broad emotional response category accounted for more than half of the responses, and many of these reactions were negative (e.g., "It's your fault" and "They don't want to touch me").

Greene and Faulkner (2002) sought to compare what reactions were expected prior to disclosure and what reactions occurred after HIV disclosure. They interviewed 10 African American girls with HIV and reported five categories of responses to HIV disclosure: different treatment, negative emotional reactions, received support, target told others, and treated no differently. Unlike Serovich et al. (1998), who reported overwhelmingly emotional responses, girls in this study reported most often that they were treated differently. This different treatment was described in both positive (e.g., "brought us closer together") and negative terms (e.g., "won't come near me"); therefore it was generally balanced. Additionally, Greene and Faulkner (2002) reported markedly similar expected and actual reactions to disclosure (they were the same categories except for an unsure category for expected, but the order of frequency was different). Adolescents in this study were generally able to anticipate (or recalled that they did) how others would respond when told about the HIV diagnosis, but they were occasionally surprised by others' responses. It is important to remember that not all disclosure goes as planned, but sometimes people can accurately estimate others' reactions.

Some of the most problematic actual responses to HIV disclosure reported involve lovers and family members. Metts and Manns (1996) reported that reactions to HIV disclosure from the first disclosure recipients were supportive, perhaps indicating people may choose to tell more supportive recipients initially, leaving more difficult ones for later. The highest proportion of unsupportive reactions were from family members, and over time people with HIV received the most support from friends and other individuals with HIV and the least from family. Similarly, Stempel et al. (1995) reported more negative reactions from male family members and primary sexual partners. Hays et al. (1993), however, argued that friends and lovers provide more helpful responses than family or colleagues (see also Kimberly & Serovich, 1996). Thus, research indicates there is a wide range of actual responses to HIV disclosure, some of which match expected reactions. We explore one specific type of response next, that of social support.

Boundary Coordination Issues with HIV Disclosure and Social Support

Social support is associated with health. It is generally "found to be health-promoting, health-restoring and associated with a decrease in mortality risk" (Sarason, Sarason, & Gurung, 1997, p. 547). Stokes (1983) explored the size of network structure, specifically how many confidants are enough? Stokes reported a curvilinear relation between life satisfaction and number of confidants, suggesting that too few or too many network members is not optimal. As CPM theory (see chap. 2) suggests, when someone is told about a person's HIV status they share the information and are linked into a set of responsibilities because they know that information (Petronio, 2002). When individuals want to support their friends, partners, or family members, instead of being reluctant they are expected to be actively engaged as confidants (Petronio, 2000a, 2000b). However, this may not always be the case. The discloser may have high expectations that the partner, friend, or family member will be an active participant in managing the information and provide needed social support. People may find, however, that confidants are not as engaged as they need them to be.

A promising finding in the literature on coping with HIV is that satisfaction with social support (one consequence of disclosure) may be associated causally with a lower probability of progressing to an AIDS diagnosis. Leserman et al. (2000) conducted a study with 82 men living with HIV who were interviewed regularly for up to 7½ years. None of the men at the beginning of the study had been diagnosed with AIDS and they had no HIV-related symptoms. Individuals with high levels of social support satisfaction were less likely to develop AIDS than those with low levels of social support satisfaction. Leserman et al.'s (2000) study did not, however, provide any data about research participants' rates of disclosure about the HIV diagnosis to significant others. The type of social support received after telling others about the HIV diagnosis is likely to affect the quality of life and physical coping with HIV disease. We next examine the types of social support that someone is likely to receive after disclosing about the HIV diagnosis and the effects on health outcomes in coping with HIV.

Types of Social Support.   There is evidence that the type of social support received may vary after the disclosure recipient learns about the HIV diagnosis.

TABLE 5.1
Summary of Types of Helpful and Unhelpful Social Support

Types of Helpful Social Support	Types of Unhelpful Social Support
Expressing love or concern	Acting in a patronizing or overprotective manner
Serving as confidant	Avoiding interaction with the person with HIV
Providing encouragement	Acting embarrassed or ashamed
Providing an opportunity for reciprocity to allow the person with HIV to feel needed and important	Avoiding directly mentioning or discussing HIV or other emotions related to the person's disease
Aiding as a role model	Expressing a pessimistic, negative, or hopeless attitude about AIDS
Interacting naturally	Breaking confidentiality
Providing information	Acting in a judgmental manner
Advice	Not accepting limitations that AIDS may place on one's abilities to do things
Material or practical assistance	Raising doubts about the effectiveness of one's medical care
Providing companionship or enjoyment	Displaying rude or insensitive comments or actions
Providing support for other network members in dealing with one's illness	Giving unsolicited advice or criticizing how they were coping with HIV

Adapted from Hays et al. (1994) with elements from Barbee et al. (1998).

Note. Adapted from "Identifying Helpful and Unhelpful Behaviors of Loved Ones: The PWA's Perspective," by R. B. Hays, R. H. Magee, and S. Chauncey, 1994, *AIDS Care, 6,* p. 382. Copyright 1994 by Taylor & Francis, Ltd: http://www.tandf.co.uk/journals.

Contrary to popular views, not all social support is necessarily helpful (e.g., it may be unwanted, inappropriate, or overwhelming). For instance, Hays et al. (1994) asked a group of MSM with advanced progression of HIV disease (a diagnosis of AIDS or AIDS-related complex [ARC[1]]) about helpful and unhelpful behaviors enacted by family or friends since the diagnosis (see Table 5.1 for examples of helpful and unhelpful social support). A related study by Barbee et al. (1998), based on Sensitive Interaction Systems Theory (SIST), asked people with HIV to recall experiences with social support provided by others. They asked about times when someone else thought they were being supportive but their behavior was actually helpful or not helpful in coping with the HIV infection. Most people could recall instances in which others had been either helpful or unhelpful. The overwhelming number of helpful acts were behaviors such as "solve" (e.g., giving information to help with a problem) and solace (e.g., showing understanding). The dominant unhelpful behaviors in Barbee et al.'s (1998) study fell into three categories: unwanted

---

[1]Kalichman (1995, p. 357) described AIDS-related complex (ARC) as "a variously defined term with little clinical value used to identify certain HIV-infected individuals prior to an AIDS diagnosis. Compared with earlier in the epidemic, ARC is used less often today."

TABLE 5.2

Examples and Percentages of Helpful and Unhelpful Behaviors
(Source: Barbee et al., 1998)

Helpful Behaviors	Unhelpful Behaviors
Solve behaviors (42% of the helpful acts)	Unwanted solve behaviors (23% of the unhelpful acts)
Asking questions about one's problems	Someone asking too many personal questions about how the disease was contracted
Giving information to help solve problems	Offers of assistance in which someone "tried to take over"
Doing something active or tangible to help solve problems	"She's overcompensated and helped me too much"
Solace behaviors (53% of the helpful acts)	Unwanted escape and dismissive behaviors (70% of the unhelpful acts)
Giving affection	Showing disinterest, minimizing what happened
Showing understanding and empathy	Refusing to talk about the HIV diagnosis and related issues
Assuring availability for helping in the future	Criticizing the way in which the person was coping with HIV
Doing things to try to lift their mood	
Asking how they felt about the problem	

solve, unwanted escape, and dismissive behaviors (see Table 5.2 for examples of helpful and unhelpful behaviors). Barbee et al. (1998) found that there were differences in who was likely to enact helpful and unhelpful support (see Table 5.3). Friends and health professionals were predominantly viewed as providing helpful social support; however, family members were seen as providing mostly unhelpful social support. Lovers or partners were reported to provide roughly equal helpful and unhelpful support.

In another study using SIST, Derlega et al. (in press) compared how people with HIV seek and receive social support from peers, parents, and partners. This study used a sample of 125 men and women with HIV who filled out questionnaires about social support by various people. Participants reported using more

TABLE 5.3

Who Enacts Helpful and Unhelpful Social Support (Source: Barbee et al., 1998)

Person	Helpful Forms (%)	Unhelpful Forms (%)
Friends	62	38
Health professionals	67	33
Lovers or partners	50	50
Family	38	62

"ask" behaviors with friends and partners than with parents. For receiving support, participants reported receiving more "approach" behaviors (solve and solace) from friends and partners compared with parents, and they received fewer avoidance behaviors from friends than parents. Additionally, Derlega et al. reported that avoidance strategies were positively correlated with depression.

These studies indicate that not all support is helpful for those with HIV. Support providers often experience anxiety and turmoil when they have ongoing interactions with someone who is under stress, chronically ill, or bereaved (Barbee & Cunningham, 1995; Lehman, Ellard, & Wortman, 1986). Family members' use of unwanted dismiss and escape behaviors in interactions with a relative with HIV (Barbee et al., 1998; Derlega et al., in press) may reflect fear of losing a loved one, an inability to cope with their own negative emotions, or conflicting attitudes about HIV disease. As one sister of a man with HIV indicated, "I've not been there for him. I couldn't handle knowing my baby brother was dying, so I just checked out." In this case, the man felt abandoned by the sister's coping behaviors. Thus, it is important to explore helpful social support. Providers may also feel uneasy because they are being asked to accept the burden of the information about someone's HIV status, thereby forcing them to accept a certain level of responsibility. They may not be able or willing to share the information because it means that they have to not only cope with knowing but may also have to manage third-party disclosure to others. Sometimes it is necessary for a confidant to relieve the burden of knowing by telling someone else.

What are the relations among social support, coping, and disease progression? Leserman et al. (2000) reported faster progression to AIDS with increased denial coping, decreased satisfaction with social support, and increased stressful life events. Pakenham, Dadds, and Terry (1994) reported adjustment was related to social support and coping, but there was no difference in adjustment and coping by disease stage. In this study (Pakenham et al., 1994), social support was related to health; specifically, lower number of physical symptoms and CD4 cell count (one estimate of an AIDS diagnosis, if less than 200) were associated with more social support. Coping was associated with psychosocial adjustment, but social support was more strongly associated with health-related variables. Fleishman and Fogel (1994) studied three coping behaviors: positive coping, seeking social support, and avoidant coping. Positive coping was related to decreased symptoms longitudinally, whereas avoidant coping was related to increased symptoms longitudinally.

There may be different types of coping with varied outcomes. Siegel et al. (1998), using a sample of 139 MSM, explored how individuals with HIV cope with stigma by disclosing selectively. Siegel et al. (1998) described proactive and reactive coping strategies based on how actively people with HIV challenge social norms and values. Reactive strategies include hiding status, presenting the illness as a less stigmatizing one (deception), and distancing self by changing attributions. Proactive strategies encompass public education and social activism. Leslie, Stein, and Rotheram-Borus (2002) studied 295 parents with HIV (mostly mothers) and examined social support, conflict with adolescent children, and emotional distress, and their effects on illness distress, health care satisfaction, and substance abuse. They found social support is associated with active coping and conflict with kids is associated with passive coping. Song and Ingram (2002) argued that satisfaction with social support is associated with decreased mood disturbance, and unsupportive social support is related to use of denial and disengagement strategies. Lutgendorf, Antoni, Schneiderman, and Fletcher (1994) reported active coping and less avoidant coping are better for both emotional and physical health.

If satisfaction is important in health, how satisfied are individuals with HIV about the support they receive? Pequegnat and Szapocznik (2000) argued that family members are significant in coping and social support, yet they may also be a source of friction. Lester et al. (1995) reported that most women with HIV were satisfied with social support from friends and family. Serovich et al. (2000) found similarities in perceptions of social support provided by family and friends. Thus, many people with HIV are satisfied with their social support.

Social Support and Coping. Although the level of social support someone is able to give depends on his or her ability to deal with the information, social support certainly helps individuals with the HIV infection cope with the disease. There is evidence that the type of social support received following HIV disclosure is associated with psychological coping for individuals living with HIV. Hays et al. (1992) asked MSM who also had HIV about their depression and satisfaction with three types of social support they received from others. The three types of social support measured were emotional (receiving emotional comfort), informational (receiving advice and information), and practical (being able to count on others for help, as in asking for money or assistance in an emergency). In addition, participants provided information indicating if, in the last 6 months, they had experienced certain physical symptoms associated with HIV disease for at least 2 weeks (e.g., night sweats, fever, unusual weight loss, enlarged glands or lymph nodes). Higher scores on satisfaction with emotional, informational, and practical support were correlated with lower scores on current depression (Time 1) and depression measured 1 year later (Time 2).

There was evidence in Hays et al.'s (1992) study that depression was higher among the men who had more physical symptoms of HIV disease. The development of HIV symptoms may have increased distress and concerns about loss of control for individuals who had been in good health for many years. What is most interesting in Hays et al.'s (1992) study is that the beneficial effects of social support were greatest among those reporting more HIV-related physical symptoms. Although greater satisfaction with emotional, informational, and practical support were each associated with lower depression, only informational social support was a buffer against the effects of HIV symptoms on depression. As the number of HIV symptoms increased, those with higher informational support were less depressed than the men with the lower informational support.

Hays et al. (1992) speculated that the onset of HIV symptoms creates a number of concerns, including the need for health services and treatment, job issues, and dealing with personal relationships. If persons with symptoms can disclose and talk with someone who knows about the HIV diagnosis and who has useful advice and information, they might be able to cope more successfully with the disease. In Hays et al.'s (1992) study, the researchers did not break down the impact of satisfaction with informational support for different providers such as family members, friends, lovers, health professionals, or others living with HIV. However, satisfaction with informational support may be more strongly related to lower depression when individuals are considering the benefits of HIV disclosure to health professionals, other persons who have similar symptoms, or anyone who keeps up with the rapidly changing knowledge base about HIV (Hays et al., 1992).

The study by Hays et al. (1992) suggests that satisfaction with support received from those who know about the HIV diagnosis affects coping. However, satisfaction with social support may not by itself indicate how helpful others were in assisting the person with HIV in coping with the disease. People who perceive high support may have a more favorable view of themselves and other people, which might account for the positive relation between perceived social support and coping with HIV in the research by Leserman et al. (2000) and Hays et al. (1992).

A study by Ingram, Jones, Fass, Neidig, and Song (1999) tested the notion that among individuals living with HIV, being the recipient of unhelpful responses influences depression beyond the impact of satisfaction or dissatisfaction with social support. The participants in Ingram et al.'s (1999) study were men and women with HIV. They completed a questionnaire to assess how much they received unsupportive or upsetting responses from others who knew about their HIV diagnosis. The unsupportive social interactions questionnaire tapped four factors: insensitivity, disconnecting, forced optimism, and blaming (items from their questionnaire are presented in Table A.12; see Appendix). Participants in Ingram et al.'s study also completed measures of satisfaction with available social support and depression. As previously discussed, higher satisfaction with social support was correlated with lower depression. More interesting, however, is that higher scores on three unsupportive social interaction measures (insensitivity, disconnecting, and blaming) were all associated with higher depression. The more unsupportive social interaction received, the more depressed the person with HIV. Only the measure of forced optimism—which Ingram et al. suggested may not have clearly described unsupportive behavior—was uncorrelated with depression.

A question may be asked though: Does the perception of social support depend on actually disclosing to someone about the HIV diagnosis? Perhaps people are satisfied with social support received regardless of disclosing or not disclosing to others about the HIV diagnosis. Data from a study by Serovich et al. (2000) addressed this question. One hundred thirty-four men with HIV completed questionnaires tapping perceived social support provided by family and friends, respectively. Participants also completed measures of the percentage of family and friends, respectively, who were personally told (note this is not the same as who knew the diagnosis, as the measure does not assess indirect disclosure) about the HIV diagnosis. Perceived social support from family and friends was positively correlated with the percentage of family and friends to whom the individuals with HIV had disclosed the diagnosis. These results suggest that the more family members and friends someone tells about the diagnosis, the more people who are potentially available to provide social support. However, as we have noted, there is also a downside to disclosure: The wider the network of people who know about someone having HIV disease, the greater the possibility of rejection and social support problems (e.g., Cline & McKenzie, 2000; Derlega & Chaikin, 1977; Derlega et al., 2000; Greene & Faulkner, 2002; Greene & Serovich, 1996). Consequently, a key in being able to tell someone about HIV and guarding against the potential danger of too many others knowing is negotiating rules to manage privacy boundaries around the information. Because someone becomes a co-owner of the information once a person has revealed, the person with HIV may work to set the parameters with the confidants so that third-party disclosure is limited by agreement to adhere to boundary rules. In addition, as CPM argues, when the expected rules regulating the privacy boundaries are violated the person with HIV may deny further disclosures or withdraw (Petronio, 2002). The best scenario is when both discloser and confidant coordinate the boundary around the diagnosis to the benefit of both parties.

Social Support and Activism Groups.   In trying to cope, how do people seek assistance? Peterson et al. (1995) found MSM in San Francisco reported seeking help about concerns regarding AIDS high-risk behavior. Most of the men sought assistance from peers and professionals and saw both as most helpful. Hays, Catania, McKusick, and Coates (1990) examined help-seeking behaviors among gay men in San Francisco, and men with AIDS sought more social support than men with HIV. For men with HIV and AIDS, peers were seen as most helpful, and family were least sought after and helpful.

The popularity of support group attendance may be related to stigma associated with a particular illness, with support seeking highest for diseases such as HIV and alcoholism that are seen as stigmatizing (Davison, Pennebaker, & Dickerson, 2000). Development of alcoholism groups (Alcoholics Anonymous) has been the most extensive in the United States; however, support groups have expanded dramatically to include issues such as eating disorders, rape, HIV, and so forth. HIV support groups and organizations are widely available currently, especially in larger cities. Forms of self-help groups are emerging online as well as in person (Davison et al., 2000). These social support groups are crucial in coping with the HIV epidemic, especially for minorities (Yep et al., 2003). For example, support groups allow people to practice telling others in a safe environment (Limandri, 1989) and provide an outlet, often when people have not told others.

These groups may be important information sources and assist with adjustment. Vázquez-Pacheco (2000) described, however, how some men with HIV attend support groups initially for a brief time to deal with changing life issues but then do not attend groups. Thus, it would be helpful to see further research on length of group membership (and disease stage) and how individuals with HIV (and their families and partners) use these groups.

Individuals with HIV must manage high levels of uncertainty and some do so by seeking information (Brashers, Neidig, et al., 2000). The nature of uncertainty changes with the course of HIV illness as people with HIV must meet ever-changing challenges (Brashers, Haas, Klingle, & Neidig, 2000; Brashers, Neidig, Reynolds, & Haas, 1998). Related research explores the role of self-advocacy of individuals with HIV and AIDS activism (e.g., AIDS Coalition to Unleash Power [ACT UP]; see Brashers, Neidig, et al., 2000). Individuals high in self-advocacy are more knowledgeable and aggressive in interactions with physicians (and perhaps choose not to adhere to all medical recommendations). If activism and self-advocacy are related, then perhaps those who are more active are more likely to disclose.

The Internet offers one option for seeking information and coping with a disease such as HIV, but there has been little evaluation of its use (some with support groups). In the case of the Internet and HIV, one issue is the range—both in quality and quantity—of health information available with relative ease. Although Internet access is now widely available, in-home access is available only to a relatively small portion of the world population (see Rice & Katz, 2001). Reeves (2000) studied the impact of the Internet on the coping ability of 10 persons with HIV. Reeves found the Internet provided a sense of empowerment and control, augmented social support (for some it functioned as primary support in the form of chat rooms etc., for others as secondary or supplemental support), and facilitated helping others (similar to our previous discussions of the roles of people with HIV as volunteers or public speakers in chap. 3). In particular, Reeves' participants utilized the Internet to find out about medications, side effects, and disease progression, things they could do without disclosing directly and risking negative consequences. One widely studied Internet HIV application has been CHESS (Comprehensive Health Enhancement Support System), a computer-based health system that focuses on interactive computer use (see Boberg et al., 1995; Pingree et al., 1996). Analyses of the CHESS system for people with HIV indicates that people tailor computer use to suit their needs (see Smaglik et al., 1998). Specifically, Smaglik et al. reported that the nature, not the amount, of the Internet information use was related to increased quality of life for people with HIV. In Smaglik et al.'s study, involvement with information tools and not the amount of discussion group use or total Internet use was related to quality of life. Clearly, Internet support is an important area for further research.

Counseling sessions and groups for individuals with HIV are also critical means of support. Counseling goals in such groups change by stage as social support and stigma affect identity (Lutgendorf et al., 1994). People may discuss specific disclosure decisions and issues in these sessions, and this could be a way to show people that they have the skills to disclose. This may be a first experience for some with any kind of counseling or support group, and they may find the experience especially troubling. One character in the Broadway show *Rent* (Larson, 1996, Act I, Scene 13) attends an HIV support group. He interrupts the group affirmation, expressing discomfort with the process: "I find some of what you teach suspect, because I'm used to relying on intellect. But I try to open up to what I don't know, because reason says I should have died three years ago." The support provided by this kind of group is significant but may be difficult to accept, as this character struggles to comprehend. Mattson (2000) argued we should reframe HIV counseling such that it becomes more empowering, focusing on self-efficacy, perhaps efficacy about disclosing skills.

Many people volunteer to help with HIV-related groups and organizations (Lindhorst & Mancoske, 1993; Omoto, Gunn, & Crain, 1998), and many are satisfied with the volunteer experience (e.g., Metts & Manns, 1996; Omoto, Snyder, & Berghuis, 1993). Snyder, Omoto, and Crain (1999) reported AIDS volunteers were more stigmatized than other volunteers, and this can prevent volunteering. In this research, stigma predicted burnout, emphasizing the social costs of volunteering in which people are "punished for good deeds" (see Snyder et al., 1999, p. 1175). Thus, volunteers seeking to support individuals with HIV encounter added difficulties. These volunteers may also disclose their volunteer work to others, perhaps contributing to decreased stigma. In this case, a positive outcome, decreased stigma, is balanced with negative outcomes of volunteering, specifically burnout and courtesy stigma.

The HIV epidemic has also resulted in the expansion of institutions and networks to provide social support for individuals with HIV. Service organizations, support groups, and educational awareness groups all become resources that can provide social support for individuals with HIV. The grassroots community organizations with HIV created a structure to fill gaps in support services. Frey and colleagues (e.g., Adelman & Frey, 1997; Frey, Query, Flint, & Adelman, 1998) have studied one such organization, an AIDS residence (Bonaventure House in Chicago, IL). This research documents how the residence serves as a mediating structure, providing social support for residents.

Individuals with HIV also volunteer or become activists, or both. Activism related to AIDS has been extensive, ranging from aggressive civil disobedience to wearing red ribbons for awareness. One important activist outcome of the AIDS epidemic has been to streamline FDA procedures for approving experimental treatments. Social activism can be considered a proactive coping strategy for people with HIV (Siegel et al., 1998). Becoming active may be a means of regaining control with the disease. Brashers, Haas, Neidig, and Rintamaki (2002) studied how activist organizations serve to educate and motivate people with HIV. In the Brashers, Haas, et al. (2002) study, activists with HIV use more problem-focused coping and less emotion-focused coping than activists without HIV. Activists also have more knowledge of treatment information sources and increased HIV social networks. We do not know at present if activists disclose more, but that would seem likely. We would expect someone who was a part of an organization would perhaps be more easily identified and disclose more. Thus, there is evidence that individuals with HIV who are activists may function better with their disease, perhaps through social support access.

Summary of Social Support.   We have discussed in this section how HIV disclosure leads to different types of social support and how the nature of the social support received is associated with coping with HIV. Satisfaction with social support is positively related to coping physically and psychologically with HIV, and unhelpful responses from others are negatively related to psychological coping. We also explored the role of support and activism.

When someone is linked into a privacy boundary because he or she is offering support, to be of some help to the person with HIV the support needs to be perceived as satisfying, that is, the kind of support the person is looking for. It is likely that the person with HIV views the support given with certain expectations that may revolve around how the information about his or her status is treated. When the person with HIV and the support provider coordinate the needs effectively, the outcome is positive for the discloser. When there is a lack of coordination, disruption occurs.

HIV Diagnosis, Psychological Health, and Identity—Implications for HIV Disclosure

What is the link between an HIV diagnosis and psychological health? People diagnosed with HIV eventually confront quality of life issues, or "living with dying," especially early and again in the later stages of AIDS (Stevens & Tighe Doerr, 1977; Wilson, Hutchinson, & Holzemer, 1997). As a result, "The number of HIV infected seeking mental health services will likely increase sharply in the future" (Kalichman, Rompa, & Cage, 2000, p. 662). Many people with HIV (especially children) have difficulty separating their illness from identity (see Wiener, Heilman, et al., 1998). Davies (1997) described the existential problems of living with HIV, including disrupted time orientation with "provisional existence"; having access to helpful social support through disclosure may be significant to help with this. The ambiguity of the disease requires individuals with HIV to adjust and reconceptualize their lives, goals, and relationships. To adapt, they focus on empowerment through identity construction, self versus other emphasis, and a moral dimension to health (Crossley, 1997). People also cope with the threat of AIDS by adopting a fighting spirit, reframing stress, planning, and seeking social support (Leserman, Perkins, & Evans, 1992). This coping and adjustment is crucial for health. For example, AIDS long-term survivors (diagnosed with AIDS more than 3 years) reconstruct their lives in the context of AIDS by focusing on normalizing, living, self-care, and relationships

(Barroso, 1997). In all of these readjustments to the diagnosis, disclosure has the potential to provide access to social support.

The question remains: Do individuals with HIV report decreased psychological health? Ciesla and Roberts (2001) meta-analyzed 10 studies of HIV and depression and concluded that individuals with HIV were at greater risk for depression. Specifically, people with HIV reported more frequent depressive but not dysthmic disorder, and this was not related to sexual orientation or disease stage. For example, Hoff, Coates, Barrett, Collette, and Ekstrand (1996) reported men with HIV were more depressed, similar to the increased anxiety and depression reported among women with HIV (Lester et al., 1995). Chuang, Devins, Hunsley, and Gill (1989) reported high psychosocial distress both early and late in disease progression. This contradicts findings by Markowitz, Rabkin, and Perry (1994) in which the majority of men with HIV were not clinically depressed, thus leading to the conclusion that individuals with HIV are not necessarily depressed. De Vroome et al. (1998) also argued that depression increased among HIV positive gay men compared with a general control population but not compared with gay men who were HIV negative controls. Kalichman et al. (2000) additionally cautioned that depression inventories may inadvertently also measure the presence of HIV somatic symptoms, which can erroneously inflate scores of persons with advanced HIV disease (29% of people with HIV were misidentified as depressed due to measure overlap). Thus, more study is needed to examine psychological health of individuals with HIV and the possibility that disclosure can decrease depression (or it may increase stress if there are interpersonal problems caused by the HIV disclosure).

HIV Progression, Self-Disclosure, and Psychological Health. Some evidence indicates individuals with HIV may be more prone to depression, but this is unclear, as more studies are needed with matched control groups. But if lower mental health is related to disease progression, might this association be reduced or reversed by HIV disclosure? Perhaps HIV disclosure assists individuals in coming to terms with advanced illness, both the physical features and end of life issues. HIV disclosure might also provide access to support at a time when declining health makes it more difficult to take care of oneself. We would expect increased disclosure to be related to increased psychological health, but more study would be useful to examine this issue.

One theme apparent in research related to mental health is the choice to end life, and this could easily be linked to disclosure at the terminal stage. If suicidal behavior is a way of coping with AIDS, the euthanasia or suicide option may be a means of exercising control (Metts & Manns, 1996; Starace & Sherr, 1998). *It's My Party* (Kleiser, 1996) is a movie in which the main character with AIDS develops brain lesions (indicating advanced disease progression), decides he is going to commit suicide, and has one last party. At the party all his friends and family come to celebrate with him (and say good-bye). The movie revolves around this one night. In this case, there was extended social support for this choice to die (and much disclosure). Further research in mental health, including end of life issues, for people with HIV would be useful.

HIV Disclosure and Stigma

In chapter 3 we explored how stigma can influence people's decisions to disclose their HIV infection. In this section of this chapter, we focus on the stigma-related consequences to disclosing. Because the potential for stigmatizing is very real, the anticipated reactions that lead to a person being stigmatized makes people with HIV cautious in choices about whom to link into their privacy boundary around the information about the disease. Individuals with HIV are very concerned about stigma, for example, 1 year after diagnosis 61% of a sample of 93 predominantly MSM in San Francisco reported concern about stigma (Stempel et al., 1995). If others find out about the HIV diagnosis then individuals with HIV may be stigmatized or discredited, encouraging the use of a variety of strategies to cope with stigma (Siegel et al., 1998). People who are known to have HIV may be marked as outsiders, which can lead to social rejection, isolation, loss of work, and internalized shame (e.g., Alonzo & Reynolds, 1995; Crawford, 1996; Goffman, 1963; Jones et al., 1984). Many diseases such as cancer, leprosy, and mental illness are stigmatizing because they may be life threatening, disfiguring, and unpredictable. However, stigma poses a somewhat more serious problem for persons with HIV because AIDS is associated with behaviors that some consider immoral or deviant (e.g., being gay men and injection drug use; Devine et al., 1999), and many people fear that HIV is contagious through casual contact (see, e.g., Crandall & Coleman, 1992; Herek, 1999a; Leary & Schreindorfer, 1998; Peters et al., 1994). For instance, individuals with HIV compared to cancer are more likely to feel socially rejected, financially threatened, ashamed, and socially isolated (Fife & Wright, 2000). We consider the consequences related to stigma of disclosing versus not disclosing the HIV diagnosis by examining consequences of stigma based on misinformation, then group bias, and finally courtesy stigma.

Stigma and Misinformation.   Many individuals with HIV can recall instances in which they felt rejected or discriminated against by someone who knew about their diagnosis. These instances often are based on others' fears about how casual contact may lead to contracting the disease (see Greene & Faulkner, 2002). Consequently, possible misunderstandings about the disease may lead to negative consequences and accentuate the caution in linking anyone else into the boundary around a person's HIV status. One woman gave the following account of how she was badly treated by her sisters when they found out about her HIV diagnosis:

> [They] didn't want me to eat out of their plates or to play with my nieces. They were just really scared. They just didn't know. Then we had a family discussion and we

talked with a doctor. The doctor taught the family about how they can be infected. After that my sisters seemed to calm down a lot ... when they got some information about the disease.

In this instance, the difficulties caused by the reaction were reduced by having the physician, a third party with credible information about the disease, address the misinformation and allow the family to restore their ability to provide support.

Another woman told her mother about the HIV diagnosis. Her mother made her keep the information about the HIV diagnosis a secret from the rest of the family, thereby limiting the possible linkages with others. Although this helped the mother cope with the information, it restrained the daughter's options to seek support from others. Nevertheless, the mother's response appeared to be produced by her fear that the daughter would infect the family:

When I got out of a drug rehabilitation program I went to visit my family. Everybody was hugging me. And my mother was just standing back and watching me. She told me, "You shouldn't kiss them kids. You shouldn't let them drink out of your cup. You sit over there [pointing away from the others]."

These fears of infection are seen repeatedly in descriptions of stigmatized reactions to HIV disclosure. This woman also described an episode when she was in the drug rehabilitation program and one of the counselors called her into his office:

I had gone to the bathroom. When I came out, I passed one counselor's office and he called me in. I asked him what did he want. He said, "What you should do is go and get some bleach and clean the toilet seat. You should clean up behind yourself. It's bad enough that you are here, but you are going to infect everybody else." That hurt my feelings.

Even those professionally in contact with individuals with HIV can be misinformed and insensitive (e.g., Crawford et al., 1991; Gerbert et al., 1991; Kelly et al., 1987a, 1987b; Pleck, O'Donnell, O'Donnell, & Snarey, 1988; Wallack, 1989). In fact, some health care workers report anxiety and fear when providing care for AIDS patients (All, 1989). Although we might assume that increased information and education about health would reduce this type of stigma, clearly this is not the case.

Besides medical personnel, close family or friends can also respond based on misinformation. A man with an AIDS diagnosis described how his grandmother would not eat anything he cooked:

My grandmother used to eat my cooking. She doesn't eat my cooking anymore. I always try to explain to her that she can't get anything from me. But I have an aunt who has brainwashed my grandmother against me because I have AIDS. I think my aunt has poisoned her mind. It's hard to deal with because I love my grandmother so much but she makes it hard for me mentally, emotionally. She makes it very hard.

This man's relationship with his grandmother changed dramatically based on her misperceptions and fears, augmented by another family member.

Finally, a woman described that although she has many friends, some of them are afraid of contracting HIV disease from her:

> I have a friend who was very close to me. She would do anything for me. But she will come to my house, and she will always bring a paper cup. She will very rarely eat something that I cook. We'll have a conversation, and we will go out doing things together. But she will say, "Yeah, but they still don't know if you can get it [HIV] from saliva." So she's not really sure about me or comfortable about me completely. I would say that 80% of my relationship with her is okay, but the other 20% she is skeptical. We do things together. We go places together. I can go to her house. I can sleep in her bed. I can use her toilet. But when she comes to my house, it's kind of reverse. She'll only use the toilet downstairs. She won't use the bathroom I have off my bedroom. So I detect all these little things.

For this woman, although the little things her friend did were based on misplaced fear of contracting the disease, the way that the friend behaved was perceived by the woman as indicators of rejection and reinforced her feelings of being stigmatized. This reaction is similar to stigmatizing responses reported by Greene and Faulkner (2002) in which adolescents reported that they were often "treated differently" after disclosing their HIV diagnosis.

These negative reactions to someone with HIV may decrease over time as family, friends, and others in the social network learn that HIV cannot be transmitted by casual contact. Persons with HIV may share educational information with family and friends about HIV and how it is contracted to combat the stigma and misinformation about the disease. Also, if others see someone coping with HIV as a medical condition (e.g., taking medications, dealing with the physical symptoms, etc.), stigmatizing attitudes toward HIV may decrease (Alonzo & Reynolds, 1995).

Stigma and Group Bias. Negative reactions to someone who discloses their HIV status are not only influenced by others' fears of contracting the disease, but reactions to HIV and AIDS may be influenced by negative attitudes about particular groups such as MSM and drug users (Capitanio & Herek, 1999; Devine et al., 1999; Herek & Capitanio, 1999; St. Lawrence et al., 1990). If people reveal that they became infected with HIV from behaviors associated with being gay men or drug use, then negative attitudes toward these behaviors may be the reason for social rejection by the recipient. A laboratory study conducted by Derlega, Sherburne, et al. (1998) demonstrated that behavioral reactions to someone who discloses having HIV are influenced by perceptions of the infected person's sexual orientation (also see St. Lawrence et al., 1990). In the Derlega, Sherburne, et al. (1998) study, college students signed up for a study on impression formation. Research participants were supposedly paired randomly with another person so that they would have a better opportunity to get to know one another. As part of the experimental procedure, the "other person" revealed to his coparticipant that he had recently found out that he was HIV positive. He wrote in a handwritten message, "I can't believe I'm telling you this. I mean, I don't know you or anything. I just found out I'm HIV positive. I still can't believe it" (Derlega, Sherburne, et al., 1998, p. 343). He also revealed that he was either homosexual or heterosexual. Participants interacted less intimately (focusing on low-intimacy facts and feelings about themselves) with the person with HIV who identified himself as homosexual than if he identified himself as heterosexual. Thus, disclosing how one was infected with HIV can influence others' reactions.

Courtesy Stigma.   This type of stigma concerns rejection and stigmatization that may extend to family and friends who fear that they will also be stigmatized by their association with the person with HIV. This phenomenon is termed *courtesy stigma* (Goffman, 1963; also see Leary & Schreindorfer, 1998), similar to the idea of "contagion." Family members, for instance, might ask the person with HIV to not disclose about the HIV diagnosis to others to protect the family's reputation. Opening boundaries may cause problems more far reaching than just for the individual. One woman with HIV mentioned how she was asked by her father not to talk to his family about her HIV. She said, "His main concern to me was if people out there found out what I had, what would they think of me? What would they think of him? I'm his daughter and I've got HIV." On the other hand, she can talk to her mother's family about the HIV diagnosis:

> My mom's family is very open-minded. You can talk to them about anything. It's always been that way. They have illnesses because they are getting up there in age. And they don't treat me any different. I'm welcomed in their house. They're not afraid to be around me, which I thought they might be. I was not the one to tell my grandmother, my mother was. And my aunt knows on my mother's side of the family, even my cousins.

For this woman's family, there was much more open access to the information. Some families have particular orientations to private information (Morr, 2002; Petronio, 2002). Consequently, in the preceding case, the family (at least on the mother's side) exercised a highly permeable family privacy boundary that allowed the members to feel comfortable disclosing even the most risky information.

Summary of Stigma.   We have discussed examples of how stigma can function to inhibit disclosure; however, stigma may also work in the opposite way to increase disclosure. Awareness of HIV stigma may embolden some individuals with HIV to "come out" in their community as persons with HIV. They may give talks to school, religious, and community groups, be active in HIV service organizations, or join social advocacy groups such as ACT UP (AIDS Coalition to Unleash Power) on behalf of social and health issues affecting people with HIV. ACT UP's New York chapter has the following statement on its home page on the World Wide Web: "ACT UP is a diverse, nonpartisan group of individuals united in anger and committed to direct action to end the AIDS crisis. We advise and inform. We demonstrate. We are not silent" (http://www.actupny.org).

Many people with HIV also disclose to correct misperceptions. One person described how his cousin was "talking trash" about people with HIV they both knew. "Because he was putting down people that I know who had AIDS. I just told him to get him straight. You know, get off these people's backs about the disease they got because your own cousin's got it, too." For this man, stigmatizing comments encouraged his disclosure rather than inhibited it, a caution not to assume that stigma functions only in one direction. Thus, stigma can have many types of influences, although the negative consequences have received more attention.

HIV Disclosure and Close Relationships

We now turn to effects of HIV disclosure on relationships. We consider how HIV disclosure affects relationship closeness, significant others as caregivers, relationships with children, and reducing risk behaviors in intimate relations. We begin by examining the effects of disclosure on relationship closeness.

Relationship Closeness

Family members or intimate partners who learn about a relative or partner with HIV may react initially with shock, disbelief, and distress about the diagnosis. The news may bring individuals closer together, it may worsen relationships, or it may have no apparent effect on current relationships (Greene & Faulkner, 2002). The impact of HIV disclosure on strengthening or weakening relationships is likely to depend on the quality of preexisting family or couple relationships as described in chapter 3 (also see Armistead et al., 1997; Kotchick et al., 1997). Indeed, Greene (2001) reported relational quality was the best predictor of willingness to disclose HIV infection to mother, father, partner, friends, and siblings (see also Greene & Serovich, 1995). In the following account, a man diagnosed with AIDS in the early 1990s believed that he was facing imminent death. He described how disclosing to his sister, with whom he felt very close, strengthened their relationship. She was the first person he called after finding out about the diagnosis:

> We have always had a good relationship. But it seems like it is improving more. For her, nothing has changed, and I am the same person that I was before. It seems like she is going out of her way for us to have a good time in the time that is left. It seems

like we are trying to do things that we have missed out on because we both had lived in different cities. We would do little things like watching movies together or playing cards or going to the store. It makes me feel good because I feel like I am still a part of everything and that I am not being shunned.

In this case, there were positive outcomes of disclosure for the relationship, and the man felt affirmed by the consistency of the relationship. As this example illustrates, when coordination of private information runs smoothly and people are able to match their efforts to manage the disclosed information, they are able to benefit from the situation as we see in the next case.

Another person described how his perceptions of a friend as being "loving and supportive and caring" led to his disclosing about the diagnosis to him:

Before I really knew, I felt perhaps I could be HIV infected because of the little sickness that came. I had this person sit down. He just happened to be visiting and I was sharing with him. [I said] "Will you be here for me?" The person was overwhelmed with me sharing that with him. He comes around. We went out to dinner last week and to a movie. Because this person was compassionate [I told him]. In this instance, you look for people with compassion.

This man also had a positive outcome for relationship closeness after disclosing, including increased contact, caring, and social support. The ability of the confidant to provide support is often predicated by his or her willingness to accept a certain level of responsibility for managing the disclosure about HIV status in a way that illustrates supportiveness. However, not everyone is able to succeed in responding in a positive way. When confidants are unable to accept this responsibility, boundary turbulence often erupts and can negatively affect the relationship (Petronio, 2002).

As suggested, disclosure to family members may, however, worsen family relations, especially if there is a prior history of family conflict. There may be overt conflict, tension, or family arguments about a wide range of issues including who should know about the diagnosis, should the person with HIV be allowed near children in the family, should he or she speak in public about the HIV diagnosis, and is HIV a punishment for one's sexual behavior or drug use (e.g., Crawford, 1996; Greene & Faulkner, 2002; Semple et al., 1997). We discussed many of these issues in the section on stigma. The following account is from a man who had numerous health problems associated with AIDS. He died several years following this interview. His parents were divorced, and his father had not been involved in his life for many years. He described how his father intervened in a heavy-handed manner to help him after he had gotten out of a hospital. He felt that his father manipulated him while he was having health problems, perhaps to be seen by the family "as some kind of hero for stepping in and taking care of me." The father's help seemed to be more like "taking over:"

My father was living with his girlfriend. They offered to take me in until I got well again. They said it would be great. I could have a whole wing of the house and come and go as I pleased. So I thought that was fine. I thought that was how they were going to help me until I was ready to take care of myself. They were going to take care of everything for me. Well, I got over there and what they really did was to completely try to take over. I wasn't allowed to make any kind of decisions. There was a big concentration on all the negative aspects of HIV and AIDS. [They said], "We are preparing for you to die very soon." They would come right out and say this and try to cut off any other ties I might have with the rest of the family. They were taking away any rights I felt I had at that point. I couldn't come and go as I please, as they said I could. They were watching over me like I was a 5-year-old. That just didn't work at all. They were after me to sign over all my power of attorney to them so they could completely run my life. In the end it just ended up completely alienating me from them.

This man had a very difficult experience with his father after disclosing, and this was complicated by the change in living situation when the father offered support (recall the previous discussion of unhelpful social support). This case illustrates a pattern seen in coordination of private information. As CPM argues (Petronio, 2002), sometimes when people are in need of support one person gives over more of his or her private information than the other person and this can lead to a power imbalance between the discloser and confidant, as we see in the case just described. The father exercises power to control the son because the son is in need of assistance. This situation is exacerbated by the fact that the father appears to want to limit boundary permeability about the private information, thereby controlling and restricting the son's contacts with other family members. The father may have been enacting these behaviors to gain control over who else was privy to the information about his son's HIV diagnosis. In the end, the father's behavior alienated the son and interfered with any functional support system for the son.

Persons with HIV and their loved ones—if they have a good relationship to begin with—may be brought closer after HIV disclosure because they are coping with a major health problem. Specifically, some couples may feel closer (despite the loss of support from others) because they form an alliance to keep the information secret (Vangelisti & Caughlin, 1997; Wegner, 1989; Wegner, Lane, & Dimitri, 1994). When people aim for tightening their privacy boundaries and restricting access, they reduce the possibility of seeking additional support from outside the relationship. However, this action may work to strengthen their relationship as the couple bonds together. A woman described how she learned from her husband in the 1980s that he had HIV. He had been sick several times with pneumonia. When he was in the hospital he called her to say, "Well ... I got the big one." She replied, "Oh, my God, you got cancer!" He said, "No, I have AIDS." She in turn tested HIV positive. This is how they coped with keeping the information about their HIV diagnoses secret until the husband became critically ill:

> He and I decided not to tell anybody, not even anyone in the family. We decided not to tell anybody because I thought my daughter-in law's not going to let my grandkids visit me, and his kids were not going to be able to visit him. We had a good marital relationship, and I really loved him very much. I stuck by him. So we just decided to keep it quiet. And we did that for 2 and a half, almost 3 years. We were dependent on each other for the privacy. ... It was a private thing between us, and both of us felt good that we kept it that way. I would always rub his head, something I never did before. I felt the need to be a little closer to him, to give him a little more, because I didn't get sick. He did.

This couple actively worked to develop privacy rules around the disclosed information and regulated the privacy boundary in a coordinated pattern (Petronio, 2002). Thus, they set the parameters for restricting any additional linkages into the boundaries. The act of co-owning the information and managing their privacy about the diagnosis functioned to bring them closer together. Similarly, gay male couples with HIV report external strains on the relationship from "heterosexism," and they focus on interpersonal commitment in the relationship to cope (see Haas, 2002; Powell-Cope, 1998). Thus, couples may draw closer to fight the disease together.

There is some research available to speculate on relationship disruption among couples in which one or both partners are diagnosed with HIV. Winstead et al.'s (2002) study reported extensive detail about relationships of 20 heterosexual women with HIV. In Winstead et al.'s study, only 4 of 20 relationships were intact at the time of the interview. There is a complex relation between HIV status and the couple's relationship success. One big question might be whether one contracted the disease while in the relationship or before the relationship started. If the HIV infection was acquired during the relationship, there may be questions about how the infection was contracted. If the infection was acquired before the relationship, then partners can weigh the relative importance or even put into perspective what happened prior to the relationship.

We can also use some literature on disabilities generally to project what might apply to couples with HIV (Braithwaite & Thompson, 2000), although there may also be dissimilarities (e.g., a partner might or might not share HIV infection; with HIV there is concern about possible transmission). It is difficult to estimate the rate of divorce for people with HIV (and not all people with HIV are married or have access to a legal marital relationship, thus relationship *disruption* is a term that can apply to many couples). Goffman (1963) noted that people with disabilities in general possess limited choices in the formation of personal relationships as a result of an "aesthetic-sexual aversion to disability that permeates society"

(p. 44). Similarly, the question can be asked if there are any gender differences in ending relationships for persons with HIV. Women with disabilities have a higher divorce rate and find it harder to establish intimate relationships than do men (one of the explanations is that nondisabled women are more willing to enter into relationships with persons with disabilities due to socializing as caretakers); this might be an analogous experience for persons with HIV (see Asch & Fine, 1988). There is a need for additional research on the impact of HIV status on couples' relationships, particularly about disruption.

There are pluses and minuses for couples (or families) who conceal information about the HIV diagnosis from everyone. Keeping a secret about the HIV diagnosis may bring couples closer if they already have a good relationship. These couples may also become isolated from others (family, friends, support groups, or community organizations) who might be able to provide social support (discussed previously in this chapter). Keeping HIV a secret from everyone may also foster feelings of guilt, shame, and stigma: The couple may feel ashamed about their partner's HIV status because they are keeping this information hidden (Bem, 1972; Fishbein & Laird, 1979; Kalichman, 2000).

Couples in committed relationships may see their relationships break apart or be severely tested if, as a consequence of HIV disclosure, a partner feels betrayed by the other (e.g., Couch, Jones, & Moore, 1999; Cranson & Caron, 1998). Some people might not have known about their partner's previous or current sexual history, drug use, or sexual orientation. In a relationship, people often assume that certain kinds of private information is considered the province of both parties and therefore should be shared between them (Petronio, 2002). When one person withholds information that the other partner sees as belonging to both partners (dyadically private), he or she may feel betrayed. For instance, many bisexual men who are in a primary relationship with a woman are unlikely to tell the woman about having sex with men (Kalichman et al., 1998; Weatherburn, Hickson, Reid, Davies, & Crosier, 1998). A woman described to us how her marriage broke up after she and her husband tested HIV positive. Her husband had kept it secret that he had sex with other men. He insisted at first that he had become HIV infected after an isolated incident with another man. He said that he had been raped after going out one night and getting drunk. The woman explained that she tried to keep the marriage from falling apart. She said, "I accepted the fact that he got drunk and was raped. Sexual relations changed, though. I was just uncomfortable after that." Then one time she heard her husband talking on the phone with another man in an explicit sexual manner. She confronted him at that point. He confessed that he had known since he was 16 that he was attracted to men. She described: "That's when I got mad, and that's when our marriage just went out the window."

One additional negative consequence for couples is the possibility of violence. Some individuals with HIV (particularly women) report physical abuse after disclosing their HIV infection (e.g., Armistead et al., 1999; Brown et al., 1994; Gielen et al., 1997; Kimerling et al., 1999; Rothenberg & Paskey, 1995; van der Straten, King, et al., 1998). At least one study though found no association between HIV disclosure and physical abuse directed at women (see Vlahov et al., 1998). Crosby (2000) reported some men experience post disclosure violence from partners, and this should also be explored in a range of samples using both men and women with varied sexual orientation and ethnicity. This fear of violence is also described in reasons for not disclosing a diagnosis. Brown et al. (1994) further argued that mandatory partner notification programs are especially problematic for women due to the possibility of physical violence (see North & Rothenberg, 1993; Golden, 2002, reviewed the efficacy of studies of HIV partner notification programs).

We have discussed the effects of HIV disclosure on relationship quality. As described, disclosing HIV can have a positive, negative, or no effect on the relationship (often depending on the relationship quality before the disclosure). As the disease progresses, a partner or family member may take over many responsibilities to assist the person with HIV. These caregiving roles are crucial in relationships in which one or both partners have significant health issues. Thus, we turn to effects of HIV disclosure on significant others as caregivers.

Significant Others as Caregivers

HIV-related health issues affect not only persons with HIV but also loved ones who are told and brought into the privacy boundary around HIV diagnosis. Knowing about the loved one's health status has implications for two reasons. First, knowing implies a certain responsibility for taking care of and dealing with the disclosure (Petronio, 2002). Second, finding out about such a diagnosis for a loved one is important for the relationship. Those who care for someone with HIV may become deeply involved in providing assistance and therefore need support for themselves. Examining the issues of medication adherence and assistance with daily care, we turn next to how significant others may become involved in caregiving after they know about the HIV diagnosis.

Promoting Medication Adherence. Since the development of antiretroviral combination therapies in 1995, the number of deaths due to AIDS-related conditions has decreased dramatically in countries where these medications are widely available. HAART reduces the HIV viral load (actively replicating HIV) in the blood to undetectable levels and improves clinical health (Carpenter et al., 1998). It is important to remember, however, that not all patients respond to HAART. Many individuals with HIV can expect to live longer and healthier lives if they are able to adhere to (and afford) the challenging treatment regimens for HAART (Greene & Cassidy, 1999; Williams, 1997). At present, however, it is unknown if these effects diminish with time (e.g., 10–20 years). Drug resistance is also a significant concern (Williams, 1997) with these demanding regimens and difficult side effects of HAART (e.g., many pills taken with a high protein meal). In contrast, Blower, Aschenbach, Gershengorn, and Kahn (2001) modeled a drug-resistant HIV strain and saw resistance as a minor issue (some drug sensitive cases do seroconvert), with low probability of occurrence. Still, there is widespread concern about drug resistance, as HAART is currently the only known effective treatment.

Many factors influence adherence to HAART regimens (Catz & Kelly, 2001; Greene & Cassidy, 1999), but one important factor is social support. Individuals who express satisfaction with their emotional support are more likely to adhere to HAART regimens (Catz, Kelly, Bogart, Benotsch, & McAuliffe, 2000). Crespo-Fierro (1997) argued there are many reasons for noncompliance with these medications and encouraged tailoring programs to individuals to increase adherence.

Women in particular may have difficulty with HIV medications, especially with compliance. Siegel and Gorey (1997) described barriers to AZT (generic name is *zidovudine*) use in 71 women with HIV; this is especially important for pregnant women (see also Misener & Sowell, 1998), as AZT use by pregnant women and infants decreases the possibility of an infant's contracting HIV (see guidelines, Mofenson, 2002). Women in particular hold negative attitudes toward AZT use (see also Greene & Cassidy, 1999). Women view AZT as toxic, prescribed indiscriminately, inadequately tested in women (and minorities), promoted for the wrong reasons, and inappropriate when feeling well (Siegel & Gorey, 1997). Women describe AZT as "poison" and "toxic waste" (these strong negative attitudes toward AZT use are also shared by men; see Perry, Ryan, Ashman, & Jacobsberg, 1992). The side effects of AZT should not be overlooked, as it is suspected, for example, of causing heart disease (Allen, 2002), especially in men in their late 30s and 40s. These dramatic possible side effects are discernable after only 5 years tracking protease inhibitors. As a consequence, the role of significant others in medication adherence for patients, especially women, deserves particular attention.

In interviews with women living with HIV (Winstead et al., 2002) individuals often reported that family members, friends, and intimate partners who knew about their HIV status were optimistic and hopeful about new HIV treatments. Significant others may educate themselves (or be educated by the person with HIV) about the medical treatment of HIV. In turn, they may encourage persons with HIV to take medications and to look after their health (e.g., to exercise, eat fruit and vegetables). Parents, children, friends, and intimate partners may become part of a team of caregivers in helping loved ones to cope with HIV. They might ask someone with HIV how they are doing with their medications. Significant others may also share information that was learned from the media about medical developments in HIV treatment. They may also ask how they can help out and what they can do to make things easier for the person with HIV. A woman who had recently begun combination retroviral therapy described how her 11-year-old son encouraged her to pursue medical treatment. He elicited disclosure by asking a question, asking about her T-cell count after she came back from a doctor's visit (T-cell count is a commonly used marker for estimating level of immune dysfunction, where higher is healthier, Bartlett & Gallant, 2001). He said, "Wow, this medicine is working. You might never be going to die. You keep going to your doctor's appointments." This type of reinforcement can have positive effects. Medical adherence assistance from significant others is an important possible benefit from HIV disclosure, and significant others can also provide daily assistance.

Providing Daily Assistance.   Significant others who know about someone's HIV infection may show love and concern by encouraging adherence to medical treatments, but a heavier emotional and physical involvement may be required of caregivers if help is needed for daily living. Research (e.g., Folkman, Chesney, & Christopher-Richards, 1994; Haas, 2002; Rosengard & Folkman, 1997; Wrubel & Folkman, 1997) illustrates the degree of responsibility caregivers may assume in looking after loved ones with AIDS-related illnesses. Folkman et al. (1994) interviewed men in the early 1990s (before HAART was available) providing daily assistance to partners with an AIDS diagnosis and in the terminal phase of illness. Most (73%) of the partners with the AIDS diagnosis died during this 2-year study. One third of the caregivers were also diagnosed with HIV. The caregivers provided a range of support including housekeeping, grocery shopping, meal preparation, emotional support, nursing care, and patient advocacy. Caregivers often felt positive about extending care, but they also experienced the stress of caring for someone who was seriously ill:

> This is a daily event, but it's absolutely the most stressful time in being a caregiver and these are the daily injections which I give my partner. I have to set up the syringe and then pick the spot on his arm to give him the shot. He's in a panic, and I'm in panic, but the job has to be done. I am personally deathly afraid of needles. I'm hurting him every morning. I hate this. I absolutely hate this. Waking up and thinking that this is your first chore of the day. My day starts after giving him his shot. He's very scared, which spills over into what I'm doing, which is supposed to be helping him. (Wrubel & Folkman, 1997, p. 699)

This quote illustrates the toll that providing assistance takes on the support provider, and this clearly will affect the relationship.

The role of caregiver for a partner with AIDS may be especially difficult for individuals who feel that caregiving is burdensome and who have little available social support. Haas (2002) reported that some families share these tasks with partners, expanding the support network, although the relational partners were the primary support for men with HIV followed by close friends and then family. Cowles and Rodgers (1997) studied the effect of AIDS on nonprimary caregivers and described how significant others of individuals with HIV function in important support roles. Rosengard and Folkman (1997) found that perceptions of caregiving burden and low social support were positively associated with the frequency of suicidal thoughts among these caregiving partners of men with AIDS. In summary, significant others serve as caregivers through promoting medication adherence and providing daily assistance; however, this can only occur after HIV disclosure and can change the relationship with the person with HIV. After describing the role of significant others, another important relationship for many with HIV is with children.

Effects of Disclosure on Children

Children are affected by HIV in multiple ways, for example, if their parents are infected, another family member such as a sibling is infected, or children live with HIV themselves (see Gewirtz & Gossart-Walker, 2000; Wiener, Septimus, et al., 1998). To date, there are more than 13 million "AIDS orphans" around the world (Sepkowitz, 2001). In some families, multiple persons are infected, and mothers often place the child's own care before their own (Gewirtz & Gossart-Walker, 2000; Wiener & Figueroa, 1998). Most individuals with HIV who are parents weigh whether or not to disclose the HIV diagnosis to their children (e.g., Armistead et al., 1999; Rotheram-Borus, Draimin, Reid, & Murphy, 1997; Schrimshaw & Siegel, 2002; Wiener, Battles, et al., 1998; Winstead et al., 2002). However, the research is mixed about the children's reactions to the HIV disclosure. For instance, Rotheram-Borus et al. (1997) found that adolescent children who were told that their parent had AIDS experienced more emotional distress and behavioral problems (e.g., substance abuse, smoking more cigarettes, and engaging in unprotected sex) compared to children of parents with HIV who were not informed. On the other hand, research by Schrimshaw and Siegel (2002) reported few lasting adverse effects and even closer relationships post disclosure; this study noted, however, that children had some very emotional reactions when they were initially told.

The short- and long-term effects of parents' HIV disclosure on children likely depend on a number of factors including the children's age, severity of HIV and AIDS symptoms, and the prior quality of the relationship between parents and children (see also Gewirtz & Gossart-Walker, 2000; Greene, 2001; Greene & Faulkner, 2002; Kimberly et al., 1995; Wiener, Septimus, et al., 1998). We also do not know what effect children's suspicions or prior knowledge about the parent's HIV status may have on their reactions when they are finally told (Schrimshaw & Siegel, 2002). When parents do disclose, telling the children may be because they did not want children to hear it from someone else, the disclosure may have been accidental (e.g., from eavesdropping), they may be told to prepare them for the parent's death, or the child may have asked (Wiener, Battles, et al., 1998). For whatever reason, when the children are told they face the burden of having this information. Being linked into a privacy boundary around their parent's HIV status means that they are also responsible for the information. They have to figure out when to tell others or when to protect the information just like anyone else would after being told. The problem is that parents may not be good at helping the children determine the privacy rules for the information and in communicating how they want the information managed with people outside the family.

Children's Reactions.   Children may express concerns about losing their parent when told that the parent has HIV (Wiener & Figueroa, 1998; Wiener, Septimus, et al., 1998). Many mothers, for instance, report that their children are afraid of the unknown, separation, and death. A woman with HIV reported the following:

> My kids were not used to seeing me lay down. They would get upset and say, "Mom, are you OK?" But I could see the fear in them that this might be it. And as a matter of fact my daughter even told me that. ... She had a conversation with me and she told me, "You don't understand, Mom. You're learning how to cope with this. But my brothers come to me every night and say, 'What happens if Mom dies?'"

This woman also recalled how her children did not want their father (her ex-husband) to know about the HIV diagnosis. They were afraid that he would take them away from her because she was HIV positive. She sat down with her three children to talk about the importance of making plans for the future:

> Now that you know about me and everything, I need to make some arrangements in case something happens to me. If I get too sick I want to make sure that you are OK. If something does happen to me, I need to talk to your father. I want to make sure he's going to be there to take care of you.

The daughter replied, "No, mom, you can't talk to dad about this. I don't know how he's going to react. He might try to take us away from you." The mother said, "Well, he can't take you away from me just because I'm [HIV] positive. I want you to understand that." This issue of future living situation is important for planning for both parents and children.

Children may also become very protective of the health of the parent or sibling with HIV, perhaps taking on inappropriate responsibilities (Gewirtz & Gossart-Walker, 2000). For instance, children may ask if the parent is taking medications or they may take on household chores to keep the parent from getting tired. One adolescent described, "Like, I never used to do the laundry before the disease. Now I want to have as much time with my momma as can be, to take any strain from her so she's well." This protectiveness may reflect children's fears that the parent might not be available for them in the future. There may be a kind of role reversal in which the child becomes the support for the parent.

Some children might be in denial or uncomfortable talking about HIV. A woman we interviewed said she had not had a "real deep conversation" about the infection with her son. She felt that when her son was ready he would approach her to initiate a conversation about HIV. Parents have different standards for what constitutes readiness; some use age requirements, whereas others use maturity guidelines.

There are cases in which parents' HIV disclosure may have little or no effect on children—particularly if family relations are poor. A woman described how her adult son, who is a drug addict, has not expressed any interest in her life for a long time:

> My son, he's a drug addict. I think he has no time to think about my sickness. He's not all there, and he could care less. If I were to say that I needed $10 for co-payment for my medicines, he probably would ask me could he borrow it. So, to him, it doesn't really matter. He has no sympathy as far as I'm concerned.

In this case the poor relational quality prior did not change after disclosure.

Knowing that a parent has HIV may stimulate children to think about and possibly disclose their feelings about life-and-death issues (Levine, 1993; Wiener & Figueroa, 1998). Planning for a child's future is an especially salient issue for women with HIV (Kimberly et al., 1995; Winstead et al., 2002). Some children have difficulty if caregiving is disrupted; for example, with a parent's hospitalization people may turn to extended families for care (Gewirtz & Gossart-Walker, 2000; Wiener, Septimus, et al., 1998). A woman who had been seriously ill from AIDS many times described the following conversation she had with her daughter while driving by a cemetery:

> [My daughter] knows what she wants on my head stone. She wants a cat. ... She's asked me if it is going to be cold or if I am going to be scared going underground. And I answer her. I told her the moment I die I'm going to be a guardian angel on her shoulder. I'm going to be there for the rest of her life. She can turn to me anytime she wants. If she is scared, she needs a friend, or if no one's around, I'll be there with her.

A child who knows the diagnosis may for the first time grapple with issues of death and dying, and the parent may be able to assist with these questions and fears. However, parents and children may not have a sense of who they can turn to seek help in managing this information.

Parents' own struggles with alcohol or drug use may have an impact on how children react to HIV disclosure. Parents' drug addiction (including time spent in jail or in a rehabilitation center) may complicate children's reactions to the disclosure of the HIV infection. If the parent is viewed as "responsible" for their illness due to drug use or gay or bisexual sex, this may affect reactions. A mother gave this account:

> For all of his [son] life, I was a drug addict. He didn't really have me. And so now I'm not a drug addict anymore, and I'm the best mother that I know how to be. But, you know, I can't make up for that time. And he doesn't say it, but I see the sadness in his eyes sometimes. It's like, "I just got my mom back, and now is she going to die on me?"

Children With HIV.   Beyond struggling with issues related to parents or other family members' HIV infection, children also may live with HIV infection. Perinatal transmission has been dramatically reduced in recent years, yet there are a number of children under age 13 infected with HIV. Not all children with HIV are told their diagnosis. "It is not unusual to find perinatally infected 10- and 11-year old children who have not been told of their diagnoses, even though they are on comprehensive medication regimens" (Gewirtz & Gossart-Walker, 2000, p. 316; see also Wiener, Septimus, et al., 1998). In some families, siblings of children with HIV are also not told (Wiener & Figueroa, 1998; Wiener, Septimus, et al., 1998). As they grow older, children are more likely to manage their disclosure decisions (Wiener, Heilman, et al., 1998). For children with HIV, there are many developmental struggles; for example, medical care or hospitalization may interfere with school attendance (and associated normal socialization processes; Wiener, Heilman, et al., 1998). The Ryan White case was an early publicized example of such an instance (see White & Cunningham, 1991). Ryan acquired HIV through contaminated blood products in the 1980s and wanted to attend school with his classmates. There was a great deal of public debate about balancing safety and compassion for the child. Children with HIV must confront unique issues such as school and recreational activities (e.g., playing sports).

Children with HIV do not generally receive the negative attributions of some other people with HIV and are often seen as "blameless." Yet Levin, Krantz, Driscoll, and Fleischman's (1995) study of neonatologists indicated they recommend less aggressive treatments for ill newborns with HIV (based on estimates of low potential life quality). Thus, it is important to continue to explore mode of transmission and responsibility attributions and how they affect perceptions of children with HIV.

Some children with HIV (and their families) go public in part to help educate others and reduce stigma. One study of these "public" families indicates the children with HIV may have more difficulty than children from nonpublic families (Wiener, Heilman, et al., 1998), a finding worth continued attention.

Summary for Children.   Increased attention to children and parents with HIV (and AIDS orphans) has occurred as people live longer and struggle with disclosure decisions (see Wiener, Septimus, et al., 1998, p. 711 for a list of books about children and HIV). A parent with HIV, anticipating possible health problems, might tell relatives who need to be prepared to assume guardianship or to watch over children of the person with HIV. For instance, a woman told her oldest son about the HIV diagnosis "Because I wanted him to oversee his brother and sister when the time comes." How (and if) parents disclose HIV to children will be an important area for continued consideration. Children's reactions are mixed, but parents clearly delay telling children until a certain age or stage of development. We have explored two important intimate relationships, significant others as caregivers and children, yet disclosure decisions can also influence risk behaviors. We turn next to the effect of HIV disclosure on safer sex and other risk behaviors, another relational consequence.

Impact on Safer Sex and Other Risk Behaviors

HIV disclosure can have numerous effects for couples in which one (serodiscordant) or both (seroconcordant) partners are HIV positive. Issues include, for example, who else to tell about the diagnosis, social support, commitment to the relationship, financial problems, loss of or changes in sexuality, health problems, reproductive decisions, raising children, and HIV-related stigma (e.g., Kalichman, 2000; Schnell et al., 1992; van der Straten, King, et al., 1998; Van Devanter et al., 1999). Yet a major issue for both individuals and couples who are sexually active is the need to practice safer sex behaviors (e.g., using condoms, choosing specific sexual behaviors) and to not share needles (or razors, toothbrushes, etc.). Definitions of safer sex vary widely, for example, not simply using condoms but questions about the level of risk for oral sex (see Scully & Porter, 2000), condoms breaking, or deep kissing (e.g., Klitzman, 1999). Safer sex behaviors are important to prevent uninfected partners from contracting HIV, yet safer sex also protects the infected partner(s) who is especially vulnerable to contracting additional strains of HIV or other sexually transmitted diseases (Kalichman, 2000). In this context, HIV disclosure serves a dual function to protect both the self and other (see Nimmons & Folkman, 1999).

Condom use is recommended broadly if not universally for many sexual encounters (Bayer, 1996; Stein et al., 1998). Recall that it is illegal in some states for people with HIV to have unprotected intercourse (cf. Burris, 2001). Yet there are mixed results in the research literature about the impact of HIV disclosure on reducing unprotected sex (e.g., Hoff et al., 1997; Stein et al., 1998). Most strikingly, Wolitski et al. (1998) reported there were no differences in self-reported sexual practices for HIV positive disclosers versus nondisclosers, and reduced risk practices were not universally adopted among either group. Especially when one partner is not infected with HIV, it may seem obvious that the couple would practice safer sex. Conversely, Elwood (1999, 2002) has described the "bug chaser" (referring to people trying to become HIV infected) phenomenon in which people deliberately expose themselves to HIV through needle sharing or unprotected sex with an infected partner in hopes of becoming infected (possible reasons include sharing HIV status with a partner, accessing health benefits, and suicide), but this phenomenon seems rather unique. Yet many persons with HIV who have disclosed their status to their partners do not use (or their partners do not use) condoms all the time when they are having vaginal or anal sex. For instance, Stein et al. (1998) studied HIV disclosure to sexual partners among men and women with HIV. Sixty percent of the research participants had told sexual partners about their HIV status. Among those who did not disclose to sexual partners about their HIV status, 43% reported using condoms all the time. Among those who did disclose to sexual partners, still only 43% also reported using condoms all the time. Although many people with HIV reported always using condoms, others did not— regardless of whether sexual partners were informed about the HIV diagnosis. Dawson et al. (1994) studied 677 MSM; in only 15% of the couples was the partner's HIV status known by both parties. Yet many people engage in high-risk behaviors but are unaware of the partner's HIV status.

Does testing HIV positive change risk behavior? Yes, there is some decrease in sexual risk (e.g., Fox, Odaka, Brookmeyer, & Polik, 1987; Green, 1994; McCusker et al., 1988; Schechter et al., 1988; Wang, Rodés, Blanch, & Casabona, 1997) and some decrease in drug risk behaviors (e.g., Deren, Beardsley, Tortu, & Goldstein, 1998) post HIV diagnosis. For instance, Wilson et al. (1999) reported heterosexual women with HIV were less sexually active and increased their condom use compared with women without HIV (the women with HIV lowered but did not eliminate risk behavior). Mayes, Elsesser, Schaefer, Handford, and Michael-Good (1992) studied a different population, women partners of hemophiliacs with HIV, and all of these women reported being sexually active but not all used condoms consistently (60% always used condoms). There were many reasons why, including some partners who were not aware of the diagnosis. Friedman et al. (1994), who described a sample of injection drug users, reported inconsistent condom use but more condom use if the partner was not an injection drug user or if the partner was known to be HIV positive. In Simoni, Walters, and Nero's (2000) study of 230 women with HIV in New York, almost all women had disclosed their HIV diagnosis to steady partners; they were more likely to have unprotected sex than women without steady partners, regardless of the partner's HIV status. HIV test counseling may influence these types of risk behaviors (Mattson, 1999), particularly if it focuses on personal relevance.

The failure to disclose about one's HIV status can place the unknowing partner at risk for HIV transmission if the couple does not practice safer sex. If someone discloses to a partner about the HIV infection then both know about the risk of transmitting the disease through unprotected sex. HIV disclosure may "put the information on the table" about HIV-related risks associated with sexual relations. However, HIV disclosure may not be sufficient by itself to guarantee the use of condoms for many couples (e.g., Fisher et al., 1998; Marks et al., 1998; Stein et al.,

1998; Yep, Lovaas, & Pagonis, 2002). For instance, a woman with HIV described the safer sex outcome of telling two sexual partners about her HIV diagnosis:

> Now, my best friend, he always used a condom [when we had sex]. But the guy I'm with now, I don't understand him because we had had sex without a condom. I'll be asleep sometimes and wake up, and he'll be in me. He won't put a condom on, and it just makes me wonder. Why would he take a chance when I have told him I am HIV positive?

In this relationship, one partner who knows the HIV diagnosis of his partner knowingly engages in unprotected sex, even at the risk of becoming infected and after being asked to use condoms. Further research with partners of individuals with HIV may assist in understanding when and why they make these choices.

Despite several studies showing little association between disclosure and condom use, it is worthwhile for individuals with HIV to disclose to sexual partners about their HIV status. Knowledge about HIV status encourages sexual partners to assess the risks of contracting HIV and to consider HIV testing for the partner who may not know her or his own HIV status (Kalichman, 2000). Final decisions about sexual behavior (especially unprotected sex), however, are likely to depend on many factors (such as perceptions of risk, pleasure of sex with or without condoms, group norms favoring safer sex, sexual negotiation between partners, length of time in the relationship) in addition to knowledge of one's partner's HIV status (Collins, 1998; Hoff et al., 1997).

Reproductive Choices.   Serodiscordant heterosexual couples may report difficulty maintaining safer sex behaviors, and even when both are aware of transmission risk they are not always practicing safer sex behaviors (Skurnick, Abrams, Kennedy, Valentine, & Cordell, 1998). Kline and VanLandingham (1994) argued that the role (and cooperation) of the partner is important in consistent condom use, and particularly how the couple reaches reproductive decisions is crucial. Virtually no research exists explaining how heterosexual couples with HIV negotiate reproductive decisions, especially the role of fathers in heterosexual couples. Recent research indicates women with HIV (following a very specific course of medical treatment) are very likely to have an HIV-negative child, so this option may be pursued intentionally by couples (e.g., Bartlett & Gallant, 2001; Mofenson, 2002). HIV disclosure, including a discussion of possible health risks to the mother and fetus during pregnancy and the issues of raising a child with HIV, are crucial features of these reproductive decisions and deserve further attention.

Pregnant women may initiate disclosure of HIV diagnoses, and this depends on both their disease and pregnancy stage. In the 1990s the public health recommendation to test all pregnant women for HIV became more prominent, and this is now a routine part of most prenatal screening. (In February 1995 the U.S. Public Health Service issued draft recommendations urging HIV testing for all pregnant women in the United States. There is some controversy over whether the testing should be required; e.g., see Rothenberg & Paskey, 1995.) In this case, pregnant women may know the HIV diagnosis much earlier in their disease stage than others (Lester et al., 1995; Sunderland, Minkoff, Handte, Moroso, & Landesman, 1992), and this also affects reproductive choices. Specifically, women with HIV are more likely to terminate pregnancy (choose abortion; e.g., De Vincenzi et al., 1997; Selwyn et al., 1989; Sunderland et al., 1992), undergo sterilization (Lindsay et al., 1995), and report fewer pregnancies (e.g., De Vincenzi et al., 1997; Sunderland et al., 1992). Many women with HIV do carry pregnancies to term (Siegel & Gorey, 1997). It is uncertain how these choices affect HIV disclosure (or if women tell others if they are aborting), and this may inhibit access to social support. This is an area for further examination, as pregnant women may know their diagnoses earlier, and if they choose to abort may or may not link sharing this information to disclosing their HIV status. Added to this, there are few long-term studies of AZT use, for example, to study the effects on children's development.

Other Complications. For other individuals with HIV, disclosure and safer sex decisions are complicated by alcohol or drug use. One bisexual woman with HIV reported how she had significantly curtailed her drinking, in addition to choosing periods of abstinence. She was committed to using condoms (or gloves or dams as appropriate) when she was sexually active if she had not told a partner, but she had several recent difficult episodes:

> I am absolutely certain about using safer sex if I am intimate, but I also realize I have to stop drinking. Twice recently I had a really hard time being safe when I was drunk. Do you have any idea how hard it is to unroll a condom when you are drunk? Unbelievable. What a mess. It's impossible. And it's not like the guy was much help, even after I reminded him why [her HIV diagnosis]. So condoms and alcohol do not mix for me any more, no sex if I'm drinking. But that's not the hardest part, it's keeping fucking latex [dental dams] in place for oral sex [with women], that slides everywhere, worse than condoms. And the women help only a little more than men. And if I'm drunk, how am I supposed to do that responsibly? So I just cannot drink if I think I might have sex, even a possibility, I can't take the chance they'll take care of it. I have to, to stop the spread.

This woman had a clear image of the behavior she wanted for herself, and she was distressed at lapses and modified her drinking as a result. She also mentioned the use of dental dams, and that crucial discussion has been absent in HIV literature with the nearly exclusive focus on male condoms. The use of dental dams or other latex barriers is especially relevant in relationships for oral sex (e.g., rimming and cunnilingus). Elwood and Greene (in press) reported that crack users showed awareness of risk of HIV infection if their gums were cracked and bleeding (one outcome of crack use), and this is significant for oral sex. Thus, alcohol and drug use can complicate disclosure and safer sex decisions.

Alternatives to Disclosure for Safer Sex.   Is it necessary to disclose an HIV diagnosis to remain safe? Klitzman's (1999) participants described how condoms are a "great substitute for talking." Some individuals with HIV choose not to disclose but to insist on safer sex (Sobo, 1997; Vázquez-Pacheco, 2000). In this way, they fulfill their sense of moral responsibility to protect the partner and themselves. In addition, they are able to maintain impermeable privacy boundaries around their HIV status. Their rules for managing privacy are clear and straightforward; they do not open the boundary that protects this information. However, while they maintain their privacy they also reframe "nondisclosure as irresponsible" to a series of relational choices negotiated between the parties. In Moneyham et al.'s (1996) study, women used safer sex behaviors but did not necessarily disclose their infection, mostly out of concern that disclosing would end their relationships.

Research indicates it is easier to discuss condoms in terms of pregnancy than HIV (e.g., Reel & Thompson, 1994), but this option cannot be utilized in all relational forms (e.g., MSM). It is encouraging to note, however, that just raising the topic of condom use—regardless of what or how it is said—results in more condom use (e.g., Reel & Thompson, 1994). For some, condom use obviates the necessity to disclose and discuss HIV status, with no obligation to tell anonymous partners if someone practices safer sex (Klitzman, 1999). Sometimes the partner wants to not use a condom, and this creates difficulties in using this safer sex method. Other problems include fatigue with maintenance of condom use (see Carballo-Diéguez, 2001). It may be especially difficult to reinitiate safer sex practices with long-term partners if someone does not disclose (Mattson & Roberts, 2001), and some HIV test counselors recommend that the person with HIV claim she or he has a yeast infection (a form of deception) if he or she is unwilling to disclose the HIV diagnosis, perhaps not wanting to admit an extra-relational affair.

Another possibility for individuals with HIV who avoid disclosure issues is decreasing or eliminating sexual contact. For some, disengagement from sexual activity is a common early reaction, yet many people with HIV do form or continue intimate relationships (Adam & Sears, 1994; Hoff et al., 1996). In Green's (1994) study men and women with HIV in Scotland reported disruption in sexual relationships, some lost libido, and some practiced no sex or periods of celibacy. Many people with HIV reported changes in particular sexual acts, but they felt these behaviors were not as fulfilling (not "real, full sex"). Post HIV diagnosis, there is often a decrease in frequency of sexual intercourse in which people are generally concerned about HIV transmission (e.g., De Vincenzi et al., 1997; Nyanjom et al., 1988). Contrary to this trend, Elwood and Williams (1999) described how some men with HIV patronize bathhouses so they can have unprotected anal intercourse, knowing silence norms facilitate it by prohibiting communication and HIV disclosure (see also Elwood, Greene, & Carter, in press).

Dating Post HIV Diagnosis. For some people with HIV, choosing not to date remains constant, but others begin dating and must confront disclosure issues later. Reentering the world of dating with HIV is difficult (Hatala, Baack, & Parmenter, 1998). Marks et al. (1991) reported 45% of participants (MSM with HIV, predominantly Hispanic) had been sexually active after learning their diagnosis. Hoff et al. (1996) reported MSM with HIV were less likely to be in primary relationships than MSM without HIV. Hoff et al. (1996) studied MSM who were with, without, and untested for HIV. Most negative or untested men preferred a romantic partner without HIV infection, but the majority of men with HIV had no serostatus preferences in a romantic partner. Additionally in this study, men also preferred seronegative friends, and this has important implications for social support.

Some men with HIV date only HIV positive men (or do not date at all; Klitzman, 1999). Hatala et al. (1998) examined 100 personal ads from gay men in San Francisco who disclosed their HIV status (positive or negative). They reported that disclosure of HIV in ads was relatively rare (less than 2% of possible ads examined). When they did disclose HIV status, men who were negative tended to mention more physical characteristics in their ads and request a negative partner. Men with HIV were more likely to mention health issues in ads and request a positive partner. Some ads of both positive and negative men requested the HIV status of the prospective partner. For people with HIV, dating can be extremely difficult. "In the dating world, HIV-positive men are still often treated as social pariahs, victims of what one frustrated ad placer referred to as 'viral apartheid'" (Hatala et al., 1998, p. 275). What little research is available on dating focuses on MSM and is very limited. It is less clear how disclosure progresses, affects relationships, and is affected by the relationship. To date, there is little research examining the couple to include the partner's perspective.

Summary of Consequences of HIV Disclosure

To this point, we have discussed the consequences of disclosing an HIV diagnosis. These outcomes occur only after disclosure and choices to open the privacy boundary around HIV status. The results are far reaching and not always expected. We first explored the social support outcomes for HIV disclosure, focusing on health outcomes for a support system and types of people who provide helpful support and then on disclosure and identity. Next, we examined the consequences related to stigma and showed how many people with HIV experienced negative reactions after sharing the diagnosis. Finally, we explored how HIV disclosure affects close relationships, particularly how it affects relationship closeness, significant others, children, and risk-behavior practices. All of these discussions have centered on the outcomes of HIV disclosure, but in many circumstances people choose not to share the diagnosis.

People with HIV disclose very selectively, managing privacy boundaries carefully. We turn next to the consequences of HIV nondisclosure.

PRIVACY PROTECTION, MANAGEMENT, AND HIV NONDISCLOSURE

Individuals with HIV live with the consequences of disclosing to others about their HIV status. However, there are also consequences of protecting HIV status by restricting the level and amount of disclosure. Unwillingness to disclose means that a person is limiting boundary permeability around his or her HIV status. The person choosing not to disclose may be defining the action as protecting privacy, but doing so may also present difficulties. Thus far we reviewed the consequences of HIV disclosure on stigma, social support, close relationships (including relationship closeness, significant others as caregivers, effect on children, and effect on safer sex and other risk behaviors). In this section, we consider some effects of not disclosing when the person with HIV decides not to tell and perhaps even to conceal information about the diagnosis from selected others. As CPM theory (Petronio, 2002) argues, at times we draw boundaries tighter, restricting access to information. There are many instances with an HIV diagnosis in which people choose to withhold information from others. In fact, it is possible that there is more nondisclosure than disclosure for many individuals with HIV. This section examines the consequences of this boundary tightening through nondisclosure.

Conflicted Feelings About Others' Right to Know

The effects of HIV nondisclosure on persons with HIV depend in part on whether the information about the diagnosis is viewed as private or secret (see Greene & Faulkner, 2002; Greene & Serovich, 1996; Kelly, 2002; Simmel, 1964/1950; Warren & Laslett, 1977). From a CPM perspective, secret information is a type of privacy. Thus, secrets represent information that is tightly guarded by a person with rules that restrict access about who knows the information. Private information is also regulated by rules determining who is a target of disclosure and when, how much, and how often others are told (Petronio, 2002). Knowledge about the HIV diagnosis may be considered private information when there are expectations that only a selected group of significant others are told but may be considered a secret when no one has a right to or need to know (see also chap. 1). The HIV diagnosis may be defined as secret information when it is perceived that the information needs to be concealed to protect oneself and others from harm. If people with HIV perceive their HIV status as private information, they are comfortable withholding this knowledge from others. However, viewing the information about the HIV diagnosis as a secret may cause inner conflicts if people with HIV perceive that others (e.g., an intimate partner, family member, friend, employer, coworker) have a right to know about the information. For instance, a man with HIV described his guilty feelings about intentionally concealing his HIV status from sexual partners, which sometimes included having unprotected sex:

> I am only human. Sometimes I got caught in a corner or boxed in. You know, I am only a man. Maybe that's how I rationalize, but I do get boxed in and reasoning sometimes goes out. I feel guilt-ridden, but you have such a need for the person at the time. You are lonely, and you know the rejection that you'll probably get if you tell. These are all messed up rationales that should not even come to play when you are jeopardizing another person's life. But I am just being honest. I have made mistakes like that. I try to use a condom. But sometimes in the heat of passion you rationalize your way through it. This is something I have to answer to God, I guess.

In this case, the man was aware of the balancing dilemma but not always comfortable with how he handled it. Elwood et al. (in press) interviewed MSM who were bathhouse patrons, and they described how norms and desire interfered with decisions to both talk about and use condoms. The "norm of silence" bathhouse patrons described included a dilemma patrons acknowledged of not talking about safer sex including condom use but still recognizing risk and at times engaging in risky practices (see also Elwood & Williams, 1999).

The desire for normal social relationships may pose an extra burden for persons with HIV who withhold information about the diagnosis for an extended time. When others eventually find out about the HIV diagnosis, they may be disappointed that they were not informed earlier or they may react angrily if they perceive that the information had been kept a secret from them (cf. Derlega et al., 1993; Greene & Faulkner, 2002; Jones & Gordon, 1972). CPM theory describes the development of individual decision rules about who is told and in what order; for example, if a parent finds out another family member knew first this may be seen as rule breaking. Family members often expect that they would be included in a privacy boundary around this kind of information and when they are excluded they perceive that it sends a message about the way the other is defining the relationship (Petronio, 2002). Greene and Faulkner (2002) labeled this phenomenon "relational violations," when a person felt they should have been told earlier and feels "left out." The following quote presents the justification of a person with AIDS for not disclosing and describes the brother's negative reactions when he found out that he was not told earlier. Their mother had disclosed to the brother when his sibling was ill:

> I said to him, "Well, being terminally ill and how I got this whole disease, and then my lifestyle [being gay]. I didn't know if you were ready for this. And it would be overwhelming for you because you have this other picture of me. And, though I was eventually going to tell you, the illness beat me. It beat me in telling you. So, I am forced, and you are forced to handle it now. Of course, I was trying to be discrete in telling you so that you could handle it easier." But he is angry with me that I didn't tell him soon enough. He said, "Well, why didn't you call me straight and tell me?"

He also said, "Well, you know I love you, and we are not supposed to keep things like this from one another." And I told him again, "There was so much to tell, and it was so overwhelming."

This person wanted to delay disclosure but disease progression changed the boundary management decision. The brother felt he should have been told earlier.

In the long run, people's concern for the health of a loved one with HIV may outweigh any disappointment about not being told directly about the diagnosis (compare to the discussion of indirect disclosure in chap. 4). However, this last example illustrates how someone who stakes a claim to the information may be upset when he or she finds out about the HIV nondisclosure.

HIV Nondisclosure as Information Control

With the success of HAART, many individuals with HIV are healthier and more physically active than they were previously (Bartlett & Gallant, 2001; Brashers, Neidig, et al., 1999; Kelly et al., 1998; Sowell, Phillips, & Grier, 1998; Trainor & Ezer, 2000). HAART may make it easier for persons with HIV to withhold information about the diagnosis from others, especially if they appear to be in good health. However, HIV nondisclosure may still be difficult if certain people are seen fairly often (e.g., family, intimate partners, friends, coworkers) or if there is a desire to initiate sexual intimacy in new relationships. It may be difficult to explain treatment side effects, multiple visits to a physician, tiredness, and pillboxes if someone does not want to disclose to others about the HIV diagnosis.

One strategy for nondisclosure might be for the person with HIV (or significant others) to ask those who know about the diagnosis to assist in concealing the information from others. In this way, they negotiate the privacy rules for the information and enter into an agreed on boundary for how to manage the disclosure. This inner circle might be asked to withhold the information from certain individuals, for instance, coworkers, distant or elderly relatives, young children, neighbors, or anyone who is known to be a "snitch" or gossip. Greene and Faulkner (2002) detailed several accounts of nondisclosure due to perceived gossip problems.

A second strategy for nondisclosure, however, might be to construct stories to mask some aspects of coping with HIV. One man described how, when visiting a friend's house, he would hide his HIV medications in a diabetes pill bottle:

I take my medication out of the original bottle when it comes, and I put it in another prescription bottle. He [the friend] knows that I am diabetic and that I take pills for diabetes. I would take my medication and put it in that bottle [for the diabetes pills]. He would think that I would be taking medication for diabetes. It's funny how people can accept cancer, they can accept a diabetic, but they can't accept a person with HIV.

Another man with AIDS-related physical problems told his parents, brothers, and sisters that he had cancer. This strategy is widely reported, and interestingly the disease of choice in this type of misdirection or privacy management seems to be cancer. He did not trust how certain family members would react if he told them about AIDS:

> I told them that I had bone cancer. I don't want to confide in them because there are members of my family that I don't want to confide in as far as certain issues are concerned. It is hard not being able to tell those people who are very close to you. It is hard not being able to share this. It is hard to go outside your family structure and reveal this and confide in someone else. But that is the way I've chosen to deal with it at this point.

For this man, it was important to not disclose, so he created a cover story to protect himself. These types of stories are widely described by individuals with HIV when they want to retain privacy.

Few studies specifically address perceived privacy or what rights people feel they have to know others' HIV related information. Greene et al. (1993) explored attitudes toward HIV and privacy. They reported perceptions of privacy were significantly correlated with willingness to release information both about who is tested for HIV and who tests HIV positive. Specifically, the more strongly people felt about protecting privacy generally the less support they reported for release of HIV information to others. Interestingly, college students reported the highest privacy perceptions, followed by parents with preschool children and parents of young adults. The Greene et al. (1993) study did not include specifically people with HIV; however, it provides an indicator of how U.S. privacy attitudes affect people's attitudes toward disclosure and access to HIV-related information (at least among those who do not have HIV). People with more protective perceptions of privacy do not as readily think they or others should have to share information. Thus, information control is an important criterion for nondisclosure of HIV.

Breakdown of Information Control

Many individuals with HIV (and their significant others) are successful in controlling who is told about the HIV diagnosis. However, there may be a host of factors that undermine information control. We consider how physical aspects of coping with HIV as well as social interactions influence the breakdown of information management.[2]

The presence of physical symptoms associated with HIV progression may make it difficult to conceal one's HIV status. Recall the scene from the film *Philadelphia* (Demme, 1993) in which the main character's (played by Tom

---

[2]We focus here on the breakdown of information control assuming that unwanted others may learn about the HIV diagnosis. However, information control may also be threatened if others are told about the HIV diagnosis but then probe intrusively for more details. For instance, there may be unwanted questions about how HIV disease was contracted (e.g., drug use, sexual partners, or both).

Hanks) lesions were a crucial part of the discrimination lawsuit (and nonvoluntary disclosure) and assumption by others that he had AIDS. We interviewed a man who had thrush, a fungal infection in the mouth associated with immune suppression (Bartlett & Gallant, 2001; Kalichman, 1995). The man was fearful of telling anyone in his family about the HIV diagnosis. However, his sister, who is a nurse, was suspicious about the white patches in his mouth. "She keeps asking me, 'What is your diagnosis?,' or 'What is wrong with you?, What did your doctor say?'" His response has been, "I give her off the wall answers, or I don't answer, or I just leave the room."

There may also be physical side effects from taking antiretroviral therapy that make it difficult to control who finds out about the HIV diagnosis. For instance, some individuals with HIV develop a condition of fat redistribution called *lipodystrophy syndrome* after taking anitiretroviral medications. Lipodystrophy may include metabolic disturbances and a redistribution of fat over the body (Collins, Wagner, & Walmsley, 2000). There may be a buildup of fat in the nape of the neck (buffalo hump) as well as in the breasts and abdomen; a bull-necked appearance caused by benign tumors; loss of fat in the face, arms, buttocks, and legs; and prominent veins caused by the loss of subcutaneous fat. For some people, these physical effects are easily identifiable.

Lipodystrophy may lower body image self-esteem, with some persons labeling themselves as "grotesque," "deformed," or "unattractive" (Collins et al., 2000), similar to some of the earliest identifiable AIDS symptoms: rapid weight loss or lesions. In a study of HIV positive men and women with lipodystrophy, one person noted that, "People in my community can tell I am HIV positive from just looking at my face. It is like the old KS [*Karposi sarcoma*] lesion on the nose" (Collins et al., 2000, p. 547). A woman we interviewed who has an enlarged abdomen told us how she was occasionally approached by acquaintances at shopping malls congratulating her for being pregnant. She had to tell these acquaintances that she was not pregnant but had some other physical ailment.

There may be social factors that influence the loss of control over who knows about the infection. Someone who knows about the diagnosis (e.g., a lover, relative, or friend) may believe that others have a right to know, leading to the spread of the information (see Greene & Faulkner, 2002). Some individuals with HIV may resign themselves to this loss of privacy if they believe others have a right to assert this claim. This notion is similar to CPM theory ideas of how boundaries are negotiated and co-owned. For instance, a man described how he had not told his mother or other members of his family about his HIV status. He did tell his brother but with the admonition not to tell their mother because he "didn't want to hurt her." A month later, the mother had assembled everyone in the family (including a relative flown in from another state) for dinner. The following happened:

She [my mother] called me over to the house. She said, "I'm going to cook dinner and we are going to talk." When she says she's going to cook dinner and wants to talk, mother has something to say that she couldn't just say any kind of way and you probably may not like it. So, here's what we do. You prepare yourself for this meeting because you know mother's going to get you. OK, I go to this dinner that all the children are at. I said, "It's not anybody's birthday. It's not a holiday. Why is momma having a dinner?" And I said to myself, "[My brother] told momma what's wrong." So she sat there after she put all the food on the table. They said grace, and we started eating. After that she said nobody can leave the house. And all of them sat down, the husbands, the children. They all sat there, and everybody looked at me in my face like they were all prepped before I got to the house. I was the last one to get there. Daddy was even there. Remember, my mother and father are separated. My father said, "You have something to tell us, don't you?" [At this point, he tells the entire family about the HIV diagnosis.]

If a confidant or someone else (such as the mother in the preceding example) is perceived to be justified in telling others, then the person with HIV may acquiesce in the loss of privacy. However, if someone with HIV believes that others have no claim to the information—whether or not they are family—then the HIV disclosure by the confidant may be seen as a privacy violation. In the following illustration, a man with HIV described how he felt violated and angry after his aunt had told other family members about his HIV status:

My family had a cookout, the fourth of July last year. I made the mistake of telling my aunt that lives in D.C. I thought when I was telling her that I could trust her. She ended up telling some people. The policy was that the information was strictly supposed to be between us. She was starting out to be helpful. She'd call and see how I was doing. Then the next thing that I knew everyone in the family I didn't tell knew about it, but they were coming to me and saying, "We heard something. Is it true?" And I was very disappointed at her and very angry because I didn't expect that from her.

We have provided examples of how confidants may be the source of unwanted disclosure about the HIV diagnosis. Situational factors, however, may also permit HIV information to pass into the hands of unwanted persons who in turn pass it along to others. One woman reported a nurse had seen her at a clinic (and supposedly looked at her chart) and shared the HIV diagnosis with friends in the community who were also neighbors of the woman with HIV. A man told us how he occasionally met an acquaintance at an ASO where they were both seeking assistance. The acquaintance told the man's sisters and niece about seeing him at the ASO, supposedly so they could provide him with support. This is how the man described what happened:

I ran into a friend of my sisters and my niece. I knew he had it [HIV], and he knew I knew he had it. My sisters and everybody knew he had it. He goes to the same church I go to that I recently joined. I think it was spiteful of him to go to my sisters and niece and tell them that he saw me at [the ASO], and that maybe I want to talk to them about it. [He said] I might want to tell them so they can give me more support. But the problem with that is I had not told them. My sister confronted me about it. I said no [I didn't have the HIV disease] because I wasn't ready or prepared to tell her or the rest of my family.

This man described how the threat to his privacy continued:

My sister started asking my mother. She told my mother somebody told her. My mother asks me a couple of times if I had it, and my sister keeps asking other people. My sister asks the lady that comes in and helps my mother. This lady and I had become very close in the last 2 years at a time when I had stopped associating with other friends. My sister asked her, and she said she didn't know. The lady told me that my sister asked her [about my HIV status].

In this situation, an entire chain of events unfolded based on seeing a person he knew at an ASO. Although the man continued to maintain his privacy and deny his diagnosis, there was great strain on the relationships with his sister and mother.

Sometimes the loss of control about HIV information occurs due to bureaucratic insensitivity or ignorance about HIV and may extend into a violation of legal rights to privacy. A homeless person with AIDS described how staff at a hotel knew he was HIV positive because his stay was subsidized by a local ASO. The hotel used rooms on only one side of the hotel for clients from the ASO and when the man was about to leave the hotel, a staff person "started bleaching the whole place down while you were there." He said:

They [the hotel staff] said it's no discrimination. But they put you all in one area where it is obvious that everybody has the AIDS there. I guess they meant well, but she [hotel staff] said that's the only rooms. And then when they help you they put it on your registration card that you got AIDS.

Thus, some people with HIV do not seek what assistance they need to avoid association with HIV and possible stigma.

Individuals may be successful in gaining others' cooperation in concealing the HIV information from others. However, keeping boundaries closed (meaning that the information about the HIV diagnosis does not leak to unwanted third parties) may be increasingly difficult over a long period of time. People who know about the information may unintentionally disclose it. The following example illustrates how information about HIV may be revealed accidentally. A woman with HIV (we call her "Margaret") had become friendly with another woman with HIV, "Maria." They met at a summer camp for kids and families with HIV. Margaret was visiting at Maria's apartment, and their daughters were playing outside. What happened next is that Margaret's daughter met a neighbor of Maria who asked how she and the other child had met. This is Margaret's description of what happened:

> She [my daughter] said, "Oh, my mommy and her mommy are in the same support group." And the neighbor said, "Support group for what?" My daughter goes, "Oh, my mommy and Maria have HIV." Just telling this neighbor, I can't believe it. I have sat down so many times with her [my daughter], and I have talked to her about not telling anybody. She just was telling this woman we were in the same support group. And Maria was just fit to be tied. I said to Maria, "You know, I am flabbergasted. We have sat down so many times to talk about this and I can't believe she did that." Of course, Maria out and out lied to the neighbors. She said to them, "I don't know where she got that from."

Here is Margaret's account of her follow-up conversation with her daughter:

> I sat down with my daughter and talked to her. I asked her why she did that. And she said, "Well, I didn't know, mom." And I said, "Well, honey, we've talked about this." I said, "You have to be careful who you talk to. Maria is very upset. She didn't want anybody else to know in the neighborhood, and now this lady is asking her."

There are occasions when privacy may break down because a confidant reveals the information about HIV to others to manipulate or hurt the person with HIV. Particularly if there are interpersonal problems in a close relationship, one partner may decide to "out" the person with HIV to ridicule or humiliate him or her in front of others (or perhaps force the person to confront issues). This is what occurred to the woman in the following account. She is a mother with HIV who has four children. Her husband repeatedly nagged her to tell the older children about her diagnosis. However, she did not feel ready to tell them yet:

> He kept pushing me, saying, "You need to tell your kids." My daughter had a friend over and the boys [my two sons] were sitting there playing Nintendo. He said, just out of the blue, "Isn't there something you need to tell your kids?" And I looked at him and my daughter. My daughter said, "What?" She said, "What do you need to tell me?" And he said, "You know. You know. You need to talk to your kids." And I said, "This is not the time. No, this is not the time to do that." The boys and my daughter thought it was kind of funny, saying, "What is it? Are we going to move? Are we going to do something?" They thought there was some big change going to happen. And for about a half an hour we went on with this little bickering.
>
> I said [to my husband], "Please don't." I started crying, and I said, "Don't do this. This is not right." Well, somehow we ended upstairs, and the baby was up in the crib. My daughter was coming up there to make sure nothing had happened. And the boys had come up there too. My husband said, "Just go ahead and tell them." So I just blurted out, "OK." I was crying, hysterical. I said, "During my pregnancy I was diagnosed HIV positive." And I said to him, "Is that what you wanted me to tell

them? Is that what you wanted me to come out and say?" And he said, "Now, don't you feel a whole lot better?"

I was crying and my daughter looked at me and she was crying. She said, "Mom, I love you. You're my mom. It doesn't matter." She went running out of the room. And I'm crying and my sons are sitting there, and they began to cry.

This woman felt pressured to disclose at a time and in circumstances not to her choosing. Her husband was insistent on her telling the children despite her desire to wait.

In many relationships, family members, friends, or intimate partners may be counted on to guard the information about the HIV diagnosis. As these anecdotes illustrate, there is no guarantee that people can be counted on to assist in concealing the HIV information from unwanted others. Keeping the information concealed from others is likely to depend on the quality of the relationship between the person with HIV and the disclosure recipient (Greene, 2001; Vangelisti & Caughlin, 1997). Concealing the information will also depend on the confidants' expectations about how much the person with HIV "owns" the information and how much this claim to ownership should be respected. On the other hand, despite everyone's best efforts, physical factors associated with the progression of HIV disease or side effects of treatment may increase the difficulty of concealing knowledge about the HIV diagnosis from others. Controlling access to information about the HIV diagnosis is not an easy task.

Privacy and Nondisclosure as Psychological Inhibition

There may be socially mediated costs of nondisclosure including social isolation, loneliness, unavailability of social support, and fear of being stigmatized if people find out about the HIV diagnosis. However, there may also be physical and psychological costs of HIV nondisclosure uniquely associated with concealing this information from significant others. We review studies from the expanding literature on psychological inhibition (e.g., Cole, Kemeny, & Taylor, 1997; Cole, Kemeny, Taylor, & Visscher, 1996; Cole, Kemeny, Taylor, Visscher, et al., 1996; Lepore & Smyth, 2002; Pennebaker, 1988, 1990, 1995; Smyth, 1998) to document how inhibiting HIV disclosure may be harmful for physical and mental health.

A study by Cole, Kemeny, Taylor, Visscher, et al. (1996) found that gay men with HIV who are in the closet about their sexual orientation are more likely to suffer from accelerated progression of HIV disease. Concealing one's homosexual identity (as a form of psychological inhibition) involves inhibiting the expression of important thoughts and feelings about the self. The failure to disclose important information about the self may increase the activity of the sympathetic division of the autonomic nervous system and weaken immune system functioning. The participants in Cole, Kemeny, Taylor, Visscher, et al. (1996) were asked to rate how much they concealed their homosexual identity compared to other gay men. HIV disease progressed more quickly for gay men who were closeted compared to those who were open about their sexual orientation. The closeted gay men suffered greater loss of CD4 cells, developed an AIDS diagnosis in a shorter time, and died sooner than those who were out about their sexual identity. The relationship between concealing sexual identity and the outcome measures was not affected by controlling for any of the potential mediating variables (social support, having a primary partner, repressive response style, and depression).[3]

From this we can speculate how HIV nondisclosure poses a direct risk to physical health. Individuals who withhold information about their HIV status from others may spend considerable time hiding this information. The inhibition of thoughts and feelings about HIV (because of HIV nondisclosure) may be a stressor on the body that accelerates AIDS progression and leads to other stress-related physical problems (Cole, Kemeny, Taylor, Visscher, et al., 1996; Cole, Kemeny, Taylor, & Visscher, 1996; Lepore & Smyth, 2002; Pennebaker, 1988, 1990, 1995). We note though that HIV nondisclosure as psychological inhibition is associated with actively concealing information about the HIV diagnosis from others. If someone with HIV considers knowledge about their HIV status as private information and not as a secret that must be hidden from others (see Warren & Laslett, 1977), then HIV nondisclosure may not increase the probability of health risks. Thus, how the individual sees the nondisclosure is critical for health.

There is other research on psychological inhibition suggesting that keeping HIV a secret has cognitive consequences (see also Cameron & Nicholls, 1998; Kelly, 2002; Kelly, Klusas, von Weiss, & Kenny, 2001). Keeping a secret from others is a deliberate process that requires mental work and energy. It may paradoxically lead to an obsessive mental preoccupation with the information that the person is trying to hide from others as well as considerable psychological distress. Wegner and colleagues (e.g., Lane & Wegner, 1995; Smart & Wegner, 1999; Wegner, 1989, 1994; Wegner & Lane, 1995) have collected considerable data indicating that working to suppress thoughts about a secret is frequently the first step in attempting to keep a secret. The person may be reminded of the secret when in the presence of other people and the thought suppression may decrease the probability of accidental disclosure. Suppressing thoughts about the secret also has the paradoxical effect of making the thoughts more accessible to consciousness. For instance, it is as if attempting to not think about the HIV diagnosis (as part of keeping this information a secret) would cause a rebound in thinking about HIV.

Smart and Wegner (1999) conducted research on the cognitive consequences of concealing information about an eating disorder (anorexia nervosa or bulimia

---

[3]We also note that concealing information about HIV status may not always be unhealthy. For instance, Cole et al. (1997) found that among gay men who were HIV positive, those who were rejection sensitive (who were uncomfortable about social situations in which their sexuality would be salient to others) and concealed their homosexual identity did not experience accelerated HIV progression (e.g., times to an AIDS diagnosis and a critically low CD4 T-cell count). Concealing one's sexual orientation among rejection-sensitive gay men may be a protective buffer from negative health effects, given that society often stigmatizes being gay.

nervosa) from another person. Some of the women (regardless of whether or not they actually had an eating disorder) were asked to play a role in an interview of someone with an eating disorder. The women who actually had an eating disorder and who role played not having one reported more thought suppression (based on "pushing thoughts of your eating habits or body image out of your mind") than did the women in the other conditions in the study. The women with an eating disorder who role played not having one also reported more intrusive thoughts about eating problems. The women who tried to keep secret from the interviewer their thoughts about eating disorder and body image were more active in trying to push these thoughts out of consciousness, and they were more likely to have intrusive thoughts about them. Additionally, Lane and Wegner (1995) found, across a wide range of secret topics (e.g., "hitting someone," "being a homosexual," "a lie I told"), positive associations between how strong the desire to keep the information secret was, how much individuals tried not to think about the topic, and how much they had intrusive thoughts about the topic of the secret.

We infer from Smart and Wegner's (1999) research that someone with HIV who keeps this information as a secret from others may become preoccupied with thoughts about this secret. Keeping the secret may initiate a process of thought suppression, which is a mental strategy designed to assist in keeping the information a secret. However, the thought suppression could cause more thinking and perhaps even a preoccupation with thoughts about HIV. This cycle of secrecy, thought suppression, and thought intrusions may cause considerable psychological distress for the person who relies on HIV nondisclosure as a strategy for concealing who has access to the HIV information.[4]

CONCLUSIONS

We have suggested how HIV nondisclosure—as psychological inhibition—may be related to poorer health outcomes as well as to an obsessive preoccupation with the secret thoughts about HIV. Someone making decisions about HIV disclosure or nondisclosure is likely to consider all the benefits and costs associated with either decision—both for oneself and significant others. For instance, HIV disclosure provides access to much-needed social support, but it increases risks associated with being stigmatized and rejected by others. Simultaneously, HIV nondisclosure reduces the risks associated with being stigmatized and rejected, but it also increases the risks of harmful effects associated with psychological inhibition. For individuals with HIV, it is important to consider the overall benefits

---

[4]We have described how HIV nondisclosure may cause individuals psychological distress, particularly by inducing them to become preoccupied by the information they are attempting to hide from others. However, there is interesting research by Stiles and colleagues (Stiles, 1987, 1995; Stiles et al., 1992, which we described in chap. 4) indicating that psychological distress may cause individuals to disclose more about themselves. According to Stiles's (1995) fever model of disclosure, "people tend to disclose more when they are psychologically distressed (anxious, depressed, frightened, angry, etc.) than when they are not and that this disclosure helps relieve the distress—by catharsis and promoting self-understanding" (p. 82).

and costs associated with disclosure and nondisclosure for oneself and others and then make decisions about to whom and under what circumstances to disclose or not disclose the HIV diagnosis. This balancing of risks and costs is explored in terms of CPM.

This chapter began by reviewing consequences of disclosing an HIV diagnosis. We first examined actual responses to HIV disclosure and then social support by looking at helpful or unhelpful social support, satisfaction, coping, and identity. Then we examined stigma that can result from disclosing a seropositive diagnosis. Finally, we looked at consequences of disclosing on a relationship including relationship closeness, caregivers, children, and risk behavior. For each of these consequences we documented both positive and negative outcomes of disclosing the diagnosis. The latter portion of the chapter explored the consequences of tightening the boundaries or nondisclosure. First, we examined others' right to know, then informational control and breakdown of informational control, and finally psychological inhibition. Thus, outcomes of these privacy management decisions are extremely complex and must be considered when disclosing.

A final word is appropriate. We are advocates of HIV disclosure, especially when there is a need for social and professional support and there is a risk of transmitting HIV via sexual behavior or sharing needles. However, there are tradeoffs associated with HIV disclosure and nondisclosure in terms of possible benefits and costs. For example, a blanket policy to disclose to all partners (such as mandatory partner notification programs) may put some people at substantial risk post disclosure (see Brown et al., 1994; Gielen et al., 1997; Rothenberg & Paskey, 1995; van der Straten, Vernon, et al., 1998). The degree of success in coping with HIV, as someone infected or affected by HIV, depends in part on the net results of balancing these benefits and costs associated with HIV disclosure and nondisclosure. It is too simplistic to recommend disclosure to everyone or no one, as individuals with HIV must assess each situation in light of issues described in this chapter and balance often competing needs.

CHAPTER SIX

Epilogue: Looking to the Future of Disclosure and HIV

In this book we have presented information about how individuals with HIV and those close to them manage disclosure decisions using a CPM perspective. We first examined the criteria or rules people develop to manage these decisions to disclose an HIV diagnosis. Next, we looked to the features of the actual HIV disclosure messages. Finally, we reviewed the consequences or outcomes for decisions to disclose an HIV diagnosis or to maintain privacy. This epilogue explores what the future may hold for research on HIV disclosure. The last section of the book (Appendix, after the Epilogue) presents resources for people dealing with these HIV disclosure issues.

HIV and AIDS Treatments

There have been dozens, possibly hundreds, of therapies explored for AIDS, but in the U.S. at present there are 15 agents in 3 classes of drugs (Sepkowitz, 2001). Since 1995, new treatments, such as HAART, hold promise for changes in life quality for some people with HIV. HAART attacks the HIV virus, allowing a person's immune system to repair itself and fight opportunistic infections (Bartlett & Gallant, 2001; Epstein & Chen, 2002; Hammer, 2002). It is important to continue to monitor HAART side effects (Allen, 2002), as the medications have not been studied long-term and the side effects likely influence medication adherence. At the XIV International AIDS Conference, many researchers presented studies on treatments, including a new class of antiretrovirals called *fusion inhibitors* (T–20) as well as other drugs such as *experimental integrease inhibitors* (see Kresge, 2002). Many individuals with HIV using HAART or other treatments are living longer with delayed or perhaps even no progression to AIDS, and this may change the way they process disclosure decisions. For some, these new treatments may decrease disclosure, as many previously only disclosed or sought help when very ill (e.g., Hays, Chauncey, et al., 1990; Hays et al., 1993). In the same vein, individuals with HIV may feel they are healthier and do not need the same level of social support because they are healthy, thus remaining more private. In contrast, it is possible to argue that new treatments will increase disclosure. This may happen because people do not feel they are disclosing about a "death sentence" and the information is less shocking. HIV stigma may also be reduced if treatments are effective over long periods. At present, what will result from these new treatments (more or less disclosure) is uncertain, but this will be an important area to monitor in the future.

We must also recognize that currently available drug therapies are not affordable in many countries (and for some in the United States), and these countries continue to have rapid increases in HIV infections and AIDS-related deaths (Sepkowitz, 2001). Unfortunately, estimates indicate less than 2% of people infected worldwide use these medications (see Altman, 2002; UNAIDS Reports, July 2002), although the figure is much higher in the United States. For example, half of HIV infections in the world currently occur in sub-Saharan Africa where these medications are virtually unavailable (UNAIDS/WHO, 2001). In areas where the medications are becoming affordable, there are monitoring problems (Stephenson, 2002). Other emerging areas of the HIV epidemic include Asia (e.g., China and India), Eastern Europe (e.g., Russia), and the Caribbean and Latin America (see Baltimore, 2002; UNAIDS, 2001). The high cost of the drugs has lead to debates concerning patents and production of generic equivalents in other countries (e.g., Brazil, Cuba; see Epstein & Chen, 2002). One response to the high cost in some countries in the Caribbean and Latin America is for the government to provide (or supplement the cost of) HIV medication . These differences in available treatments also affect decision making surrounding the HIV diagnosis. Confounding these differences between the U.S. and global epidemic are differences in the structure of social support for individuals (e.g., families and institutions such as service organizations). Many families worldwide have multiple infections and/ or the infected person is the family's source of income, leaving the family destitute when the person dies (Epstein & Chen, 2002).

AIDS Vaccine

Development of an AIDS vaccine has received a great deal of attention in the past 5 years (former U.S. President Bill Clinton called for research on a vaccine in 1997), as it has promise to slow the epidemic significantly (Haney, 2002). At present, AIDSVAX is in the third and final stage of clinical testing, which began in 1998, and there is some promise for this vaccine. The vaccine does not stop HIV infection; rather, it holds the virus in check (Haney, 2002). At the 9th Annual Retrovirus Conference in Seattle in 2002, the pharmaceutical company Merck reported preliminary human testing. Any vaccine is probably at least several years (maybe even beyond 2010) from general use, and it may face the same global distribution challenges as HAART.

If a vaccine becomes widely available in the near future, the epidemic could change dramatically after the point when the vaccine is available. It would be difficult to know, however, if those with HIV would then be more or less likely to disclose their infection. With fewer expected infections, we could see a decrease in disclosure if HIV becomes relatively infrequent. It is also possible to see increased disclosure if attribution of responsibility for infection changes. For example, a person who was vaccinated yet still contracted HIV might be held less "accountable" for the infection (see chaps. 3 and 5). Compared with HAART treatment, the effect of a vaccine on HIV disclosure is unknown; nevertheless, it is a prospect worth speculating about.

The XIV International AIDS Conference held July 7 to 12, 2002, in Barcelona, was closed jointly by former Presidents Bill Clinton and Nelson Mandela, attesting to the importance of this event. The topics of HAART and vaccines featured prominently in conference discussions. At the conference, there were calls for significant increases in global HIV funding (beyond the 500 million dollars the United States pledged to fight mother–infant transmission in a dozen African nations and the Caribbean, announced by G. W. Bush on June 19, 2002; see Stolberg, 2002).

Changes in Stigma

Linked to both HAART treatment and an AIDS vaccine is the possibility that HIV and AIDS stigma will change in the future. Despite some changes (e.g., legal), it remains true that "the most significant obstacle to progress in the AIDS epidemic is discrimination" (Mondragon et al., 1991, p. 1137; see also Blendon & Donelan, 1988). We described in chapter 3 how different types of stigma affect willingness to disclose an HIV diagnosis, and in chapter 5 we documented a wide range of stigmatizing responses people reported to HIV disclosure. Stigma is a crucial feature of HIV disclosure (e.g., Alonzo & Reynolds, 1995; Derlega, Winstead, et al., 2002). Studies by Herek et al. (2002), for example, demonstrate that knowledge of HIV transmission and awareness of AIDS have both increased. Unfortunately, other aspects related to stigma, specifically the perception that individuals with HIV are responsible for their infection, may not have decreased (Herek et al., 2002). In the public perception there is still an association of HIV and AIDS with specific behaviors and groups (e.g., Herek et al., 2002; Kennedy & Fulton, 1998; Leary & Schreindorfer, 1998). The CDC (http://www.cdc.gov), among others, has invested tremendous effort in campaigns targeting HIV and AIDS perceptions and risk behaviors, but at present stigma persists. It is not possible to anticipate all the changes in stigma, but one possible outcome of both HAART and an AIDS vaccine might be to shift perception of HIV from a fatal to a chronic long-term illness. If such a change occurs, disclosure of HIV may become more similar to disclosure of other illnesses.

The emphasis of this book has been on HIV, but it is useful to consider how stigma affects other disclosure topics besides HIV. For example, to what degree does stigma influence decisions to disclose about sensitive topics such as epilepsy, sexual orientation, or rape? There are literally dozens, even hundreds, of health-related topics alone that people may choose to disclose about (beyond nonhealth topics such as a job change or financial difficulties; see Kelly, 2002; Wegner & Lane, 1995). Do the processes described for decision making about HIV apply in other contexts? The answer may lie in the degree of stigma. For example, it would seem comparatively easy to share with someone that you had a tooth filled compared with sharing that you have lupus (an autoimmune disorder) or sickle-cell anemia. The previous discussion of aspects of stigma may again be of use here. Three important considerations (among others) are the possibility of contagion, the severity, and finally the attributed role of responsibility for contracting the disease or illness. Take the case of the common cold, for example. For many, a cold is contagious, not severe (even temporary), and generally contracted without perception of responsibility. Today, lung cancer and STDs (and even unfortunately rape) are conditions in which people may be seen as having some responsibility for the "condition," and thus they may be less likely to disclose. The disclosure findings presented in this book can potentially be extended to other conditions, but HIV is unique in many ways—combining the type of illness (i.e., chronic, debilitating, stigmatizing), transmission mode (i.e., fluid exchange, sexual in nature, needle sharing), and populations affected (e.g., IDUs, MSM, etc.).

Related to stigma, people with HIV have concerns over who might find out or have access to their medical information, and new HIPAA standards mandate safeguards for storage, maintenance, transmission, and access to individual health information (Committee on Maintaining Privacy, 1997; Rada, 2002). HIPAA is a complex set of regulations with many parts, and it is important to recognize the difference between the recommendations and rules adopted. These national standards have the potential to better protect the privacy of medical information. With better safeguards in place, there may be some lessening of stigma-related concerns especially in disclosing to health care workers.

Relationships

One added consequence of changes in stigma is the attention to the relationships of individuals with HIV (e.g., Derlega & Barbee, 1998a; Derlega, Greene, et al., 2002; Kalichman, 2000). Individuals with HIV are living longer than earlier in the epidemic and must manage their relationships with those who know or do not know about their HIV diagnosis. If others do not know the diagnosis, the person with HIV must take care to monitor this information. If others are aware, another set of issues may arise such as caretaking, planning, and so on. In this book, we highlighted family relationships (including, e.g., parents and siblings), relationships with a partner or lover, friends, and children. We also discussed relationships with health care workers and coworkers or supervisors. Beyond all these important relationships, more work would be beneficial examining extended family disclosure and relationships such as to grandparents and aunts or uncles, as well as relations with health professionals and religious advisors.

FUTURE RESEARCH

The material presented in this book highlights the importance of continued examination of HIV disclosure. The outcomes—both for the individual and others—are significant. We present here specific areas for future research on HIV disclosure, disclosure, and CPM theory.

Future Research on HIV Disclosure

Some responses to HIV disclosure can be labeled unhelpful, and this should continue to be examined (Barbee et al., 1998; Derlega et al., in press; Ingram et al., 1999). For example, are individuals with HIV able to identify beforehand what kind of responses they would want to a disclosure, perhaps even to share this request with the other? Or is it the case that it becomes easier to identify unhelpful social support after the fact? More work understanding the perspective of the help provider would also be useful. Are people aware they are being unhelpful (or helpful) in their response, and what are the stressors experienced by support providers that make it difficult to render effective assistance (cf. Lehman et al., 1986)? What content of disclosure may be helpful or unhelpful? Even the form that HIV disclosure takes (e.g., silence, direct sharing, and misrepresentation) could in turn affect negative responses. Important questions still remain regarding social support, for example, the role of personal relationships in social support processes (Sarason et al., 1997).

At present there is extremely limited information available to couples about reproductive decisions when one or both of them have been diagnosed with HIV infection. With new HAART treatments, people may be more likely to choose to have children. If this is the case, does the couple make the decision together? Are both partners aware of the HIV diagnosis and the necessity for a mother with HIV (and later the child) to strictly adhere to the medication schedule so the child will not become infected (see Mofenson, 2002)? Are these children more likely to be told the parent's HIV diagnosis at a younger age? These are all questions that may be raised in the future.

The possibility of physical and sexual violence in response to HIV disclosure is especially troubling (e.g., Brown et al., 1994; Gielen et al., 1997; Kimerling et al., 1999; Rothenberg & Paskey, 1995; van der Straten, King, et al., 1998; but see Vlahov et al., 1998, for a different view of the effects of HIV disclosure on victimization). Some women—and several men—in our interviews reported either knowing of instances in which people were beaten in response to disclosing an HIV infection or fearing or experiencing this for themselves. This fear of violence will complicate recommendations to disclose to partners (see North & Rothenberg, 1993). Service providers must be aware of this potential and have resources to assist these women and men. There may be cases in same-sex relationships in which this violence also occurs. An additional report by several individuals was of HIV disclosure recipients (such as brothers or uncles) wanting to hurt the source of infection (Greene & Faulkner, 2002), and this should also be of concern and explored further.

The reports of relationship disruption after an HIV diagnosis should also be studied further. Individuals with HIV have reported fears that their relationships will break up (cf. Winstead et al., 2002). It is true, however, that starting new relationships is complicated and raises disclosure issues (e.g., Adam & Sears, 1994; Hatala et al., 1998; Klitzman, 1999). Many individuals with HIV inevitably begin or continue dating relationships and must consider both disclosure and decisions regarding sexual behavior (Winstead et al., 2002). The association of disclosure with decreased risky behavior may be a crucial mechanism to help stop the spread of HIV. If individuals with HIV disclose to their partners, there may be two people who, it is hoped, are working together to reinforce safer behavior. This relation between disclosure and risk behavior is complex, as some couples in which both are aware of the HIV infection continue to practice riskier behaviors.

The role of ethnicity and gender will also be relevant in HIV disclosure. The reports of different rates of HIV disclosure by gender and ethnicity were clear throughout the book. Women were most likely to be recipients of disclosure compared to men in roles of parent and sibling. This did not hold true for lovers or partners, as men may be more likely to be told by women (or perhaps there is no difference). At present, however, the conclusions are not definitive and warrant added consideration. In the same way, ethnicity affects HIV disclosure decisions, and this may still be tied to lingering (and incorrect) stereotypes in the United States of AIDS as a "gay, White man's disease" (see also immigration restrictions[1]). Minorities may have particular difficulty accessing support services and may disclose less if they perceive these stigmatizing beliefs about HIV. Other efforts could explore how different relational types affect HIV disclosure, for example, lesbians or people in open relationships (relationships in which partners may have sexual partners outside the relationship and this is known). Female to female sexual behavior risk for STDs is generally unrecognized (Bauer & Welles, 2001; Mays, 1996; Rich, Back, Tuomala, & Kazanjian, 1993; Troncoso, Romani, Carranza, Macias, &

---

[1]The U.S. Immigration and Naturalization Service (similar to some other countries) policy severely restricts immigration of people with HIV (see 1987 ban, modified in 1993 summary at www.amfar.org/cgi-bin/iowa/news). HIV infection is also a possible criterion to deport noncitizens, and in the wake of the September 11, 2001 attacks this may be an important issue as restrictions are tightened. Additionally, it is worthwhile noting the exclusions in all immigration policies of recognition of same-sex partnerships. For further information about immigration, see the American Foundation for AIDS Research Web site (www.amfar.org) section "News" (2001).

Masini, 1995). If women who have sex with women (WSWs) are at risk for contracting HIV but do not perceive themselves to be at risk (Bauer & Welles, 2001), this could interfere with disclosure processes in ways different from MSM or heterosexual women.

There is a need for expanded exploration for women and minorities and unique features of their coping with HIV. There is also little research with hemophiliacs and those infected through transfusions (many who were infected prior to blood screening for HIV implemented in March, 1985). It might be possible to target subgroups with tailored health prevention messages; unfortunately, this is not currently practiced to a large extent. Several content analyses of HIV public service announcements (PSAs) show they appeal to very broad audiences, missing this opportunity to segment to specific groups (e.g., DeJong, Wolf, & Austin, 2001; Freimuth, Hammond, Edgar, & Monahan, 1990). Further critiques of these public health efforts include absence of discussion of barriers to recommended behaviors such as condom use; the messages could address, for example, embarrassment or negotiation skills. This type of specific targeted message is more likely to have beneficial effects for disclosure.

Future Research on Disclosure

Research on disclosure itself must continue to expand to incorporate the complexities of this process. As Dindia (1997) noted, "disclosure is currently conceived of and studied as a static phenomenon" (p. 411). Disclosure is often studied as a one-shot event or even an individual personality trait. Research presented in this book does not lend support to either of those positions. There are further opportunities to explore levels of self-disclosure, moving beyond disclosure as a dichotomous one-time event. Disclosure—about HIV or some other topic—is not a single event; it is returned to, sometimes as part of an ongoing discussion. Beyond the process aspect, disclosure is not linear, as people may modify, change, and/or reframe previous comments. Perhaps the disclosure process occurs in phases or stages or through an unlayering process (see Altman & Taylor, 1973; Limandri, 1989). This kind of approach to disclosure lends itself to focus group research or interviews to better understand the interpersonal process perspective of disclosure. Additional longitudinal studies of disclosure and relationships would also be helpful.

Future Research on CPM

To understand the literature on disclosure and HIV, we used CPM theory that focuses on how people develop and use privacy rules to share or withhold information (Petronio, 2002). This theory has proved useful in determining the way that many people with HIV navigate making decisions about who, when, and how they should give access to the sensitive information about their health status. The theory of CPM is uniquely helpful in explaining not only the perceptions and development of privacy rules for disclosure but also expectations about the way others should treat the information once disclosed. There is still a great deal to be learned about how people coordinate their privacy boundaries so that each person linked into such a boundary can synchronize a collective regulation of the disclosure about a person's HIV status. Further research is needed to understand the successful coordination of privacy rules that all people within the boundary adhere to as well as when coordination fails. Because people often assume that others will use the same rules as they do, the person with HIV may not discuss the constraints of additional disclosures about the illness. There are many situations in which individuals do not coordinate third-party disclosures. However, not doing so sometimes means that trusts are violated and others are told about the disease without the consent of the person with HIV. This type of violation, or in CPM terms boundary turbulence, causes further difficulties for those who are living with HIV. Turbulence may erupt when individuals tell others about the illness even when they do not want to know, when family members are not told about the illness and feel entitled, or when people with HIV draw others into their confidence against their wishes. Because we know less about situations that lead to turbulence than we do about the reasons people might disclose, more research is needed.

Although there is a ready body of research about self-disclosure, taking a look at dyadic and family interactions has been less often considered. CPM gives us a ready way to examine how and why people coordinate disclosure occurrences, however, more research is needed to explore the way that coordination specifically works for people with HIV. When boundary coordination works well, all parties are able to endorse collectively determined privacy rules. Thus, when rules are synchronized, trust increases and those who are privy to the information about the illness can function as a reliable support system for the person with HIV. Future research is needed to determine how people can more effectively coordinate privacy boundaries and the rules governing disclosure to achieve the ultimate level of assistance needed from others. In addition, research is essential to understand the conditions under which those people linked into privacy boundaries surrounding information about someone's HIV status are unable to coordinate privacy rules. When rule violations take place and boundary turbulence results, we need to know why that happens, under what conditions these violations are likely to take place, and how we can implement change to help individuals with HIV achieve successful disclosure experiences. Through positive regulation of privacy boundaries, it is more likely that people with HIV will rely on others and tell them about the illness. In turn, they will benefit in being able to acquire the needed care to cope with the illness. Further, learning the best ways to manage privacy may also mean that the spread of this disease will decrease because those infected might be more able and willing to make decisions to disclose about the illness making it less detrimental to all parties. CPM theory offers a structure and process to organize the information we already know about HIV disclosure issues as we have seen in this book. For the future, CPM sets the stage for a more clearly identifiable way to address important and significant investigations into the puzzle of disclosure about HIV.

CONCLUSIONS

Throughout this book, we have highlighted how people balance the risks and benefits in decisions to disclose an HIV diagnosis. This is not an easy task; in fact it is a source of tremendous distress for those with HIV. As Vázquez-Pacheco (2000) noted, "it isn't really the time or the place that is the problem. It's the subject. Having that serostatus discussion is never easy" (p. 22). We have documented the beneficial effects of disclosing for both physical and psychological health as well as relationships. For some, however, the decision to disclose about the HIV diagnosis carries too much risk and they choose to be silent about their condition (Kelly, 2002). We recommend HIV disclosure to selected confidants if, after careful consideration, the possible physical and psychological benefits are perceived to outweigh the disadvantages.

Resources for Individuals Living With HIV, Their Significant Others, Researchers, and Health Professionals

The appendix of this book brings together a variety of resources for individuals living with HIV, their family and friends, and people who work with them. The book has described a number of ways to understand HIV disclosure decisions, disclosure messages, and disclosure outcomes; in the end, individuals with HIV continue to struggle with these disclosure choices. This appendix provides assistance with many issues related to HIV disclosure (e.g., coping, support, and self-advocacy). We hope that using the exercises, filling out the scales, or accessing other resources presented in this appendix may help individuals get in touch with issues influencing how well or poorly they may be coping with HIV. Researchers and students may also find the measures useful to further explore the disclosure area.

This appendix contains three major sections. The appendix first presents personal exercises and resources that have been adapted for use with HIV (see Table A.1). These exercises can be used by people with HIV to explore disclosure decisions. The second part of the appendix focuses on measures of disclosure-related variables referred to previously in chapters 2 to 4 (see Table A.2 for a list of tables A.3-A.20). The scales were developed for research comparing groups of people;

TABLE A.1
List of Personal Exercises Presented

Exercise	Page
Writing task	183
Recording task	184
Role playing	184
Thought listing	185

TABLE A.2

List of Measures Presented

Table	Measure	Page
A.3	Privacy and HIV Testing	187
A.4	Reasons For and Against HIV Disclosure	188
A.5	Disclosing Feelings Associated With HIV and/or AIDS Symptoms	190
A.6	Parental HIV Disclosure Interview (PDI) Format	191
A.7	Distress Disclosure Index (DDI)	192
A.8	Self-Disclosure in Conversation	193
A.9	Self-Concealment Scale (SCS)	194
A.10	Self-Perceptions of HIV Stigma	195
A.11	Stigma Impact of HIV	196
A.12	Unsupportive Social Interactions Inventory (USII)	198
A.13	Social Support Questionnaire (Short; SSQ6)	200
A.14	Stressors and Related Stress for HIV	202
A.15	Center for Epidemiologic Studies Depression Scale (CES–D)	204
A.16	Adequacy of Personal Resources	205
A.17	HIV Symptoms Scale/Functional Health Status	206
A.18	Multidimensional Health Locus of Control Scale (MHLC) Form C	208
A.19	Patient Self-Advocacy Scale (PSAS)	210
A.20	HIV Knowledge Questionnaire (HIV–K–Q)	211

nevertheless, it might still be beneficial for individuals to fill them out to assist in understanding how they are coping with HIV. Some technical information is presented with the description of scales for health professionals, researchers, and students. This information, however, should not affect the usefulness of the questionnaires for general readers. There may be methodological problems using and interpreting some scales (e.g., depression) unless certain issues are confronted (such as common overlap between measures of HIV physical symptoms and depression), which we point out for the readers. Finally, the third part of the appendix incorporates additional suggested readings, contact information (Web sites, magazines, journals, and toll-free numbers), and social artifacts (plays and films) for those who would like to explore further. The selection presented here is not exhaustive but represents some measures and exercises useful in the context of disclosure of an HIV diagnosis.

PERSONAL EXERCISES

Individuals with HIV struggle with issues related to disclosure, but to this point there have been limited resources to assist with this decision-making process. Four exercises are presented next: a writing task, a recording task, a role-playing exercise, and a thought listing technique. The use of imagined interactions provides a setting in which a person can practice disclosing information and examine the potential outcome (Rosenblatt & Meyer, 1986). The exercises are presented from the perspective of the person with HIV, but they can easily be adapted for partners, other family members, or friends of an individual with HIV. There are additional techniques used in therapy and support group contexts, but our focus here is on the personal resources for individuals with HIV.

Writing Task

Several researchers have demonstrated that disclosure of stressful experiences to oneself through writing may have physical and psychological benefits (Lepore & Smyth, 2002; Pennebaker, 1988, 1995; Smyth, 1998), and it may be useful for persons living with HIV. Journal writing is generally thought to be therapeutic; for example, parents encourage their children to write down their feelings as a way to understand and cope. Wiener and Figueroa (1998) presented stories and drawings by children with HIV, focusing on the therapeutic benefit of writing and drawing for children in particular. There is mixed research on the benefits of disclosure (via writing about facts and feelings about stressful experiences) compared with disclosure with a focus on writing about how to cope with one's difficulties. As Cameron and Nicholls (1998) stated, "Writing is therapeutic when participants write about their thoughts and emotions in ways that enable them to make sense of their experiences and to identify ways to resolve conflicts" (p. 84). Thus, the writing task presented focuses on both disclosure and coping with HIV. As a final qualification, disclosing to oneself by writing about stressful thoughts and feelings is not the same as disclosing to others about these experiences. There may be direct physical and psychological benefits of expressing previously inhibited thoughts and feelings, but disclosing as a part of writing tasks will not by itself gain the same socially mediated benefits of disclosure such as accessing social support or professional help.

This writing task is adapted from Pennebaker, Colder, and Sharp (1990), and Cameron and Nicholls (1998). The duration is 20 min. Supplies include paper, pencil, private space, and a timer.

Instructions.   This exercise will take about 20 min. For the first 15 min, let go and write about your very deepest thoughts and feelings about disclosing HIV-related problems and challenges. For the last 5 min, list three things that you can do that will help you deal with one or more of these problems or challenges.

Adaptations.

1. You can change the specific focus of the writing to issues such as social support for HIV, stigma related to HIV, and so forth.
2. You can think about the writing in terms of a specific target person, for example, a new sexual partner or a brother.

3. You can write for several days in a row, also changing the topic, target, re-reading, and refining your writing.
4. You can show this writing to another person and discuss it.

Use caution with the writing because another person could find it—regardless of whether or not you wanted them to have access to this private information.

Recording Task

Researchers have argued that speaking about feelings is much more powerful than writing about feelings (e.g., Kelley, Lumley, & Leisen, 1997), but this kind of exercise has not been studied with HIV. The motivation for such a task is similar to the writing task, but the recording task focuses more on experiencing the affect or feelings while talking about stressful experiences. Thus, the recording task presented next is similar to the first writing task. This task is adapted from Kelley et al. (1997). The duration is 15 min. Supplies include a recorder (audio or video), private space, and a timer.

Instructions. Talk into the audio recorder (or video recorder) for 15 min. Talk about an HIV disclosure-related trauma or upheaval that you may be experiencing right now or that you experienced at some other time. When you talk about the event, discuss the facts surrounding it, and talk about your deepest feelings related to the issue. Try to make your memories as vivid as possible, including thoughts, emotions, and bodily sensations that you experienced.

Adaptations.

1. You can change the specific focus of the talking to issues such as social support for HIV, stigma related to HIV, and so forth.
2. You can think about the talking in terms of a specific target person, for example, a new friend or a sister.
3. You can continue the talking exercise for several days in a row, also changing the topic, target, and refining the talking.
4. You can share the tape to another person and discuss it.

As before, use caution with the audio or video tape because another person could find it—regardless of whether or not you wanted them to have access to this private information.

Role Playing

Many health risk prevention programs now incorporate a role-playing component in their curriculum. For example, drug resistance programs such as "Just Say

No" and some abstinence-based programs have participants practice imagined behavior in a potentially risky situations (e.g., being offered drugs or dealing with a partner who desires more sexual intimacy than you do). We adapt this role play strategy to disclosure of HIV. The duration is 10 to 20 min. A private space is needed to role play with another person who knows your HIV diagnosis.

Instructions.   This exercise will take 10 to 20 min. First, select a target person to whom you want to practice disclosing (and think about how they might respond); share information with your practice partner so they will be able to "play" this role. Then, practice disclosing your HIV diagnosis; try to imagine your practice partner as the actual target or recipient. You can practice several times, targeting the disclosure to a few different individuals. The practice partner should try to respond to simulate actual disclosure.

Adaptations.

1. Write a letter to the target person disclosing your HIV diagnosis.
2. Practice disclosing with the role-playing partner reacting positively and negatively.
3. You may want to also practice asking a third party to disclose on your behalf (see chap. 3), practicing with the third person.

Thought Listing

Many therapists and mental health workers incorporate various forms of thought-listing techniques in treatment plans for clients. Table 1.1 and Table A.4 in this appendix present benefits and risks associated with disclosing an HIV diagnosis. Reviewing these lists may be useful if you have difficulty with this exercise. We adapt this thought-listing strategy to disclosure of HIV. The duration is 10 to 15 min. Supplies include paper, pencil, and private space.

Instructions.   This exercise will take about 10 to 15 min. First, select a target person (such as your father, daughter, or a coworker) to whom you want to think about disclosing your HIV diagnosis. Think specifically about how this person might respond or react to your sharing the HIV diagnosis. Take a sheet of paper and draw a line down the middle. Then label one side "benefits of telling" (or positives), and label the other side "risks of telling" (or negatives). Write down, on the appropriate side, all the good and bad things that could possibly come from sharing your diagnosis with this person.

Adaptations.

1. Think about another specific target person, for example, a new sexual partner or a cousin and repeat the exercise.

2. Take the lists and rank order each (most important to least important) and compare the benefits to risks.
3. Show the list to a person who knows your HIV diagnosis and discuss it.
4. Show the list to the target person and use it to discuss your HIV diagnosis.

Use caution with the list because another person could find it—regardless of whether or not you wanted them to have access to this private information.

MEASURES RELATED TO DISCLOSURE AND HIV

This second section presents measures or scales tapping many issues discussed in previous chapters. A list of the scales is provided in Table A.2, which lists tables A.3-A.20. Each scale is presented for ease of use. You can fill it out yourself, and directions for scoring are presented along with information about how individuals in previous studies have scored. You can talk about the questions with others or you could compare your responses with another person's. We provide a brief description of each measure, the source, and some information (if available) about previous use, including means. Information about psychometrics is presented for those who want to use the scale in research or other settings. The summary information for each measure is provided in the manner prepared by the authors of the scale to help in potential comparisons. If summed scores are reported, they can also be modified in terms of the original scale continuum, dividing by the number of points on the continuum.

A note of caution to readers who use these scales: Many of the scales presented in this appendix were developed for research on groups of individuals. It can be a useful exercise to complete the questionnaires, as this can provide some information. It is not appropriate, however, to diagnose oneself or make a diagnosis about someone based on an individual's score.

TABLE A.3
Privacy and HIV Testing

Please respond to the following statements about privacy and HIV and AIDS according to this scale:

1 = Strongly disagree
2 = Disagree
3 = Neutral
4 = Agree
5 = Strongly agree

_____ 1. Access to information about AIDS testing violates individuals' right to privacy.
_____ 2. Public good should come before individuals' right to privacy with regard to HIV testing.
_____ 3. If I were tested for AIDS, I believe that the information would remain confidential.
_____ 4. I would feel that my privacy had been invaded if I were asked if I had been tested for HIV.
_____ 5. I would feel my privacy had been invaded if I were asked if I tested HIV positive.

Note. Greene et al. (1993) examined attitudes toward privacy and HIV testing. Their sample ($N = 367$) consisted of college students, parents with young children, and parents with college age children. Individuals' perceptions of privacy predicted anticipated willingness to disclose results of HIV tests and specific knowledge of who has been HIV tested. The reliability reported by Greene et al. (1993) was .78. They reported the following means: college students, 3.55; parents with young children, 3.05; parents with college age children, 3.17. The measure was also significantly correlated with attitude toward homosexuality in Greene et al.'s (1993) study.

Scoring. The five items are summed and averaged (after recoding Item 2). Recoding, or reverse scoring, indicates the item is worded opposite the other items, so you have to adjust this score. To recode, 5 = 1, 4 = 2, 3 = 3, 2 = 4, and 1 = 5. After the recoding, sum and average the items (add them up and divide by 5 in this case). A higher score indicates more perceptions of protecting privacy for HIV information.

Description. This measure taps attitudes toward privacy and HIV testing information. It was developed with a sample of people not tested for HIV. The measure specifically addresses perceptions that access to information or asking about about HIV testing violates privacy.

From "Privacy, HIV Testing, and AIDS: College Students' Versus Parents' Perspectives," by K. Greene, R. Parrott, and J. M. Serovich, 1993, *Health Communication, 5*, p. 64. Copyright 1993 by Lawrence Erlbaum Associates, Inc.

Reasons For and Against HIV Disclosure

The following questionnaire examines your reasons for disclosing and not disclosing to someone about your HIV diagnosis. Think of someone you know but who does not already know about your HIV diagnosis. Indicate how much each statement might influence your decision to tell or not tell about the diagnosis.

1 = Not at all important
2 = Slightly important
3 = Moderately important
4 = Very important
5 = Extremely important

Reasons for Self-Disclosure

Catharsis
_____ 1. I didn't want to have to carry this information about inside me all by myself.
_____ 2. I would be able to get the information off my chest.
_____ 3. It would be "cathartic" (releasing pent-up feelings) to be able to tell my friend.

Duty to Inform / Educate
_____ 4. I felt obligated to tell my friend.
_____ 5. I didn't want to risk any health problems for me or my friend.
_____ 6. This person had the right to know what is happening to me.
_____ 7. I felt a sense of duty to tell my friend.
_____ 8. I wanted to prepare my friend for what might happen to me.
_____ 9. I wanted to educate my friend about what the disease is like.
_____ 10. My goal was to teach my friend about the disease.
_____ 11. I wanted to make sure that my friend knew how serious this disease is.

Test Other's Reactions
_____ 12. I wanted to see how my friend would feel about me after I told him or her.
_____ 13. I wanted to find out if my friend still wanted to be with me after I told him or her.
_____ 14. I wanted to see how my friend would react when I told him or her the information.

Close and Supportive Relationship
_____ 15. We loved one another.
_____ 16. We had a mutually supportive relationship.
_____ 17. We had a close relationship.
_____ 18. I trusted my friend.
_____ 19. My friend could be of help.
_____ 20. My friend would be able to provide support.
_____ 21. My friend would provide me with assistance.

Similarity
_____ 22. We had a lot in common.
_____ 23. We both had similar types of experiences.
_____ 24. We tended to think alike about things.

Reasons for Nondisclosure

Privacy
_____ 1. Some people have big mouths and my friend might go running around telling people.
_____ 2. Information about the diagnosis is my own private information.
_____ 3. I don't have to tell my friend if I don't want to.
_____ 4. I have a right to privacy.

(continued)

Self-Blame and Self-Concept Difficulties
_____ 5. I had difficulty accepting that I was HIV positive.
_____ 6. I felt ashamed about being HIV positive.
_____ 7. I felt bad about myself.

Communication Difficulties
_____ 8. I would get tongue-tied when I tried to say what happened.
_____ 9. I didn't know how to start telling my friend about the diagnosis.
_____ 10. I didn't know how to put into words what happened to me.
_____ 11. I just couldn't figure out how to talk about the diagnosis.

Fear of Rejection or Being Misunderstood
_____ 12. I was concerned that my friend wouldn't understand what I was going through.
_____ 13. I worried that my friend would no longer like me if he or she knew about my HIV diagnosis.
_____ 14. I was concerned about how my friend would feel about me after hearing the information.
_____ 15. I didn't feel my friend would be supportive.

Protecting the Other
_____ 16. I didn't want my friend to have to make sacrifices for me.
_____ 17. I didn't want to put my friend's life into an uproar.
_____ 18. I didn't want my friend to worry about me.
_____ 19. I didn't want my friend to experience any pain over things I was going through.

Superficial Relationship
_____ 20. Our relationship wasn't very serious.
_____ 21. We weren't very close to one another.
_____ 22. Our relationship was pretty casual.

Note. These statements are written with a friend as the prospective target for disclosure or nondisclosure. However, in the original research, the statements were written with a friend, intimate partner, and a parent as the prospective disclosure targets. You could easily fill out the scales with different individuals in mind. Derlega et al. (2002) sampled 145 (predominantly male) participants with HIV from several areas of the United States. They presented means for subscales and by gender.

Scoring. Items are summed and averaged to form scales for each type of reason. You can compare your scores across reasons for disclosure or nondisclosure or between subscales. Higher scores indicate a reason was more important for disclosing or not disclosing. The scale could be used to help individuals evaluate the pros and cons of disclosing to a specific person.

Description. This measure explores how much specific reasons might have influenced disclosing or not disclosing to a friend, intimate partner, and a parent. The statements focus on decision making when participants first learn of their HIV diagnosis, asking them to recall why they did or did not disclose.

TABLE A.5
Disclosing Feelings Associated With HIV and/or AIDS Symptoms

The following questions ask how much you have told your partner about the following issues. The responses for each question are the following:

$$1 = \text{Told partner nothing}$$
$$2 = \text{Told partner some things}$$
$$3 = \text{Told partner most things}$$
$$4 = \text{Told partner everything}$$

_____ 1. Frustration about not being able to do the things you want to do.

_____ 2. Anger because medical treatment was unable to help you enough.

_____ 3. Sad because you have HIV/AIDS at all or are currently ill.

_____ 4. Worry over changes in your physical appearance.

_____ 5. Sad that you have a chronic illness for which there is no cure.

_____ 6. Fear about the future course of disease (e.g., fear of dying).

_____ 7. Hopeless about your future.

Note. Druley, Stephens, and Coyne (1997) studied 74 heterosexual women with lupus. They examined the effect of illness episodes on intimacy and relationship satisfaction and described dilemmas in balancing intimacy and illness. Druley et al. reported women who disclosed more information and illness symptoms and women who concealed more information about feelings and symptoms experienced the highest negative affect. Disclosure of feelings was positively related to frequency and initiation of affectionate behavior. The reliability reported for the scale was .88 ($M = 2.3$) for the lupus sample. This measure of disclosure of feelings is adapted here for HIV.

Scoring. Items are summed and averaged to form one scale, with a higher score indicating more disclosure of feelings associated with HIV and AIDS symptoms. The scale can be used to form two measures (by adding an experiencing feelings column), one Experience of Feelings and the other Disclosure of Feelings. Also, it is possible to change the target of disclosure of feelings, for example from partner to sister, coworker, and so forth.

Description. This measure taps disclosure of feelings pertaining to HIV illness. It focuses on the positive and negative effects of disclosing feelings related to HIV symptoms.

From "Emotional and Physical Intimacy in Coping With Lupus: Women's Dilemmas of Disclosure and Approach," by J. A. Druley, M. A. P. Stephens, and J. C. Coyne, 1997, *Health Psychology, 16*, p. 509. Copyright 1997 by the American Psychological Association. Reprinted with permission.

TABLE A.6

Parental HIV Disclosure Interview (PDI) Format

Disclosure

Who did you tell first about your HIV infection?

Do any of the respondent's children know about her HIV infection?

Did you tell your child that you are HIV positive?

Have you told any of your children over 18 years of age about your HIV infection?

Plans for Children's Future

If you went to the hospital for a week or two right now, who would care for your children?

Have you asked anybody to make a commitment to take care of your children if you became too sick to care for them or if you passed away?

Please respond to the reasons for HIV disclosure and nondisclosure according to the following scale:

> 1 = Not important
> 2 = A little important
> 3 = Important
> 4 = Very important

Reasons for Disclosure

_____ 1. Child told because parent wants to make guardianship arrangements.

_____ 2. Child told because parent cannot bear to keep her HIV infection secret.

_____ 3. Child told because he or she will realize sooner or later that his or her parent is HIV infected.

Reasons for Nondisclosure

_____ 4. Child not told because parent does not want him or her to worry.

_____ 5. Child not told because he or she may not understand.

_____ 6. Child not told because he or she may not tell other people.

Note. Pilowsky, Sohler, and Susser (1999) studied parental disclosure of HIV to children and developed a standard interview measure, the PDI. The PDI was developed using a sample of 29 mothers with HIV (predominantly African American). They proposed using the PDI to assist mothers in making decisions about disclosure of HIV to children. Kappas reported ranged from .41 to 1.0 on test–retest about 1 week apart.

Scoring. No scoring was reported (it was developed as an interview guide), but reasons for disclosure and nondisclosure could be summed and averaged. This scale might be especially suited to generating discussion with another person about disclosure issues.

Description. The PDI was developed as an interview guide for parents and caregivers with HIV. The three disclosure sections focus on disclosure to spouse or parent and other adults, disclosure to children, and disclosure to adult children. The measure emphasizes family disclosure but does not contain a wide variety of family relationships. The scale also taps reasons, timing, and future plans for children. The scale could be adapted for use by fathers by changing some pronouns.

From "The Parent Disclosure Interview," by D. J. Pilowsky, N. Sohler, and E. Susser, 1999, AIDS Care, 11, p. 450. Copyright 1999 by Taylor & Francis, Ltd: http://www.tandf.co.uk/journals.

TABLE A.7
Distress Disclosure Index (DDI)

Please read each of the following items carefully. Indicate the extent to which you agree or disagree with each item according to the following rating scale:

1 = Strongly disagree
2 = Disagree
3 = Neutral
4 = Agree
5 = Strongly agree

_____ 1. When I feel upset, I usually confide in my friends.
_____ 2. I prefer not to talk about my problems.
_____ 3. When something unpleasant happens to me, I often look for someone to talk to.
_____ 4. I typically don't discuss things that upset me.
_____ 5. When I feel depressed or sad, I tend to keep those feelings to myself.
_____ 6. I try to find people to talk with about my problems.
_____ 7. When I am in a bad mood, I talk about it with my friends.
_____ 8. If I have a bad day, the last thing I want to do is talk about it.
_____ 9. I rarely look for people to talk with when I am having a problem.
_____ 10. When I'm distressed I don't tell anyone.
_____ 11. I usually seek out someone to talk to when I am in a bad mood.
_____ 12. I am willing to tell others my distressing thoughts.

Note. The DDI described by Kahn and Hessling (2001) was validated with several samples of undergraduate college students (see also Kahn, Achter, & Shambaugh, 2001). Reliabilities for the DDI have ranged from .92 to .95 in several studies, and the scale is unidimensional. The DDI also showed stability across 2 months. Means are higher for women (42.2) than men (36.6). The DDI is associated with changes in self-esteem, life satisfaction, and perceived social support, but it has not yet been applied specifically in a health sample.

Scoring. The twelve items are summed and averaged (after recoding Items 2, 4, 5, 8, 9, and 10). Recoding, or reverse scoring, indicates the item is worded opposite the other items, so you have to adjust this score. To recode, $5 = 1, 4 = 2, 3 = 3, 2 = 4$, and $1 = 5$. After the recoding, sum the items (add them up), with a possible score ranging from 12 to 60. A higher score reflects more tendency to disclose distress.

Description. The DDI is a measure of a unidimensional construct tapping concealment versus disclosure of distress. One important conclusion regarding distress disclosure was that statistical models show concealment and disclosure of distress are not separate dimensions. The DDI includes several content areas (and has equally positively and negatively worded items): if disclosure was proactive or reactive, disclosure audiences, severity of distress, and type of distress.

From "Measuring the Tendency to Conceal Versus Disclose Psychological Distress," by J. H. Kahn and R. M. Hessling, 2001, *Journal of Social and Clinical Psychology, 20,* p. 62. Copyright 2001 by The Guilford Press.

TABLE A.8

Self-Disclosure in Conversation

Think of a same-sex friend and a same-sex stranger. Indicate for the items following the extent to which you have disclosed to each person:

0 = No discussion of topic
1 = Little discussion
2 = Some discussion
3 = A lot of discussion
4 = Full and complete discussion

	Same-sex friend	Same-sex stranger
1. My personal habits.	_____	_____
2. Things I have done which I feel guilty about.	_____	_____
3. Things I wouldn't do in public.	_____	_____
4. My deepest feelings.	_____	_____
5. What I like and dislike about myself.	_____	_____
6. What is important to me in life.	_____	_____
7. What makes me the person I am.	_____	_____
8. My worst fears.	_____	_____
9. Things I have done which I am proud of.	_____	_____
10. My close relationships with other people.	_____	_____

Note. Miller, Berg, and Archer (1983) developed the Self-Disclosure in Conversation Scale using 740 undergraduate college students. The scale was unidimensional with good reliability ($\alpha = .93$, test–retest = .69). There were both gender and target differences, with most disclosure to women friends ($M = 27.85$), next highest to men friends ($M = 23.01$), less disclosure to men strangers ($M = 15.65$), and least to women strangers ($M = 15.04$).

Scoring. You can obtain your overall self-disclosure score for each target person by adding up the scores across the 10 items (separate for friend and stranger). The higher the score the more likely you have disclosed to the target person. If a large number of individuals filled out the questionnaire, it might be possible to test some questions about differences in self-disclosure to friends and strangers. You could also examine gender differences by comparing disclosure to same and opposite gender friend (or stranger).

Description. The Self-Disclosure in Conversation Scale is useful for examining self-reports of disclosure to various persons including the gender and the level of acquaintance of a possible disclosure recipient. It could also be used to examine self-disclosure to other potential target persons such as to friends, family, coworkers, health professionals, and intimate partners.

From "Openers: Individuals Who Elicit Intimate Self-Disclosure," by L. C. Miller, J. H. Berg, and R. L. Archer, 1983, *Journal of Personality and Social Psychology, 44*, p. 1236. Copyright 1983 by the American Psychological Association. Reprinted with permission.

TABLE A.9
Self-Concealment Scale (SCS)

Please respond to these items according to the following scale:

1 = Strongly disagree
2 = Disagree
3 = Neutral
4 = Agree
5 = Strongly agree

_____ 1. I have an important secret that I haven't shared with anyone.
_____ 2. If I shared all my secrets with my friends, they'd like me less.
_____ 3. There are lots of things about me that I keep to myself.
_____ 4. Some of my secrets have really tormented me.
_____ 5. When something bad happens to me, I tend to keep it to myself.
_____ 6. I'm often afraid I'll reveal something I don't want to.
_____ 7. Telling a secret often backfires and I wish I hadn't told it.
_____ 8. I have a secret that is so private I would lie if anybody asked me about it.
_____ 9. My secrets are too embarrassing to share with others.
_____10. I have negative thoughts about myself that I never share with anyone.

Note. Larson and Chastain (1990) examined the construct of self-concealment separate from self-disclosure. They reported psychometrics for the new scale (SCS). The 10 items form three areas; keeping things to self, distressing secret, and apprehension. Reliability overall was $\alpha = .83$ with three different samples ($N = 306$; mailed to a human service worker list, distributed at a professional training conference, and given to graduate psychology students). Means for items ranged from 2.33 (Item 6) to 3.00 (Item 3), with an overall summed $M = 25.92$.

Scoring. The 10 items are summed to form one scale, with a higher score indicating more self-concealment or less sharing.

Description. The variable taps active concealment from others of information one sees as negative or distressing. The scale refers to self-reported tendency to keep things to self, possession of a distressing secret that is not shared, and apprehension about disclosure of concealed information. The SCS is distinct from self-disclosure but correlated with anxiety, depression, and symptoms.

From "Self-concealment: Conceptualization, Measurement, and Health Implications," by D. G. Larson and R. L. Chastain, 1990, *Journal of Social and Clinical Psychology, 9,* p. 445. Copyright 1990 by The Guilford Press.

TABLE A.10
Self-Perceptions of HIV Stigma

Indicate for the statements following how living with HIV has influenced the way in which you feel, think, and behave. Give yourself a score of 1 to 4 for each statement:

> 1 = Not at all
> 2 = Rarely
> 3 = Sometimes
> 4 = Often

_____ 1. Felt blamed by others for having HIV.
_____ 2. Felt ashamed of having HIV.
_____ 3. Thought HIV was punishment for things done in past.
_____ 4. Feared I would lose my job if someone found out.
_____ 5. Felt compelled to change residence because I am HIV positive.
_____ 6. Avoided getting treatment because someone might find out.
_____ 7. Feared people would hurt my family if they learned I am HIV positive.
_____ 8. Thought other people were uncomfortable being with me.
_____ 9. Felt people avoided me because I am HIV positive.
_____ 10. Feared I would lose friends if they learned I am HIV positive.
_____ 11. Feared my family would reject me if they learned I am HIV positive.
_____ 12. Felt I wouldn't get as good health care if people learned I am HIV positive.
_____ 13. People who know I am HIV positive treat me with kid gloves.

Note. Sowell et al. (1997) examined adequacy of resources and stigma in a sample of 82 rural women with HIV (predominantly African Americans in Georgia). Half of the women reported feeling stigmatized, yet they disclosed highly.

Scoring. Scoring was not reported (they reported frequencies by item). The items could be summed or summed and averaged. You can obtain an overall score on perceptions of HIV stigma by adding up the scores across the 13 items. The higher the score, the more likely someone perceives themselves as stigmatized living with HIV. It might be useful in a group discussion to have a number of individuals complete the questionnaire and then discuss to what degree individuals might feel stigmatized living with an HIV positive diagnosis. There is no absolute meaning to a particular individual's score on the questionnaire. The HIV stigma scores would be useful in comparing responses across a large number of individuals who might complete the questionnaire.

Description. The variable taps self perception of HIV stigma. Sowell et al. (1997) did not report factor structure or groupings of items into dimensions.

From "Resources, Stigma, and Patterns of Disclosure in Rural Women with HIV Infection," by R. L. Sowell, A. Lowenstein, L. Moneyham, A. Demi, Y. Mizumo, and B. F. Seals, 1997, *Public Health Nursing, 14,* p. 308. Copyright 1997 by Blackwell Science, Inc. Reprinted by permission of Blackwell Science, Inc.

Stigma Impact of HIV

Please respond to the following statements regarding your experience with HIV according to the following scale:

$$1 = \text{Strongly disagree}$$
$$2 = \text{Disagree}$$
$$3 = \text{Agree}$$
$$4 = \text{Strongly agree}$$

Experiences of Rejection and Stigma

Social Rejection

_____ 1. My employer/co-workers have discriminated against me.

_____ 2. Some people act as though I am less competent than usual.

_____ 3. I feel I have been treated with less respect than usual by others.

_____ 4. I feel others are concerned they could "catch" my illness through contact like a handshake or eating food I prepare.

_____ 5. I feel others avoid me because of my illness.

_____ 6. Some family members have rejected me because of my illness.

_____ 7. I feel some friends have rejected me because of my illness.

_____ 8. I encounter embarrassing situations as a result of my illness.

_____ 9. Due to my illness others seem to feel awkward and tense when they are around me.

Financial Insecurity

_____ 10. I have experienced financial hardship that has affected how I feel about myself.

_____ 11. My job security has been affected by my illness.

_____ 12. I have experienced financial hardship that has affected my relationship with others.

Social Psychological Feelings Regarding Stigma

Internalized Shame

_____ 13. I feel others think I am to blame for my illness.

_____ 14. I do not feel I can be open with others about my illness.

_____ 15. I fear someone telling others about my illness without my permission.

_____ 16. I feel I need to keep my illness a secret.

_____ 17. I feel I am at least partially to blame for my illness.

Social Isolation

_____ 18. I feel set apart from others who are well.

_____ 19. I have a greater need than usual for reassurance that others care about me.

_____ 20. I feel lonely more often than usual.

_____ 21. Due to my illness, I have a sense of being unequal in my relationships with others.

_____ 22. I feel less competent than I did before my illness.

_____ 23. Due to my illness, I sometimes feel useless.

_____ 24. Changes in my appearance have affected my social relationships.

Note. Fife and Wright (2000) examined the impact of stigma by illness (cancer vs. HIV). They specifically looked at how stigma affects self-esteem, body image, and personal control. Their sample included 130 people with HIV (pre- dominantly male) and 76 cancer patients. Reported reliability ranged

(continued)

from .85 to .90 on the subscales. For the HIV sample, the means and reliabilities were Social Rejection, $M =$ 19.95, $\alpha = .90$; Financial Insecurity, $M = 8.12$, $\alpha = .86$; Internalized Shame, $M = 13.74$, $\alpha = .85$; and Social Isolation, $M = 13.74$, $\alpha = .85$. The HIV sample scored significantly higher than the cancer sample on each of the 24 items except one (No. 24, changes in appearance). The four subscales are correlated (with a range), but there are indicators of four distinct dimensions.

Scoring. The items are summed for each of the four subscales providing four stigma scores. Because the subscales contain different number of items, it is difficult to compare across the subscales. If, however, you sum and average each subscale score, then you can compare across the four to see which subdimension is highest. Higher scores indicate more perceived HIV stigma.

Description. This measure looks at the impact of HIV as a stigmatizing condition. The scale measures the social and personal consequences of living with the HIV positive diagnosis. The scale focuses of four aspects of being stigmatized by HIV, including social rejection, financial insecurity, internalized shame, and social isolation.

From "The Dimensionality of Stigma: A Comparison of Its Impact on the Self of Persons with HIV/AIDS and Cancer," by B. L. Fife and E. R. Wright, 2000, *Journal of Health and Social Behavior, 41*, p. 57. Copyright 2000 by American Sociological Association.

TABLE A.12

Unsupportive Social Interactions Inventory (USII)

Rate how much of this reaction you have received:

0 = None
1 = A little
2 = Some
3 = Quite a bit
4 = A lot

Insensitivity

_____ 1. After becoming aware of my having HIV, someone avoided me or had less contact than usual.

_____ 2. Acted cold, aloof or nasty toward me.

_____ 3. Understood it was a difficult situation, but did not understand how much of an impact it was having on me.

_____ 4. Talked with another person about it, in spite of my request for confidentiality or without checking with me first.

_____ 5. From voice tone, expression or body language, I got the feeling he/she was uncomfortable talking about my having HIV.

_____ 6. Outlook about my having HIV was so pessimistic/depressing that it made me feel even worse.

Disconnecting

_____ 7. When I was talking about my having HIV, person didn't give me enough time, or made me feel like I should hurry.

_____ 8. Refused to provide the type of help/support I was asking for.

_____ 9. Changed the subject before I wanted to.

_____ 10. Didn't seem to know what to say, or seemed afraid of saying/doing the "wrong" thing.

_____ 11. Felt that I was over-reacting.

_____ 12. Didn't seem to want to hear about it.

Forced Optimism

_____ 13. Felt that I should focus on present and/or future, and should forget about what's happened and get on with my life.

_____ 14. Told me to be strong, to keep my chin up, or that I shouldn't let it bother me.

_____ 15. Tried to cheer me up when I wasn't ready to.

_____ 16. Said I should look on the bright side.

_____ 17. Felt that it could've been worse or wasn't as bad as I thought.

_____ 18. Felt that I should stop worrying about having HIV and just forget about it.

Blaming

_____ 19. Told me that I had gotten myself into the situation in the first place, and now must deal with the consequences.

_____ 20. "I told you so," or similar comment.

_____ 21. Blamed me, tried to make me feel responsible for having HIV.

_____ 22. Seemed disappointed in me.

_____ 23. Asked "why" questions about my role in having HIV.

_____ 24. Discouraged me from expressing feelings such as anger, hurt or sadness.

Note. Ingram et al. (1999) studied negative social interactions, developing the USII using a sample of 271 individuals with HIV (predominantly White men). They reported four dimensions to the USII:

(continued)

insensitivity ($M = 1.35$), disconnecting ($M = 1.13$), forced optimism ($M = 1.44$), and blaming ($M = .86$). Final reliabilities for the dimensions ranged from .77 to .89. The USII predicts depression beyond physical functioning and social support.

Scoring.   Scores on each of the four subscales are summed and averaged with a higher score indicating more received negative or unsupportive social interactions.

Description.   The USII examines HIV as a stressful life event and is stressor specific. It looks at the nature and effects of negative social interactions. The USII is designed to assess upsetting responses a person receives from others who know about someone's HIV positive diagnosis.

From "Social Support and Unsupportive Social Interactions: Their Association with Depression Among People Living with HIV," by K. M. Ingram, D. A. Jones, R. J. Fass, J. L. Neidig, and Y. S. Song, 1999, *AIDS Care, 11*, p. 320. Copyright 1999 by Taylor & Francis, Ltd: http://www.tandf.co.uk/journals.

TABLE A.13
Social Support Questionnaire (Short; SSQ6)

The following questions ask you about individuals in your environment who provide you with help or support. Each question has two parts. For the first part, list all the individuals you know, excluding yourself, whom you can count on for help or support in the manner described. Give the person's initials and their relationship to you (e.g., brother, coworker). For the second part, rate how satisfied you are with the overall support you have. If you have no support for a question, check "No one" but still rate your level of satisfaction. Do not list more than nine persons per question.

1. Who can you really count on to distract you from your worries when you feel under stress?

No one
1. _____ 4. _____ 7. _____
2. _____ 5. _____ 8. _____
3. _____ 6. _____ 9. _____

How satisfied?

Very satisfied	Fairly satisfied	A little satisfied	A little dissatisfied	Fairly dissatisfied	Very dissatisfied
6	5	4	3	2	1

2. Who can you really count on to help you feel more relaxed when you are under pressure or tense?

No one
1. _____ 4. _____ 7. _____
2. _____ 5. _____ 8. _____
3. _____ 6. _____ 9. _____

How satisfied?

Very satisfied	Fairly satisfied	A little satisfied	A little dissatisfied	Fairly dissatisfied	Very dissatisfied
6	5	4	3	2	1

3. Who accepts you totally, including both your worst and your best points?

No one
1. _____ 4. _____ 7. _____
2. _____ 5. _____ 8. _____
3. _____ 6. _____ 9. _____

How satisfied?

Very satisfied	Fairly satisfied	A little satisfied	A little dissatisfied	Fairly dissatisfied	Very dissatisfied
6	5	4	3	2	1

4. Who can you really count on to care about you, regardless of what is happening to you?

No one
1. _____ 4. _____ 7. _____
2. _____ 5. _____ 8. _____
3. _____ 6. _____ 9. _____

How satisfied?

Very satisfied	Fairly satisfied	A little satisfied	A little dissatisfied	Fairly dissatisfied	Very dissatisfied
6	5	4	3	2	1

(continued)

TABLE A.13
(continued)

5. Who can you really count on to help you feel better when you are feeling generally down-in-the dumps?

No one   1. _____ 4. _____ 7. _____

              2. _____ 5. _____ 8. _____

              3. _____ 6. _____ 9. _____

How satisfied?

Very satisfied	Fairly satisfied	A little satisfied	A little dissatisfied	Fairly dissatisfied	Very dissatisfied
6	5	4	3	2	1

6. Who can you count on to console you when you are very upset?

No one   1. _____ 4. _____ 7. _____

              2. _____ 5. _____ 8. _____

              3. _____ 6. _____ 9. _____

How satisfied?

Very satisfied	Fairly satisfied	A little satisfied	A little dissatisfied	Fairly dissatisfied	Very dissatisfied
6	5	4	3	2	1

Note. I. Sarason, Levine, Basham, and B. Sarason (1983) conducted a series of studies to develop the original Social Support Questionnaire. The original 27-item scale has extensive psychometric information using college samples (reliability = .94), and presented here is the short version (SSQ6). Mean for Number (N) = 4.25, mean for Satisfaction (S) = 5.38. The SSQ6 (Sarason, Sarason, Shearin, & Pierce, 1987) has also been used with an HIV positive sample (Ingram et al., 1999) with reported mean for N = 4.71 and mean for S = 4.58 (note the lower satisfaction with HIV but similar availability or N).

Scoring. There are two scores created from the SSQ6. First, the N (number) score is created by summing all the persons listed (across each question). The total N score is divided by 6. The S is created by summing and averaging the six satisfaction scores. A higher N indicates more support people available, and a higher S score indicates more satisfaction with social support.

Description. The SSQ6 taps global perceptions of available social support in a variety of situations. It assesses the number of people participants believe they can rely on and satisfaction with social support available in that situation.

From "A Brief Measure of Social Support: Practical and Theoretical Implications," by I. G. Sarason, B. R. Sarason, E. N. Shearin, and G. R. Pierce, 1987, *Journal of Social and Personal Relationships, 4,* p. 503. Copyright 1987 by Sage Publications Ltd. Reprinted by permission of Sage Publications Ltd.

Stressors and Related Stress for HIV

Check which of the following items have happened to you in the past month (Yes/No). If the event occurred, rate how much it stressed you:

$1 =$ Not at all stressful
$2 =$ Caused only a very little stress or worry
$3 =$ Moderately stressful
$4 =$ Very stressful
$5 =$ Exceptionally stressful and difficult to deal with

Relationship Stressors

Happened? Stressed?

Yes/No	_____	1. Problems in relationship with spouse or lover.
Yes/No	_____	2. Problems with family.
Yes/No	_____	3. Problems in relationship with friends.
Yes/No	_____	4. Revealed HIV status to friend, family, or lover.
Yes/No	_____	5. Sexual difficulties.
Yes/No	_____	6. Break-up of friendship.
Yes/No	_____	7. Friend/lover diagnosed as HIV positive.
Yes/No	_____	8. Break-up of relationship with spouse or lover.
Yes/No	_____	9. Having no sex.
Yes/No	_____	10. Not having a partner.

Medical Care Stressors

Happened? Stressed?

Yes/No	_____	11. Bureaucratic (red tape) problems.
Yes/No	_____	12. Problems with health care provider.
Yes/No	_____	13. Lost health insurance.
Yes/No	_____	14. Changed physician.
Yes/No	_____	15. Getting to/waiting for medical appointments.
Yes/No	_____	16. Problems with medication.

Grief/Illness of Others

Happened? Stressed?

Yes/No	_____	17. Illness of close friend.
Yes/No	_____	18. Death of close friend.
Yes/No	_____	19. Stresses of caregiving.
Yes/No	_____	20. Illness of family member.
Yes/No	_____	21. Death of family member.
Yes/No	_____	22. Death of spouse or lover.
Yes/No	_____	23. Dealing with a suicidal friend.

Financial/Housing Stressors

Happened? Stressed?

Yes/No	_____	24. Financial problems.
Yes/No	_____	25. Decrease in income.
Yes/No	_____	26. Moved to a new residence.
Yes/No	_____	27. Lost job.
Yes/No	_____	28. Lost housing.

(continued)

TABLE A.14
(continued)

Job-Related Stressors

Happened? Stressed?

Yes/No	_____	29. Problems at work.
Yes/No	_____	30. Problems with co-workers.

Other Stressors

Happened? Stressed?

Yes/No	_____	31. Time management problems.
Yes/No	_____	32. Trying to keep up your appearance so you don't look sick.
Yes/No	_____	33. Other (please list) _____

Note. Thompson et al. (1996) studied stressors in 105 men with HIV. They reported relationship, finance, and illness of others were most closely associated with depression for men with HIV. Increased stress was also associated with increased alcohol consumption. Their scale taps negative life events with five areas: relationships, medical care, grief or illness of others, finance or housing, and work. They report an average 6.5 strains and perceived stress 2.4 (one point higher than Cohen & Williamson 1988 for men in a general population). People with more stressors and distress were somewhat more likely to engage in unhealthy practices. Remember when comparing means, the scale presented here includes seven added items suggested by Thompson et al. (items 10, 15, 16, 23, 31–33).

Scoring. Two scores are computed after summing: a number score (did this happen to you, 1 point for each "Yes") and how much it stressed. A higher number or strain score indicates more stressors experienced, and a higher perceived stress score indicates the stressor affected you more.

Description. A major illness is a source of a great deal of stress. The measure focuses on negative events that might be linked to living with HIV.

From "The Stressors and Stress of Being HIV-Positive," by S. C. Thompson, C. Nanni, and A. Levine, 1996, *AIDS Care*, 8, p. 9. Copyright 1996 by Taylor & Francis, Ltd: http://www.tandf.co.uk/journals.

Center for Epidemiologic Studies Depression Scale (CES–D)

Below is a list of the ways you might have felt or behaved recently. Please report how often you have felt this way during the past week. During the past week I was:

> 0 = Rarely or none of the time (less than 1 day)
> 1 = Some or a little of the time (1–2 days)
> 2 = Occasionally or a moderate amount of time (3–4 days)
> 3 = Most or all of the time (5–7 days)

_____ 1. I was bothered by things that usually don't bother me.
_____ 2. I did not feel like eating; my appetite was poor.
_____ 3. I felt that I could not shake off the blues even with help from my family or friends.
_____ 4. I felt that I was just as good as other people.*
_____ 5. I had trouble keeping my mind on what I was doing.
_____ 6. I felt depressed.
_____ 7. I felt that everything I did was an effort.
_____ 8. I felt hopeful about the future.*
_____ 9. I thought my life had been a failure.*
_____ 10. I felt fearful.
_____ 11. My sleep was restless.
_____ 12. I was happy.*
_____ 13. I talked less than usual.*
_____ 14. I felt lonely.*
_____ 15. People were unfriendly.*
_____ 16. I enjoyed life.*
_____ 17. I had crying spells.*
_____ 18. I felt sad.*
_____ 19. I felt that people dislike me.*
_____ 20. I could not get "going."

Note. Radloff (1977) developed the CES–D to measure current frequency of depressive symptoms; the measure emphasizes depressive mood or affect. Radloff reported reliability (α = .90, test–retest lower) and validity information for the CES–D. It was initially used to compare psychiatric patients with a household sample, but it has also been used with HIV (Kalichman et al., 2000). The CES–D and Beck Depression Inventory (Beck & Steer, 1993) are the most widely used measurement instruments to assess depression. The asterisk indicates an item tapping a cognitive-affective subscale of the CES–D according to Kalichman et al. (2000). Kalichman et al.'s (2000) study focused on the overlap between symptoms of HIV disease and measures of depression. They demonstrated that depression scores can be artificially inflated for people with HIV. Based on the results, they suggested using only the Cognitive-Affective subscale (items with *) to avoid this overlap (removing the somatic items). Reliability was adequate (α = .81) for this 11-item subscale (M = .94) (see also chap. 5).

Scoring. The 20 items are summed (possible range 0–60) after recoding (reverse scoring) items 4, 8, 12, and 16. To recode these items, 3 = 0, 2 = 1, 1 = 2, and 0 = 3, and use these new scores when adding up all items. Higher scores indicate more depressive symptoms.

Description. The CES–D taps depression in the general population, not just in a clinical sample. It is designed to assess mild depression, not just severe depression.

From "The CES–D Scale: A Self-Report Depression Scale for Research in the General Population," by L. S. Radloff, 1977, *Applied Psychological Measurement, 1,* p. 387. Copyright 1977 by Sage Publications, Inc. Reprinted by permission of Sage Publications, Inc.

TABLE A.16
Adequacy of Personal Resources

The following items ask about your access to things. Please respond using the following scale:

$$1 = \text{Always adequate}$$
$$2 = \text{Sometimes adequate}$$
$$3 = \text{Not at all adequate}$$

_____ 1. Food for two meals/day.
_____ 2. Clothing.
_____ 3. Housing.
_____ 4. Heating.
_____ 5. Telephone.
_____ 6. Dependable transportation.
_____ 7. Day care/child care.
_____ 8. Money to pay bills.
_____ 9. Medical care.
_____ 10. Dental care.

Note. Sowell et al. (1997) examined adequacy of resources and stigma in a sample of 82 rural women with HIV (predominantly African Americans in Georgia). The majority of women reported adequate resources, but there was a group in which basic needs were not adequate (and this was worse for women with HIV and not AIDS). Sowell et al. reported percentages by item for the personal resources scale but not means.

Scoring. Scoring is not reported, but the items could be summed (or summed and averaged) with a lower score indicating more access to resources. Thus, a higher score reflects poorer functioning or resources.

Description. This measure assesses what resources are available (e.g., money, medical care, and personal products) in living with HIV. With stressful health situations it is important to determine if basic needs are met.

From "Resources, Stigma, and Patterns of Disclosure in Rural Women with HIV Infection," by R. L. Sowell, A. Lowenstein, L. Moneyham, A. Demi, Y. Mizuno, and B. F. Seals, 1997, *Public Health Nursing, 14,* p. 307. Copyright 1997 by Blackwell Science, Inc. Reprinted by permission of Blackwell Science, Inc.

HIV Symptoms Scale and Functional Health Status

This scale includes two subscales: Frequency and Interference. For Frequency (the first column), respond according to how often you have experienced each of the following symptoms during the past 2 weeks. For interference (second column), respond according to how much each symptom has bothered you during the past 2 weeks. Both columns use the following scale:

1 = Not at all
2 = Somewhat
3 = Most of the time
4 = All of the time

Frequency	Interference	
_____	_____	1. Decreased sleep.
_____	_____	2. Increased sleep.
_____	_____	3. Diarrhea.
_____	_____	4. Constipation.
_____	_____	5. Nausea.
_____	_____	6. Vomiting.
_____	_____	7. Weight loss.
_____	_____	8. Weight gain.
_____	_____	9. Decreased appetite.
_____	_____	10. Increased appetite.
_____	_____	11. Pain (any type).
_____	_____	12. Fevers.
_____	_____	13. Coughing.
_____	_____	14. Difficulty swallowing.
_____	_____	15. Breathing difficulties.
_____	_____	16. Sore throat/mouth.
_____	_____	17. Skin changes (rashes, blisters, etc.).
_____	_____	18. Visual problems.
_____	_____	19. Difficulty concentrating.
_____	_____	20. Tire easily.
_____	_____	21. Hair loss.
_____	_____	22. Numbness/tingling in hands, feet, etc.
_____	_____	23. Urinary difficulties.
_____	_____	24. Decreased ability to walk.
_____	_____	25. Decreased ability to do self-care activities (bathe, comb hair, cook, etc.).
_____	_____	26. Inability to drive a car.
_____	_____	27. Decreased activities outside home.
_____	_____	28. Difficulty with memory.
_____	_____	29. Problems with sexual functioning.
_____	_____	30. Night sweats.
_____	_____	31. Memory loss/forgetfulness.

Note. Fife and Wright (2000) examined the impact of stigma by illness (cancer vs. HIV). They specifically looked at how stigma affects self-esteem, body image, and personal control. Their sample included 130 people with HIV and/or AIDS (predominantly male) and 76 cancer patients. Reported reliability for Frequency was .87 (M HIV = 51.1, M cancer = 49.5) and .90 for Interference (M HIV = 52.3, M cancer = 48.6). The measure is more than a list of frequency or presence of symptoms because it includes participants' subjective perceptions

(continued)

of the severity of symptoms. Note the similarity in Frequency scores by disease but the higher Interference score for HIV. We speculate that interference could increase with HIV symptoms and disease course.

Scoring. Two scores are created, a Frequency and an Interference score. For frequency, sum the numbers in column 1 (possible range 31–124). For interference, sum the numbers in column 2 (possible range 31–124). Higher scores for both indicate more frequency or interference of HIV symptoms.

Description. The measure taps participants' frequency and subjective perceptions of the severity of their HIV symptoms. It is a measure of functional health status or a symptomatology scale that may affect participation in social life and social interactions.

From "The Dimensionality of Stigma: A Comparison of Its Impact on the Self of Persons With HIV/AIDS and Cancer," by B. L. Fife and E. R. Wright, 2000, *Journal of Health and Social Behavior, 41*, p. 64. Copyright 2000 by American Sociological Association.

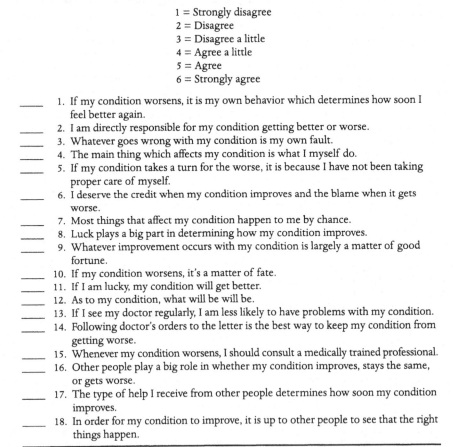

TABLE A.18
Multidimensional Health Locus of Control Scale (MHLC) Form C

Each item following is a belief statement about your medical condition (HIV and/or AIDS) with which you may agree or disagree. Beside each statement is a scale that ranges from 1 (*Strongly disagree*) to 6 (*Strongly agree*). For each item we would like you to record the number that represents the extent to which you agree or disagree with that statement. The more you agree with a statement, the higher will be the number you write. The more you disagree with a statement, the lower will be the number you write. Please make sure that you answer every item and that you record only one number per item. This is a measure of your personal beliefs; obviously, there are no right or wrong answers. Remember, when you see "condition," think HIV and/or AIDS in responding to each of the items.

$$1 = \text{Strongly disagree}$$
$$2 = \text{Disagree}$$
$$3 = \text{Disagree a little}$$
$$4 = \text{Agree a little}$$
$$5 = \text{Agree}$$
$$6 = \text{Strongly agree}$$

_____ 1. If my condition worsens, it is my own behavior which determines how soon I feel better again.

_____ 2. I am directly responsible for my condition getting better or worse.

_____ 3. Whatever goes wrong with my condition is my own fault.

_____ 4. The main thing which affects my condition is what I myself do.

_____ 5. If my condition takes a turn for the worse, it is because I have not been taking proper care of myself.

_____ 6. I deserve the credit when my condition improves and the blame when it gets worse.

_____ 7. Most things that affect my condition happen to me by chance.

_____ 8. Luck plays a big part in determining how my condition improves.

_____ 9. Whatever improvement occurs with my condition is largely a matter of good fortune.

_____ 10. If my condition worsens, it's a matter of fate.

_____ 11. If I am lucky, my condition will get better.

_____ 12. As to my condition, what will be will be.

_____ 13. If I see my doctor regularly, I am less likely to have problems with my condition.

_____ 14. Following doctor's orders to the letter is the best way to keep my condition from getting worse.

_____ 15. Whenever my condition worsens, I should consult a medically trained professional.

_____ 16. Other people play a big role in whether my condition improves, stays the same, or gets worse.

_____ 17. The type of help I receive from other people determines how soon my condition improves.

_____ 18. In order for my condition to improve, it is up to other people to see that the right things happen.

Note. The MHLC (Wallston, Stein, & Smith, 1994) is a measure of control beliefs about health, specifically about control over health. It contains four dimensions: personal control or internality (Items 1–6), the role of chance in determining one's health status (Items 7–12), and the effectiveness of powerful others with scales for doctor (Items 13–15) and other people (Items 16–18). The MLHC has been used with many different health conditions (in the 1994 study rheumatoid arthritis, chronic pain patients, Type I and II

(continued)

diabetes, and two samples of cancer patients). The factor structure has been replicated, and reliabilities have been adequate (both alphas and test–retest).

Scoring. The 18 items are summed to form four scales (see previously), with possible scores ranging from 6 to 36 for internal and chance and 3 to 18 for doctor and other people. There is no recoding necessary. Higher scores for each scale are more of the specific dimension.

Reported means for dimensions varies by disease. For internal, means were as follows: rheumatoid arthritis (17.50), chronic pain (19.24), diabetes (28.67), and cancer (18.49); for the chance dimension, rheumatoid arthritis (16.60), chronic pain (15.95), diabetes (12.46), and cancer (19.81); for the doctors dimension, rheumatoid arthritis (13.43), chronic pain (11.19), diabetes (15.99), and cancer (15.91); and for the other people dimension, rheumatoid arthritis (7.48), chronic pain (9.18), diabetes (8.48), and cancer (10.96).

Description. The MHLC measures beliefs about how much one has control over the progress of a medical condition such as HIV. It assesses beliefs about control related to internality (such as personal responsibility for one's condition getting better or worse), chance, a doctor, and other people.

From "Form C of the MHLC Scales: A Condition-Specific Measure of Locus of Control," by K. A. Wallston, M. J. Stein, and C. A. Smith, 1994, *Journal of Personality Assessment, 63,* pp. 539–540. Copyright 1994 by Lawrence Erlbaum Associates, Inc.

TABLE A.19
Patient Self-Advocacy Scale (PSAS)

The following questions ask about your feelings about your health care. For each question, indicate your level of agreement according to the following scale:

1 = Strongly agree
2 = Agree
3 = Neutral
4 = Disagree
5 = Strongly disagree

_____ 1. I believe it is important for people with HIV or AIDS to learn as much as they can about their disease and treatments.

_____ 2. I actively seek out information on my disease.

_____ 3. I am more educated about HIV or AIDS than most U.S. citizens.

_____ 4. I have full knowledge of the health problems of people with HIV or AIDS.

_____ 5. I don't get what I need from my physician because I am not assertive enough.

_____ 6. I am more assertive about my health care needs than most U.S. citizens.

_____ 7. I frequently make suggestions to my physician about my health care needs.

_____ 8. If my physician prescribes something I don't understand or agree with, I question it.

_____ 9. Sometimes there are good reasons not to follow the advice of a physician.

_____ 10. Sometimes I think I have a better grasp of what I need medically than my doctor does.

_____ 11. If I am given a treatment by my physician that I don't agree with, I am likely to not take it.

_____ 12. I don't always do what my physician or health care worker has asked me to do.

Note. Brashers, Haas, and Neidig (1999) studied patient self-advocacy and developed a scale to tap patient activism. They sampled 174 individuals with HIV and 218 adults from a general population. The PSAS forms three dimensions: mindful nonadherence ($\alpha = .82$, Items 9–12), education ($\alpha = .60$, Items 1–4) and assertiveness ($\alpha = .67$, Items 5–8). The factor analysis of the scale indicated items 3 and 4 loaded on both education and assertiveness dimensions. The overall reliability for the HIV sample was .78. Means for the scales are presented for the dimensions based on activist organization membership (or not) and by self-identification as an activist (or not).

Scoring. The 12 items are summed and averaged to form one scale after recoding item 5. To recode item 5, 5 = 1, 4 = 2, 3 = 3, 2 = 4, and 1 = 5; use this recoded score when summing and averaging (add all 12 items and divide by 12). A lower score indicates more self-advocacy and a higher score indicates less self-advocacy.

Description. The PSAS taps individuals' desire for information about and involvement in the health care process. People vary in their ability and willingness to be active patients, and this measure assesses how or if people behave in more participatory ways.

From "The Patient Self-Advocacy Scale: Measuring Patient Involvement in Health Care Decision-Making Interactions," by D. E. Brashers, S. M. Haas, and J. L. Neidig, 1999, _Health Communication_, 11, p. 101. Copyright 1999 by Lawrence Erlbaum Associates, Inc.

HIV-Knowledge Questionnaire (HIV–K–Q)

The following questions present a statement about some aspect of HIV and AIDS. Please respond to each based on whether you think it is true or false.

Circle one

TRUE	FALSE	1. HIV and AIDS are the same thing.
TRUE	FALSE	2. There is a cure for AIDS.
TRUE	FALSE	3. A person can get HIV from a toilet seat.
TRUE	FALSE	4. Coughing and sneezing DO NOT spread HIV.
TRUE	FALSE	5. HIV can be spread by mosquitoes.
TRUE	FALSE	6. AIDS is the cause of HIV.
TRUE	FALSE	7. A person can get HIV by sharing a glass of water with someone who has HIV.
TRUE	FALSE	8. HIV is killed by bleach.
TRUE	FALSE	9. It is possible to get HIV when a person gets a tattoo.
TRUE	FALSE	10. A pregnant woman with HIV can give the virus to her unborn baby.
TRUE	FALSE	11. Pulling out the penis before a man climaxes keeps a woman from getting HIV during sex.
TRUE	FALSE	12. A woman can get HIV if she has anal sex with a man.
TRUE	FALSE	13. Showering, or washing one's genitals after sex keeps a person from getting HIV.
TRUE	FALSE	14. Eating healthy foods can keep a person from getting HIV.
TRUE	FALSE	15. All pregnant women infected with HIV will have babies born with AIDS.
TRUE	FALSE	16. Using a latex condom or rubber can lower a person's chance of getting HIV.
TRUE	FALSE	17. A person with HIV can look and feel healthy.
TRUE	FALSE	18. People who have been infected with HIV quickly show serious signs of being infected.
TRUE	FALSE	19. A person can be infected with HIV for 5 years or more without getting AIDS.
TRUE	FALSE	20. There is a vaccine that can stop adults from getting HIV.
TRUE	FALSE	21. Some drugs have been made for the treatment of AIDS.
TRUE	FALSE	22. Women are always tested for HIV during their pap smears.
TRUE	FALSE	23. A person cannot get HIV by having oral sex, mouth-to-penis, with a man who has HIV.
TRUE	FALSE	24. A person can get HIV even if she or he has sex with another person only one time.
TRUE	FALSE	25. Using lambskin condom or rubber is the best protection against HIV.
TRUE	FALSE	26. People are likely to get HIV by deep kissing, putting their tongue in their partner's mouth, if their partner has HIV.
TRUE	FALSE	27. A person can get HIV by giving blood.
TRUE	FALSE	28. A woman cannot get HIV if she has sex during her period.
TRUE	FALSE	29. You can usually tell if someone has HIV by looking at them.
TRUE	FALSE	30. There is a female condom that can help decrease a woman's chance of getting HIV.
TRUE	FALSE	31. A natural skin condom works better against HIV that does a latex condom.
TRUE	FALSE	32. A person will NOT get HIV if she or he is taking antibiotics.
TRUE	FALSE	33. Having sex with more than one partner can increase a person's chance of being infected with HIV.

(continued)

TABLE A.20

(continued)

TRUE	FALSE	34. Taking a test for HIV 1 week after having sex will tell a person if she or he has HIV.
TRUE	FALSE	35. A person can get HIV by sitting in a hot tub or a swimming pool with a person who has HIV.
TRUE	FALSE	36. A person can get HIV through contact with saliva, tears, sweat, or urine.
TRUE	FALSE	37. A person can get HIV from a woman's vaginal secretions (wetness from her vagina).
TRUE	FALSE	38. A person can get HIV if having oral sex, mouth on vagina, with a woman.
TRUE	FALSE	39. If a person tests positive for HIV, then the test site will have to tell all of his or her partners.
TRUE	FALSE	40. Using Vaseline or baby oil with condoms lowers the chance of getting HIV.
TRUE	FALSE	41. Washing drug-use equipment with cold water kills HIV.
TRUE	FALSE	42. A woman can get HIV if she has vaginal sex with a man who has HIV.
TRUE	FALSE	43. Athletes who share needles when using steroids can get HIV from the needles.
TRUE	FALSE	44. Douching after sex will keep a woman from getting HIV.
TRUE	FALSE	45. Taking vitamins keeps a person from getting HIV.

Note. Carey, Morrison-Beedy, and Johnson (1997) developed the HIV–K–Q from 62 items and reported a single factor 45-item measure. The reliability was very good ($\alpha = .91$) and stable across time. They also reported validity information with a variety of samples ($N = 669$). The measure takes less than 7 min to complete, represents several knowledge domains (transmission, nontransmission, prevention methods, and consequences of infection), and only requires sixth grade reading level. The measure emphasizes sexual over other modes of transmission.

Scoring. Items 4, 8, 9, 10, 12, 16, 17, 19, 21, 24, 30, 33, 37, 38, 42, and 43 are true (the rest are false). Give yourself 1 point for each correct score, 0 for incorrect (range possible 0–45). If you divide the number correct by 45, you will have the percentage correct. No means were reported for individuals with HIV, but percentages of correct knowledge for other groups (see Carey et al., 1997) were 69% for a primary care sample, 74% for a community sample, 72% for a community women sample, 82% and 85% for college samples, 91% for experts, and 52% for community couples.

Description. The HIV–K–Q is an objective measure of knowledge related to HIV and AIDS. The knowledge measure is distinct from measures of attitudes (such as homophobia or attitudes toward interacting with people with HIV) or behaviors (such as condom use).

From "The HIV-Knowledge Questionnaire: Development and Evaluation of a Reliable, Valid, and Practical Self-Administered Questionnaire," by M. P. Carey, D. Morrison-Beedy, and B. T. Johnson, 1997, *AIDS and Behavior, 1*, pp. 64–65. Copyright 1997 by Kluwer Academic/Plenum Publishers.

Other Measures

To this point in the appendix we have presented a range of exercises and scales that individuals can fill out to assess various aspects of their living with HIV. It is hoped that a person can select among relevant ones to help assess their strengths and weaknesses in living with HIV. There are a number of additional measures we lacked the space to present in this section, but the scale names, descriptions, and references are provided following. These can also be adapted for use in a number of ways.

Additional HIV Disclosure Scales.   There are several other studies tapping related HIV disclosure constructs. Greene et al. (1993) measured disclosure with two sets of nine items each, with 5-point Likert responses ranging from (Strongly agree) to (Strongly disagree). They used parallel sets of items to compare attitudes toward disclosure of HIV tests results and disclosure of who has been tested for HIV. For example, "Employers should have access to information about results of employees' HIV tests" versus "Employers should have access to information that employees have had HIV tests." Serovich and Greene (1993) expanded these to 18 items focusing solely on family members. For example, "Spouses should have access to information about results of HIV tests." Greene and Serovich (1996) expanded these two studies and used 26 Likert items targeting results of HIV tests to various targets. Greene and Serovich (1996) also measured actual HIV disclosure by asking "Does X know you are HIV-positive?" (X were 10 target persons). Greene and Faulkner (2002) expanded on this and asked items such as "Have you told X that you are HIV positive?" and "Does X know you are HIV positive?" (unlimited number of target persons). These questions better assess the direct versus indirect disclosure described in chapter 3 as a person might know the HIV diagnosis but was not told by the person with HIV. One important distinction not yet well established in HIV disclosure research is how many people know an HIV diagnosis compared with how many people have been disclosed to by the person with HIV.

Communication and HIV.   Several researchers have been interested in how individuals with HIV communicate regarding HIV. Brown and Bocarnea (1998) developed a measure of AIDS-related communication behavior. It consists of nine items with 7-point responses, for example, "How much have you discussed AIDS." Snell and Finney (1990) developed a measure of AIDS discussion strategies. It consists of 72 items with five responses, for example, "I would tell my partner I want to talk about AIDS."

HIV and AIDS Attitudes.   Attitudes toward HIV have been widely studied in relation to stigma, and there are many measures (we describe a few here). Ernst, Francis, Perkins, Britton-Williams, and Kang (1998) developed a measure of attitudes toward AIDS-related issues (the Meharry questionnaire). It consists of 13 items with six Likert responses, for example, "AIDS epidemic is a fulfillment of biblical prophecy." O'Donnell, O'Donnell, Pleck, Snarey, and Rose (1987) and Pleck et al. (1988) developed a measure of AIDS phobia. It consists of 16 items with 7-point responses, for example "AIDS patients offend me morally." Finney and Snell (1989) and Snell and Finney (1996) developed a measure of AIDS anxiety. It consists of 50 items with 5-point responses, for example, "Thinking about AIDS makes me feel anxious." Snell, Fisher, and Miller (1991) developed a measure of stereotypes about AIDS. It consists of 115 items, four sections with 5-point Likert responses. For example, one item reads, "Homosexuality is the cause of AIDS."

Knowledge of HIV and/or AIDS.   Knowledge of AIDS was measured early in the epidemic as a health promotion strategy. There was an assumption that if knowledge increased, people would increase their preventive behavior (e.g., use condoms or not share needles) and decrease stigma (e.g., about transmission misperceptions). The traditional format of the knowledge of HIV measures includes dichotomous responses ("true," "false," "don't know"). The measures developed by DiClemente and colleagues (1986, 1987) are the most widely used instruments to measure knowledge of HIV. Their instrument content as well as the format dominated subsequent measurement of this construct. One version of their knowledge of HIV instrument contained 30 items (DiClemente, Zorn, & Temoshok, 1987) and another contained 28 items (DiClemente, Zorn, & Temoshok, 1986). DiClemente and colleagues proposed three subscales: knowledge of cause, transmission, and treatment of HIV and AIDS. Many researchers utilizing the knowledge of AIDS construct have used some modification of the DiClemente et al. (1986, 1987) measure, often adding several of their own items (e.g., Dorman & Rienzo, 1988; Gray & Saracino, 1989; Koopman, Rotheram-Borus, Henderson, Bradley, & Hunter, 1990; Roscoe & Kruger, 1990; Sunenblick, 1988). Others measures are available (e.g., Price, Desmond, & Kukulka, 1985; Stall & McKusick, 1988), but they have neither been widely used nor referenced. More recently, Carey et al. (1997) presented a 45-item measure in this format (included in this appendix as Table A.20). An innovative format for measuring knowledge of HIV and AIDS has been presented by Yarber and Torabi (1990–1991; 1998); they presented 30 multiple choice items with four responses for each. It is possible there will be a shift away from true–false knowledge items to multiple choice. The rapid changes in available information about HIV in the epidemic make revisions to content of knowledge scales constant.

ADDITIONAL RESOURCES

This appendix first provided exercises related to disclosing an HIV diagnosis. The second section presented measures or scales used to assess disclosure-related issues. Finally, this last section presents additional resources for those who want further information. There are four parts of these additional resources:

Web sites, national associations and hotlines, other readings, and social artifacts. It is beyond the scope of this book to present resources at the community or statewide level, and there are many organizations that are local in nature providing support for HIV. Many of these organizations can be located by calling local health departments, religious organizations, or by checking local phone listings.

HIV and AIDS Related Web Sites

Given the development of the Internet, many organizations now produce Web sites. The quality of these sites vary, and content (and location) changes. We present next a selection of HIV related Web sites. This list is not intended to be exhaustive; rather, it is a sample of what kinds of resources are available on the World Wide Web. Some people may not have access to computers to connect to these sites and for them we have two suggestions. First, local libraries increasingly have Internet access free of charge (as do many universities and colleges); second, some AIDS service organizations have computer terminals available for clients' use.

- ACT UP (http://www.actupny.org) is a diverse, non-partisan group of individuals united in anger and committed to direct action to end the AIDS crisis. The site includes a variety of resources including information about demonstrations and donations.
- AIDS Action Committee (http://www.aac.org/) is a resource designed to help support people with HIV, to educate the public, and advocate funding for research, treatment, and education.
- AIDS Clinical Trials Information (http://www.actis.org/index.html) includes resources for information about private and federally funded AIDS medical trials. The site also has information about treatment, vaccines, and other resources.
- AIDS Research Information Center (http://www.critpath.org/aric) is a medical information service that concentrates on patient empowerment through information. The site includes research, publications, services, and hotlines.
- AVERT- Averting AIDS and HIV (http://www.avert.org) focuses on education about HIV infection and information for people with HIV. The site includes statistics, information for young people, personal stories, history, information on becoming infected, and other free resources including details of AVERT's publications.
- The Body (http://www.thebody.com) is an AIDS information resource that uses the Web to lower barriers between patients and clinicians, demystify HIV and its treatment, improve patients' quality of life, and foster community through human connection.
- Business Responds to AIDS (BRTA) and Labor Responds to AIDS (LRTA; http://www.brta-lrta.org) are programs that provide materials and assistance

to help workplaces set up effective HIV programs. The site includes policy development, manager or labor leader training, employee education, education for employees' families, and community service and volunteerism.

- The CDC (http://www.cdc.gov) is recognized as the leading federal agency for protecting the health and safety of people in the United States. CDC serves as the national focus for developing and applying disease prevention and control, environmental health, and health promotion and education activities designed to improve the health of the people of the United States. Also see the following sites for HIV statistics: MMWR (www.cdc.gov/hiv/pubs/mmwr.htm) and HIV/AIDS Surveillance (www.cdc.gov/hiv/stats/hasrlink.htm).
- Managing Desire (information on safer sex, testing and counseling, etc.) (http://www.managingdesire.org). The Web site goal is to identify HIV prevention, knowledge, and practice through peer-to-peer communication.
- National Minority AIDS Council (NMAC; http://www.nmac.org) is the premier national organization dedicated to developing leadership within communities of color to address the challenge of HIV.
- Physician Assistant AIDS Network (PAAN; http://www.paan.org) was formed to promote networking, continuing medical education, and symposia for physician assistants working in HIV and AIDS care.
- Project Inform (http://www.projinf.org) provides information, inspiration, and advocacy for people living with HIV. Project Inform's mission is to help in the diagnosis and treatment of HIV for infected individuals, their caregivers, and their health care and service providers and advocate for affecting the development of, access to, and delivery of effective treatments, as well as to fund innovative research opportunities and inspire people to make informed choices.
- Office of National AIDS Policy (http://www.whitehouse.gov/onap/text/aids.html) offers information from the Office of National AIDS Policy at the White House. Its topics include prevention, education, care, hotlines, treatment, and general information.
- Treatment Action group (TAG; http://www.aidsinfonyc.org/tag/index.html) is the homepage for TAG, an organization dedicated to the advancement of research efforts for finding a cure for AIDS. It focuses on research, drug development, and the nation's health care delivery systems.
- United Nations Educational Scientific and Cultural Organization (UNESCO; http://www.unesco.org/education/educprog/pead/index.html) offers education for prevention of drug abuse and HIV.
- UNAIDS (http://www.unaids.org), the leading advocate for worldwide action against HIV and AIDS, has a global mission to lead, strengthen, and support an expanded response to the epidemic that will prevent the spread of HIV, provide care and support for those infected and affected by the dis-

ease, reduce the vulnerability of individuals and communities to HIV, and alleviate the socioeconomic and human impact of the epidemic.

- WHO (http://www.who.int) is the directing, coordinating authority on international health work.

National HIV and AIDS Associations

Many national associations have developed in the past 20 years, and they have resources such as Web sites, toll-free hotlines, grants, print brochures, and so forth. Many of these associations coordinate programs in communities (e.g., Meals on Wheels®, transportation, support groups), offer client services, and even fund basic science research (often through grants). Again, the list provided is a selection of national associations. It is in no way meant to be exhaustive.

1. The National Association of People with AIDS (NAPWA) advocates on behalf of all people living with HIV and AIDS to end the pandemic and the human suffering caused by HIV. Their Web site is devoted to ongoing mission to educate, inform, and empower people living HIV.

Contact: http://www.napwa.org
National Association of People with AIDS
1413 K Street, NW, 7th Floor
Washington, DC 20005
Phone: (202) 898–0414

2. National Association on HIV over Fifty (NAHOF) seeks to promote the availability of a range of educational, prevention, service, and health care programs for persons over age 50 affected by HIV.

Contact: http://www.hivoverfifty.org
56 Joy Street, Apartment 3E
Boston, MA 02210
Phone: (617) 233–7107 or (617) 523–2942

3. National Association for Victims of Transfusion-Acquired AIDS (NAVTA) is an organization for people who contracted HIV through contaminated blood or transplant tissues. The group provides support, information, and advocacy for people with transfusion-acquired HIV infection.

Contact: http://www.navta.org
NAVTA, Inc.
8721 Burdette Drive
Bethesda, MD 20817
Phone: (301) 365–8750

4. The American Foundation for AIDS Research (AmFAR) is an organization dedicated to the support of HIV research, prevention, treatment education, and the advocacy of sound HIV-related public policy.

Contact: http://www.amfar.org
AmFAR
120 Wall Street, 13th Floor
New York, NY 10005-3902
Phone: (212) 806–1600 or 1–800–39–AmFAR

5. Gay Men's Health Crisis (GMHC), founded in 1981, provides compassionate care to New Yorkers with AIDS, educates to keep people healthy, and advocates for fair and effective public policies.

Contact: http://www.gmhc.org
The Tisch Building
199 West 24th Street
New York, NY 10011
1–800–AIDS–NYC (243–7692)

National Telephone Hotlines

One early response to the HIV epidemic was to establish toll-free hotlines (in addition to printed brochures). In fact, many campaigns and early HIV prevention messages focused on seeking information as the goal, encouraging people to find out more about HIV. These hotlines are a relatively cost-efficient means of providing information to the general public, and there have been periods of extensive use of these hotlines (e.g., when Magic Johnson announced his infection). Again, what follows is a sample of available numbers including both treatment and service groups. Specific access may vary by state:

AIDS Clinical Trials Information Service (ACTIS) National TRIALS Hotline
800–TRIALS–A

Civil Rights Hotline
800–368–1019

Centers for Disease Control and Prevention
404–639–3311 or 800–311–3435

HIV Treatment Information Services
800–448–0440

National AIDS Clearinghouse
800–458–5231

National AIDS Hotline
800–342–AIDS or 800–344–SIDA (Spanish)

National Institute on Drug Abuse
 800–662–HELP

National STD and AIDS Hotline (CDC)
 800–227–8922

National Prevention Information Network (CDC)
 800–458–5231

Project Inform
 800–822–7422

Teens Tap
 800–234–TEEN

Other Readings

We are now into the 3rd decade of the HIV epidemic, and there have been many publications presented on the topic. In this section we highlight books, magazines, academic journals, and special issues of journals. This summary overlooks, for example, art, but we focus here on things that can be easily accessed by a range of people.

Books.   There are literally dozens of books on HIV published at this time, and we point out several here. These represent a range of topics and approaches:

Bartlett, J. G., & Gallant, J. E. (2001). *Medical management of HIV infection (2001–2002).* Baltimore: Johns Hopkins University, Division of Infectious Diseases.

Derlega, V. J., & Barbee, A. P. (Eds.). (1998). *HIV and social interaction.* Thousand Oaks, CA: Sage.

Elwood, W. N. (Ed.). (1999). *Power in the blood: A handbook on AIDS, politics, and communication.* Mahwah, NJ: Lawrence Erlbaum Associates, Inc.

Hampton Crockett, P. (1997). *HIV law: A survival guide to the legal system for people living with HIV.* New York: Three Rivers Press.

Kalichman, S. C. (1998). *Understanding AIDS: Advances in treatment and research* (2nd ed.). Washington, DC: American Psychological Association.

Kelly, A. E. (2002). *The psychology of secrets.* New York: Kluwer Academic/Plenum.

Lepore, S. J., & Smyth, J. M. (Eds.). (2002). *The writing cure: How expressive writing promotes health and emotional well-being.* Washington, D.C.: American Psychological Association.

Monette, P. (1988). *Borrowed time: An AIDS memoir.* New York: Avon Books.

Powell, J. (1996). *AIDS and HIV Related diseases: An educational guide for professionals and the public.* New York: Insight Books.

Schoub, B. D. (1999). *AIDS & HIV in perspective: A guide to understanding the virus and its consequences.* Cambridge, England: Cambridge University Press.

Watney, S. (2000). *Imagine hope: AIDS and gay identity.* New York: Routledge.

Watstein, S. B., & Chandler, K. (1998). *The AIDS dictionary.* New York: Facts on File.

Magazines. Besides books, several magazines have emerged dealing exclusively with HIV (different from the hundreds of magazines with special features or stories about HIV and AIDS). Many ASOs subscribe to these magazines and make them available for clients. Several of the more widely distributed HIV magazines include the following:

A&U (http://www.a&umag.org): America's AIDS magazine includes a variety of articles and features.

Body Positive (http://www.thebody.com): A magazine for people with AIDS.

Poz Magazine (http://www.poz.com): This magazine includes articles and features on HIV and AIDS.

Safersex.org (http://www.safersex.org): An online journal of safer sex.

Today's Caregiver (http://www.caregiver.com:) This is a resource for those caring for loved ones with AIDS and other illnesses.

Academic Journals. Beyond books and magazines, another mechanism for gaining information about HIV is research in the area. The majority of academic research is published in journals, and several HIV-specific journals have emerged. These journals, published several times a year, provide original data on HIV issues. For many of the journals, the publisher's Web site includes article abstracts. Often the articles themselves can be obtained through University libraries. Again, this list is not exhaustive:

AIDS and Behavior
Kluwer Academic/Plenum Publishers
233 Spring Street
New York, NY 10013–1578
http://www.kluweronline.com

AIDS Care
Carfax Publishing
c/o Taylor and Francis Group
29 West 35th Street, 10th floor
New York, NY 10001
http://www.taylorandfrancis.com

AIDS Clinical Review
  Marcel Dekker, Inc.
  270 Madison Avenue
  New York, NY 10016
  E-mail: intellprop@dekker.com

AIDS Education and Prevention
  Guilford Publications
  72 Spring Street
  New York, NY 10012
  E-mail: kathy.kuehl@guilford.com

AIDS/STD Health Promotion Exchange
  Royal Tropical Institute
  Postbus 95001
  1090 HA Amsterdam
  The Netherlands
  E-mail: pr@kit.nl

AIDS Patient Care and STDs
  Mary Ann Liebert, Inc.
  2 Madison Avenue
  Larchmont, NY 10538
  E-mail: info@liebertpub.com

AIDS and Public Policy Journal
  University Publishing Group
  17100 Cole Road, Suite 312
  Hagerstown, MD 21740
  E-mail: editorial@upgbooks.com

AIDS Research and Human Retroviruses
  Mary Ann Liebert, Inc.
  2 Madison Avenue
  Larchmont, NY 10538
  E-mail: info@liebertpub.com

Journal of HIV/AIDS Prevention & Education for Adolescents & Children
  The Haworth Press Inc.
  10 Alice Street
  Binghamton, NY 13904
  E-mail: getinfo@haworthpressinc.com

Journal of the Association of Nurses in AIDS Care
  Sage Publications
  2455 Teller Road
  Thousand Oaks, CA 91320
  800–499–8721

Special Issues of Journals.   A number of special issues of journals have focused exclusively on HIV. These may provide more focused information about special topics, and people may be able to access them through Web sites or perhaps a University library:

> *American Behavioral Scientist,* April 1999, Volume 42, Number 7: Special issue focusing on AIDS and stigma in the United States.
>
> *Illness, Crisis & Loss,* January 1998, Volume 6, Number 1: Special issue on how people construct meaning from illness and trends in the epidemic.
>
> *Journal of Social and Personal Relationships,* Winter 2002, Volume 19, Number 1: Special issue focusing on relationships of individuals with HIV. The articles include discussion of social support, self-disclosure, coping, and social activism.
>
> *Qualitative Health Research,* February 1997, Volume 7, Number 1: Special issue focusing on living with HIV, especially concerns for minorities.
>
> *Western Journal of Nursing Research,* August 1998, Volume 20, Number 4: The special issue focuses on unique concerns for women (e.g., antiretroviral decisions, infant feeding, symptoms) and gay couples.
>
> *Women's Health: Research on Gender,* 1996, Volume 2, Numbers 1 and 2: The special issue focuses HIV risk in lesbian and bisexual women (or WSW, women who have sex with women).

Social Artifacts

One final resource presented is a collection of social artifacts. These artifacts, in some ways, reflect social attitudes toward HIV. One outcome of such social artifacts is increased attention to HIV (e.g., consider the AIDS Quilt). The categories of social artifacts presented are plays and films or movies. What is presented here is a sample of what is available in the categories, focusing primarily on national level examples.

Plays.   Many plays have been written about HIV, including several with national tours or Broadway productions:

> 1. *Angels in America* by Tony Kushner (1992)
> 2. *Love! Valor! Compassion* by Terrence McNally (1995)
> 3. *Patient A* by Lee Blessing (1995)
> 4. *Queen of Angels* by James Carroll Pickett (1992)
> 5. *Rent* by Jonathan Larson (1996)
> 6. *Zero Patience* by John Greyson (1993)

Films.   Many films have been made about HIV, including several widely released in theatres, network specials, and documentaries. This is the broadest category, and we focus on U.S. rather than foreign language films:

1. And The Band Played On, 1993
2. Boys on the Side, 1995
3. Breaking the Surface: The Greg Louganis Story, 1997
4. Common Threads, Stories from the Quilt, 1989
5. It's in the Water, 1997
6. It's My Party, 1996
7. Love, Valour, Compassion!, 1997
8. Philadelphia, 1993

CONCLUSIONS

This appendix presented a variety of resources to assist individuals with HIV and
others who know or work with them. First we described exercises to assist with
disclosure decisions. Next we presented scales or measures used in research that
could be helpful in understanding various aspects of living with HIV. Finally we
provided a selection of other resources such as books, Web sites, and social artifacts. One of the most positive outcomes of the AIDS epidemic has been mobili-
zation of resources for those with HIV. In this appendix, we strove to point to
some of those resources. With all the difficulty surrounding disclosure decisions
described in this book, accessing such resources becomes critical.

References

Adam, B. D., & Sears, A. (1994). Negotiating sexual relationships after testing HIV-positive. *Medical Anthropology, 16*, 63–77.

Adam, B. D., & Sears, A. (1996). *Experiencing HIV: Personal, family, and work relationships.* New York: Columbia University Press.

Adelman, M. B., & Frey, L. R. (1997). *The fragile community: Living together with AIDS.* Mahwah, NJ: Lawrence Erlbaum Associates, Inc.

Afifi, W. A., & Weiner, J. L. (2002). Information seeking across contexts. *Human Communication Research, 28*, 207–212.

Agne, R. R., Thompson, T. L., & Cusella, L. P. (2000). Stigma in the line of face: Self-disclosure of patients' HIV status to health care providers. *Journal of Applied Communication Research, 28*, 235–261.

Albert, E. (1986). Illness and deviance: The response of the press to AIDS. In D. A. Feldman & T. M. Johnson (Eds.), *The social dimensions of AIDS: Method and theory* (pp. 163–178). New York: Praeger.

Albrecht, T. L., & Adelman, M. B. (1984). Social support and life stress: New directions for communication research. *Human Communication Research, 11*, 3–32.

All, A. (1989). Health care workers' anxieties and fears concerning AIDS: A literature review. *Journal of Continuing Education in Nursing, 20*, 162–165.

Allen, J. E. (2002, February 4). AIDS drugs may cause other illnesses. *Los Angeles Times*, p. S1.

Allman, J. (1998). Bearing the burden or baring the soul: Physicians' self-disclosure and boundary management regarding medical mistakes. *Health Communication, 10*, 175–197.

Alonzo, A. A., & Reynolds, N. R. (1995). Stigma, HIV and AIDS: An exploration and elaboration of a stigma trajectory. *Social Science and Medicine, 41*, 303–315.

Altman, I. (1975). *Environment and social behavior: Privacy, personal space, territory, and crowding.* Monterey, CA: Brooks/Cole.

Altman, I. (1977). Privacy regulation: Culturally universal or culturally specific? *Journal of Social Issues, 33*(3), 66–84.

Altman, I., Brown, B. B., Staples, B., & Werner, C. M. (1992). A transactional approach to close relationships: Courtship, weddings, and placemaking. In W. B. Walsh, K. H. Craik, & R. H. Price (Eds.), *Person–environment psychology: Models and perspectives* (pp. 193–241). Hillsdale, NJ: Lawrence Erlbaum Associates, Inc.

Altman, I., & Taylor, D. A. (1973). *Social penetration: The development of interpersonal relationships.* New York: Holt, Rinehart & Winston.

Altman, I., & Werner, C. M. (Eds.). (1985). *Home environments.* New York: Plenum.

Altman, L. K. (2002, July 3). U.N. forecasts big increase in AIDS death toll. *New York Times*. Retrieved July 4, 2002, from http://www.nytimes.com/2002/01/03/health.

Americans With Disabilities Act of 1990, 42 U.S.C.A. § 12101 ct seq. (West, 1993).

Andrews, S., Williams, A. B., & Neil, K. (1993). The mother–child relationship in the HIV-1 positive family. *Image: The Journal of Nursing Scholarship, 25,* 193–198.

Archer, R. L., & Burleson, J. A. (1980). The effects of timing and responsibility of self-disclosure on attraction. *Journal of Personality, 38,* 120–130.

Argyle, M., & Henderson, M. (1984). The rules of friendship. *Journal of Social and Personal Relationships, 1,* 211–237.

Argyle, M., & Henderson, M. (1985). The rules of relationships. In S. Duck & D. Perlman (Eds.), *Understanding personal relationships: An interdisciplinary approach* (pp. 63–84). London: Sage.

Argyle, M., Henderson, M., & Furnham, A. (1985). The rules of social relationships. *British Journal of Social Psychology, 24,* 125–139.

Armistead, L., Klein, K., Forehand, R., & Wierson, M. (1997). Disclosure of parental HIV infection to children in the families of men with hemophilia: Description, outcomes, and the role of family process. *Journal of Family Psychology, 11,* 49–61.

Armistead, L., Morse, E., Forehand, R., Morse, P., & Clark, L. (1999). African American women and self-disclosure of HIV infection: Rates, predictors, and relationship to depressive symptomatology. *AIDS and Behavior, 3,* 195–204.

Asch, A., & Fine, M. (1988). Introduction: Beyond pedestals. In M. Fine & A. Asch (Eds.), *Women with disabilities: Essays in psychology, culture, and politics* (pp. 1–37). Philadelphia: Temple University Press.

Ashe, A., & Rampersad, A. (1993). *Days of grace: A memoir.* New York: Ballantine.

Atkinson, J. M., & Heritage, J. (1984). *Structures of social action: Studies in conversation analysis.* Cambridge, England: Cambridge University Press.

Baltimore, D. (2002, June 28). Steering a course to an AIDS vaccine. *Science,* p. 2997.

Barbee, A. P., & Cunningham, M. R. (1995). An experimental approach to social support communications: Interactive coping in closed relationships. In B. R. Burleson (Ed.), *Communication Yearbook 18* (pp. 381–413). Thousand Oaks, CA: Sage.

Barbee, A. P., Derlega, V. J., Sherburne, S. P., & Grimshaw, A. (1998). Helpful and unhelpful forms of social support for HIV-positive individuals. In V. J. Derlega & A. P. Barbee (Eds.), *HIV and social interaction* (pp. 83–105). Thousand Oaks, CA: Sage.

Bargh, J. A., & Chartrand, T. L. (1999). The unbearable automaticity of being. *American Psychologist, 54,* 462–479.

Barnes, D. B., Gerbert, B., McMaster, J. R., & Greenblatt, R. M. (1996). Self-disclosure experience of people with HIV infection in dedicated and mainstreamed dental facilities. *Journal of Public Health Dentistry, 56,* 223–225.

Barroso, J. (1997). Reconstructing my life: Becoming a long-term survivor of AIDS. *Qualitative Health Research, 7,* 57–74.

Bartlett, J. G., & Gallant, J. E. (2001). *Medical management of HIV infection (2001–2002).* Baltimore: Johns Hopkins University, Division of Infectious Diseases.

Bauer, G. R., & Welles, S. L. (2001). Beyond assumptions of negligible risk: Sexually transmitted diseases and women who have sex with women. *American Journal of Public Health, 91,* 1282–1286.

Bauman, L. J., Camacho, S., Forbes-Jones, E., & Westbrook, L. (1997, May). *Correlates of personal and social stigma among women with HIV/AIDS.* Paper presented at the annual meeting of the National Conference on Women and AIDS, Los Angeles, CA.

Bauman, L. J., Draimin, B., Levine, C., & Hudis, J. (2000). Who will care for me? Planning the future care and custody of children orphaned by HIV/AIDS. In W. Pequegnat & J. Szapocznik (Eds.), *Working with families in the era of HIV/AIDS* (pp. 155–188). Thousand Oaks, CA: Sage.

Baxter, L. A., & Wilmot, W. (1984). Secret tests: Social strategies for acquiring information abut the state of the relationship. *Human Communication Research, 11,* 171–202.

Bayer, R. (1996). AIDS prevention: Sexual ethics and responsibility. *New England Journal of Medicine, 334,* 1540–1542.

Beck, A. T., & Steer, R. A. (1993). *BDI: Beck Depression Inventory manual*. New York: Psychological Corporation.

Bem, D. (1972). Self-perception theory. In L. Berkowitz (Ed.), *Advances in experimental social psychology* (Vol. 6, pp. 1–62). New York: Academic.

Berger, C. R. (1973, November). *The acquaintance process revisited: Explorations in initial interaction*. Paper presented at the meeting of the Speech Communication Association, New York.

Berger, C. R. (1987). Communicating under uncertainty. In M. E. Roloff & G. E. Miller (Eds.), *Interpersonal processes: New directions in communication research* (pp. 39–62). Newbury Park, CA: Sage.

Berger, C. R. (2002). Strategic and nonstrategic information acquisition. *Human Communication Research, 28,* 272–286.

Berger, C., & Kellerman, K. (1989). Personal opacity and social information gathering: Explorations in strategic communication. *Communication Research, 16,* 314–351.

Blau, P. (1964). *Exchange and power in everyday life*. New York: Wiley.

Blendon, R. J., & Donelan, K. (1988). Discrimination against people with AIDS. *New England Journal of Medicine, 319,* 1022–1026.

Bloom, F. R. (1997). Searching for meaning in everyday life: Gay men negotiating selves in the HIV spectrum. *Ethos, 25,* 454–479.

Blower, S. M., Aschenbach, A. N., Gershengorn, H. B., & Kahn, J. O. (2001). Predicting the unpredictable: Transmission of drug-resistant HIV. *Nature Medicine, 7,* 1016–1020.

Boberg, E., Gustafon, D., Hawkins, R., Peressini, T., Bricker, E., Pingree, S., et al. (1995). Development, acceptance and use patterns of a computer-based education and social support system for people living with AIDS/HIV infection. *Computers in Human Behavior, 11,* 289–311.

Boerum, S. J. (1998). AIDS: An unconventional perspective. *Journal of Social Distress and the Homeless, 7,* 1–27.

Bok, S. (1984). *Secrets: On the ethics of concealment and revelation*. New York: Vintage.

Booth, R. J., & Petrie, K. J. (2002). Emotional expression and health changes: Can we identify biological pathways? In S. J. Lepore & J. M. Smyth (Eds.), *The writing cure: How expressive writing promotes health and emotional well-being* (pp. 137–175). Washington, DC: American Psychological Association.

Bor, R., Miller, R., & Goldman, E. (1993). HIV/AIDS and the family: A review of research in the first decade. *Journal of Family Therapy, 15,* 187–201.

Braithwaite, D. O. (1991). "Just how much did that wheelchair cost?" Management of privacy boundaries and demands for self-disclosure by persons with disabilities. *Western Journal of Speech Communication, 55,* 254–274.

Braithwaite, D. O., & Thompson, T. L. (Eds.) (2000). *Handbook of communication and people with disabilities: Research and application*. Mahwah, NJ: Lawrence Erlbaum Associates, Inc.

Brashers, D. E. (2001). Communication and uncertainty management. *Journal of Communication, 51,* 477–497.

Brashers, D. E., Goldsmith, D. J., & Hsieh, E. (2002). Information seeking and avoiding in health contexts. *Human Communication Research, 28,* 258–271.

Brashers, D. E., Haas, S. M., Klingle, R. S., & Neidig, J. L. (2000). Collective AIDS activism and individuals' perceived self-advocacy in physician–patient communication. *Human Communication Research, 26,* 372–402.

Brashers, D. E., Haas, S. M., & Neidig, J. L. (1999). The patient self-advocacy scale: Measuring patient involvement in health care decision-making interactions. *Health Communication, 11,* 97–121.

Brashers, D. E., Haas, S. M., Neidig, J. L., & Rintamaki, L. S. (2002). Social activism, self-advocacy, and coping with HIV illness. *Journal of Social and Personal Relationships, 19,* 113–133.

Brashers, D. E., Neidig, J. L., Cardillo, L. W., Dobbs, L. K., Russell, J. A., & Haas, S. M. (1999). "In an important way, I did die": Uncertainty and revival in persons living with HIV or AIDS. *AIDS Care, 11,* 201–219.

Brashers, D. E., Neidig, J. L., Haas, S. M., Dobbs, L. K., Cardillo, L. W., & Russell, J. A. (2000). Communication in the management of uncertainty: The case of persons living with HIV or AIDS. *Communication Monographs, 67*, 63–84.

Brashers, D. E., Neidig, J. L., Reynolds, N. R., & Haas, S. M. (1998). Uncertainty in illness across the HIV/AIDS trajectory. *Journal of the Association of Nurses in AIDS Care, 9*, 66–77.

Brouwer, D. C. (2000). Nonverbal vernacular tactics of HIV discovery among gay men. In S. Petronio (Ed.), *Balancing the secrets of private disclosures* (pp. 97–108). Mahwah, NJ: Lawrence Erlbaum Associates, Inc.

Brown, P., & Levinson, S. (1987). *Politeness: Some universals in language use.* Cambridge, England: Cambridge University Press.

Brown, V. B., Melchior, L. A., Reback, C. J., & Huba, G. J. (1994). Mandatory partner notification of HIV test results: Psychological and social issues for women. *AIDS and Public Policy Journal, 9*, 82–96.

Brown, W. J., & Bocarnea, M. C. (1998). Assessing AIDS-related concern, beliefs, and communication behavior. In C. M. Davis, W. L. Yarber, R. Bauserman, G. Schreer, & S. L. Davis (Eds.), *Handbook of sexuality-related measures* (pp. 310–312). Thousand Oaks, CA: Sage.

Burris, S. (1999). Studying the legal management of HIV-related stigma. *American Behavioral Scientist, 42*, 1229–1243.

Burris, S. (2001). Clinical decision making in the shadow of law. In J. R. Anderson & B. Barret (Eds.), *Ethics in HIV-related psychotherapy: Clinical decision making in complex cases* (pp. 99–129). Washington, DC: American Psychological Association.

Button, G., & Casey, N. (1984). Topic organization. In J. M. Atkinson & J. Heritage (Eds.), *Structures of social action: Studies in conversation analysis* (pp. 165–190). Cambridge, England: Cambridge University Press.

Buunk, B. P., & Gibbons, F. X. (1997). *Health, coping and well-being.* Mahwah, NJ: Lawrence Erlbaum Associates, Inc.

Cameron, L. D., & Nicholls, G. (1998). Expression of stressful experiences through writing: Effects of a self-regulation manipulation for pessimists and optimists. *Health Psychology, 17*, 84–92.

Capitanio, J. P., & Herek, G. M. (1999). AIDS-related stigma and attitudes toward injecting drug users among black and white Americans. *American Behavioral Scientist, 42*, 1148–1161.

Cappella, J. N. (1994). The management of conversational interaction in adults and infants. In M. L. Knapp & G. R. Miller (Eds.), *Handbook of interpersonal communication* (2nd ed., pp. 380–418). Thousand Oaks, CA: Sage.

Carballo-Diéguez, A. (2001). Alternatives to male condoms for men who have sex with men. *Focus: A Guide to AIDS Research and Counseling, 16*, 1–4.

Carey, M. P., Morrison-Beedy, D., & Johnson, B. T. (1997). The HIV-knowledge questionnaire: Development and evaluation of a reliable, valid, and practical self-administered questionnaire. *AIDS and Behavior, 1*, 61–74.

Carpenter, C. C. J., Fischl, M. A., Hammer, S. M., Hirsch, M. S., Jacobsen, D. M., Ketzenstein, D. A., et al. (1998). Antiretroviral therapy for HIV infection in 1998: Updated recommendations of the International AIDS Society, U.S. Panel. *Journal of the American Medical Association, 280*, 78–86.

Castro, R., Orozco, E., Eroza, E., Manca, M. C., Hernandez, J. J., & Aggleton, P. (1998). AIDS-related illness trajectories in Mexico: Findings from a qualitative study in two marginalized communities. *AIDS Care, 10*, 583–598.

Catz, S. L., & Kelly, J. A. (2001). Living with HIV disease. In A. Baum, T. A. Revenson, & J. E. Singer (Eds.), *Handbook of health psychology* (pp. 841–849). Mahwah, NJ: Lawrence Erlbaum Associates, Inc.

Catz, S. L., Kelly, J. A., Bogart, L. M., Benotsch, E. G., & McAuliffe, T. L. (2000). Patterns, correlates, and barriers to medication adherence among persons prescribed new treatments for HIV disease. *Health Psychology, 19*, 124–133.

Centers for Disease Control and Prevention. (1999). *HIV/AIDS surveillance report, 11*. Atlanta, GA: U.S. Department of Health and Human Services.

Centers for Disease Control and Prevention. (2001). Cumulative AIDS cases reported to CDC through June 2001. Retrieved July 14, 2002, from http://www.cdc.gov/hiv/stats.htm.

Centers for Disease Control and Prevention. (2002). HIV and AIDS—United States, 1981-2000. *Morbidity and Mortality Weekly Report, 50*, 430-434.

Chaikin, A. L., & Derlega, V. J. (1974). *Self-disclosure*. Morristown, NJ: General Learning Press.

Charbonneau, A., Maheux, B., & Beland, F. (1999). Do people with HIV/AIDS disclose their HIV-positivity to dentists? *AIDS Care, 11*, 61-70.

Chelune, G. J., Robinson, J. T., & Kommor, M. J. (1984). A cognitive interactional model of intimate relationships. In V. J. Derlega (Ed.), *Communication, intimacy, and close relationships* (pp. 11-40). Orlando, FL: Academic Press.

Chelune, G. J., Sultan, R. F., & Williams, C. L. (1980). Loneliness, self-disclosure, and interpersonal effectiveness. *Journal of Counseling Psychology, 27*, 462-468.

Chesney, M. A., & Smith, A. W. (1999). Critical delays in HIV testing and care: The potential role of stigma. *American Behavioral Scientist, 42*, 1162-1174.

Chidwick, A., & Borrill, J. (1996). Dealing with a life-threatening diagnosis: The experience of people with the human immunodeficiency virus. *AIDS Care, 8*, 271-284.

Chuang, H. T., Devins, G. M., Hunsley, J., & Gill, M. J. (1989). Psychosocial distress and well-being among gay and bisexual men with human immunodeficiency virus infection. *American Journal of Psychiatry, 146*, 876-880.

Chung, J. Y., & Magraw, M. M. (1992). A group approach to psychosocial issues faced by HIV-positive women. *Hospital and Community Psychiatry, 43*, 891-894.

Ciesla, J. A., & Roberts, J. E. (2001). Meta-analysis of the relationship between HIV infection and risk for depressive disorders. *American Journal of Psychiatry, 158*, 725-730.

Clark, K. A. (1999). Pink water: The archetype of blood and the pool of contagion. In W. N. Elwood (Ed.), *Power in the blood: A handbook on AIDS, politics, and communication* (pp. 9-24). Mahwah, NJ: Lawrence Erlbaum Associates, Inc.

Clement, U., & Schonnesson, N. (1998). Subjective HIV attribution theories, coping, and psychological functioning among homosexual men with HIV. *AIDS Care, 10*, 355-363.

Cline, R. J. W., & Haynes, K. M. (2001). Consumer health information seeking on the Internet: The state of the art. *Health Education Research, 16*, 671-692.

Cline, R. J. W., & McKenzie, N. J. (1996). Women and AIDS: The lost population. In R. Parrott & C. Condit (Eds.), *Evaluating women's health messages: A resource book* (pp. 382-401). Thousand Oaks, CA: Sage.

Cline, R. J. W., & McKenzie, N. J. (2000). Dilemmas of disclosure in the age of HIV/AIDS: Balancing privacy and protection in the health care context. In S. Petronio (Ed.), *Balancing the secrets of private disclosures* (pp. 71-82). Mahwah, NJ: Lawrence Erlbaum Associates, Inc.

Cohen, S., & Williamson, G. M. (1988). Perceived stress in a probability sample of the United States. In S. Spacapan & S. Oskamp (Eds.), *The social psychology of health* (pp. 31-67). Newbury Park, CA: Sage.

Cole, S. W., Kemeny, M. E., & Taylor, S. E. (1997). Social identity and physical health: Accelerated HIV progression in rejection-sensitive gay men. *Journal of Personality and Social Psychology, 72*, 320-335.

Cole, S. W., Kemeny, M. E., Taylor, S. E., & Visscher, B. R. (1996). Elevated physical health risk among gay men who conceal their homosexual identity. *Health Psychology, 15*, 243-251.

Cole, S. W., Kemeny, M. E., Taylor, S. E., Visscher, B. R., & Fahey, J. L. (1996). Accelerated course of human immunodeficiency virus infection in gay men who conceal their homosexual identity. *Psychosomatic Medicine, 58*, 219-231.

Collins, E., Wagner, C., & Walmsley, S. (2000). Psychosocial impact of the lipodystrophy syndrome in HIV infection. *AIDS Reader, 10*, 546-551.

Collins, N. L., & Miller, L. C. (1994). The disclosure-liking link: From meta-analysis toward a dynamic reconceptualization. *Psychological Bulletin, 116,* 457–475.

Collins, R. L. (1998). Social identity and HIV infection: The experiences of gay men living with HIV. In V. J. Derlega & A. P. Barbee (Eds.), *HIV and social interaction* (pp. 30–55). Thousand Oaks, CA: Sage.

Committee on maintaining privacy and security in health care applications of national information infostructure. (1997). *For the record: Protecting electronic health information.* Washington, DC: National Academy Press.

Couch, L. L., Jones, W. H., & Moore, D. S. (1999). Buffering the effects of betrayal: The role of apology, forgiveness, and commitment. In J. M. Adams & W. H. Jones (Eds.), *Handbook of interpersonal commitment and relationship stability* (pp. 451–469). New York: Kluwer Academic/Plenum.

Cowles, K. V., & Rodgers, B. L. (1997). Struggling to keep on top: Meeting the everyday challenges of AIDS. *Qualitative Health Research, 7,* 98–120.

Cozby, P. (1973). Self-disclosure: A literature review. *Psychological Bulletin, 79,* 73–91.

Crandall, C. S., & Coleman, R. (1992). AIDS-related stigmatization and the disruption of social relationships. *Journal of Social and Personal Relationships, 9,* 163–177.

Cranson, D. A., & Caron, S. L. (1998). An investigation of the effects of HIV on the sex lives of infected individuals. *AIDS Education and Prevention, 10,* 506–522.

Crawford, A. M. (1996). Stigma associated with AIDS: A meta-analysis. *Journal of Applied Social Psychology, 26,* 398–416.

Crawford, I., Humfleet, G., Ribordy, S. C., Ho, F. C., & Vickers, V. L. (1991). Stigmatization of AIDS patients by mental health professionals. *Professional Psychology: Research and Practice, 22,* 357–361.

Crespo-Fierro, M. (1997). Compliance/adherence and care management in HIV disease. *Journal of the Association of Nurses in AIDS Care, 8,* 43–54.

Crocker, J., & Major, B. (1989). Social stigma and self-esteem: The self-protective properties of stigma. *Psychological Review, 96,* 608–630.

Crocker, J., Major, B., & Steele, C. (1998). Social stigma. In D. T. Gilbert, S. T. Fiske, & G. Lindzey (Eds.), *The handbook of social psychology* (pp. 504–553). Boston: McGraw-Hill.

Crosby, G. M. (2000). *HIV serostatus disclosure in a sexual context among gay men in San Francisco: Truths, lies and guesses.* Unpublished manuscript, Center for AIDS Prevention Studies, University of California, San Francisco.

Crossley, M. L. (1997). "Survivors" and "victims": Long-term HIV positive individuals and the ethos of self-empowerment. *Social Science and Medicine, 45,* 1863–1873.

Crossley, M. L. (1999). Making sense of HIV infection: Discourse and adaptation to life with a long-term HIV positive diagnosis. *Health, 3,* 95–119.

D'Angelo, R. J., McGuire, J. M., Abbott, D. W., & Sheridan, K. (1998). Homophobia and perceptions of people with AIDS. *Journal of Applied Social Psychology, 28,* 157–170.

Davies, M. L. (1997). Shattered assumptions: Time and the experience of long-term HIV positivity. *Social Science and Medicine, 44,* 561–571.

Davison, K. P., Pennebaker, J. W., & Dickerson, S. S. (2000). Who talks? The social psychology of illness support groups. *American Psychologist, 55,* 250–217.

Dawson, J. M., Fitzpatrick, R. M., Reeves, G., Boulton, M., McLean, J., Hart, G. J., et al. (1994). Awareness of sexual partners' HIV status as an influence upon high-risk sexual behaviour among gay men. *AIDS, 8,* 837–841.

DeJong, W., Wolf, R. C., & Austin, S. B. (2001). U.S. federally funded television public service announcements (PSAs) to prevent HIV/AIDS: A content analysis. *Journal of Health Communication, 6,* 249–263.

Demme, J. (Producer/Director), Saxon, E. (Producer), & Nyswaner, R. (Writer). (1993). *Philadelphia* [Motion Picture]. United States: TriStar Pictures.

Deren, S., Beardsley, M., Tortu, S., & Goldstein, M. F. (1998). HIV serostatus and changes in risk behaviors among drug infectors and crack users. *AIDS and Behavior, 2,* 171–176.

Derlega, V. J., & Barbee, A. P. (1994). *Unpublished transcripts of interviews with HIV-infected persons about self-disclosure and social support.* Unpublished manuscript, Old Dominion University, Norfolk, VA.

Derlega, V. J., & Barbee, A. P. (Eds.). (1998a). *HIV and social interaction.* Thousand Oaks, CA: Sage.

Derlega, V. J., & Barbee, A. P. (1998b). *Unpublished transcripts of interviews with HIV-infected mothers about HIV and personal relationships.* Unpublished manuscript, Old Dominion University, Norfolk, VA.

Derlega, V. J., & Chaikin, A. L. (1977). Privacy and self-disclosure in social relationships. *Journal of Social Issues, 33*(3), 102–115.

Derlega, V. J., Greene, K., & Frey, L. R. (Eds.). (2002). Personal and social relationships of individuals living with HIV and/or AIDS [Special issue]. *Journal of Social and Personal Relationships, 19*(1).

Derlega, V. J., & Grzelak, J. (1979). Appropriateness of self-disclosure. In G. J. Chelune (Ed.), *Self-disclosure: Origins, patterns, and implications of interpersonal relationships* (pp. 151–176). San Francisco: Jossey-Bass.

Derlega, V. J., Lovejoy, D., & Winstead, B. A. (1998). Personal accounts of disclosing and concealing HIV-positive test results. In V. J. Derlega & A. P. Barbee (Eds.), *HIV and social interaction* (pp. 147–164). Thousand Oaks, CA: Sage.

Derlega, V. J., Metts, S., Petronio, S., & Margulis, S. T. (1993). *Self-disclosure.* Newbury Park, CA: Sage.

Derlega, V. J., Sherburne, S. P., & Lewis, R. J. (1998). Reactions to an HIV-positive man: Impact of his sexual orientation, cause of infection, and research participants' gender. *AIDS and Behavior, 2,* 239–348.

Derlega, V. J., & Winstead, B. A. (2001). HIV-infected persons' attributions for the disclosure and nondisclosure of the seropositive diagnosis to significant others. In V. Manusov & J. H. Harvey (Eds.), *Attribution, communication behavior, and close relationships* (pp. 266–284). New York: Cambridge University Press.

Derlega, V. J., Winstead, B. A., & Folk-Barron, L. (2000). Reasons for and against disclosing HIV-seropositive test results to an intimate partner: A functional perspective. In S. Petronio (Ed.), *Balancing the secrets of private disclosures* (pp. 53–69). Mahwah, NJ: Lawrence Erlbaum Associates, Inc.

Derlega, V. J., Winstead, B. A., Greene, K., Serovich, J. M., & Elwood, W. N. (2002). Perceived HIV-related stigma and HIV disclosure to relationship partners after finding out about the seropositive diagnosis. *Journal of Health Psychology, 7,* 415–432.

Derlega, V. J., Winstead, B. A., Oldfield, E. C., & Barbee, A. P. (in press). Close relationships and social support in coping with HIV: A Test of Sensitive Interaction Systems Theory. *AIDS and Behavior.*

Derlega, V. J., Winstead, B. A., Wong, P. T. P., & Greenspan, M. (1987). Self-disclosure and relationship development: An attributional analysis. In M. E. Roloff & G. E. Miller (Eds.), *Interpersonal processes: New directions in communication research* (pp. 172–187). Newbury Park, CA: Sage.

Derse, A. R. (1995). HIV and AIDS: Legal and ethical issues in the emergency department. *Emergency Clinics of North America, 13,* 213–223.

De Vincenzi, I., Jadand, C., Couturier, E., Brunet, J., Gallais, H., Gastaut, J., et al. (1997). Pregnancy and contraception in a French cohort of HIV-infected women. *AIDS, 11,* 333–338.

Devine, P. G., Plant, E. A., & Harrison, K. (1999). The problem of "us" versus "them" and AIDS stigma. *American Behavioral Scientist, 42,* 1212–1228.

de Vroome, E. M., de Wit, J. B., Stroebe, W., Sandfort, T. G., & Griensven, G. J. (1998). Sexual behavior and depression among HIV-positive gay men. *AIDS and Behavior, 2,* 137–149.

Diaz, R. M. (1998). *Latino gay men and HIV: Culture, sexuality, and risk behavior.* New York: Routledge.

DiClemente, R. J., Zorn, J., & Temoshok, L. (1986). Adolescents and AIDS: A survey of knowledge, beliefs, and attitudes about AIDS in San Francisco. *American Journal of Public Health, 76,* 1443–1445.

DiClemente, R. J., Zorn, J., & Temoshok, L. (1987). The association of gender, ethnicity, and length of residence in the Bay area to adolescents' knowledge and attitudes about acquired immune deficiency syndrome. *Journal of Applied Social Psychology, 17,* 218–230.

Dindia, K. (1997). Self-disclosure, self-identity, and relationship development: A transactional/dialectical perspective. In S. Duck (Ed.), *Handbook of personal relationships* (pp. 411–426). New York: Wiley

Dindia, K. (1998). "Going into and coming out of the closet": The dialectics of stigma disclosure. In B. M. Montgomery & L. A. Baxter (Eds.), *Dialectical approaches to studying personal relationships* (pp. 83–108). Mahwah, NJ: Lawrence Erlbaum Associates, Inc.

Dindia, K. (2002). Self-disclosure research: Knowledge through meta-analysis. In M. Allen, R. W. Preiss, B. M. Gayle, & N. A. Burrell (Eds.), *Interpersonal communication research: Advances through meta-analysis* (pp. 169–185). Mahwah, NJ: Lawrence Erlbaum Associates, Inc.

Dindia, K., & Allen, M. (1992). Sex-differences in self-disclosure: A meta-analysis. *Psychological Bulletin, 112,* 106–124.

Dindia, K., Fitzpatrick, M. A., & Kenny, D. A. (1997). Self-disclosure in spouse and stranger interaction: A social relations analysis. *Human Communication Research, 23,* 388–412.

Dindia, K., & Tieu, T. (1996, November). *Self-disclosure of homosexuality: The dialectics of "coming out."* Paper presented at the Speech Communication Association Convention, San Diego, CA.

Doll, L. S., Harrison, J. S., Frey, R. L., McKirnan, D., Bartholomew, B. N., Douglas, J. M., et al. (1994). Failure to disclose HIV risk among gay and bisexual men attending sexually transmitted disease clinics. *American Journal of Preventive Medicine 10,* 125–129.

Dorman, S. M., & Rienzo, B. R. (1988). College students' knowledge of AIDS. *Health Values, 12,* 33–38.

Druley, J. A., Stephens, M. A. P., & Coyne, J. C. (1997). Emotional and physical intimacy in coping with lupus: Womens' dilemmas of disclosure and approach. *Health Psychology, 16,* 506–514.

Elwood, W. N. (1999). Burden of sin: Transmitting messages and viruses in a stigmatized plague. In W. N. Elwood (Ed.), *Power in the blood: A handbook on AIDS, politics, and communication* (pp. 3–8). Mahwah, NJ: Lawrence Erlbaum Associates, Inc.

Elwood, W. N. (2002). "The head that doesn't speak one calls a cabbage": HIV, AIDS, risk, and social support in the 21st century. *Journal of Social and Personal Relationships, 19,* 143–149.

Elwood, W. N., & Greene, K. (in press). Desperately seeking skeezers: Downward comparison theory and the implications for STD/HIV prevention among illegal drug users. *Journal of Ethnicity in Substance Abuse.*

Elwood, W. N., Greene, K., & Carter, K. K. (in press). Gentlemen don't speak: Communication rules, condom use, and the theory of reasoned action. *Journal of Applied Communication Research, 31.*

Elwood, W. N., & Williams, M. L. (1999). The politics of silence: Communicative rules and HIV prevention issues in gay male bathhouses. In W. N. Elwood (Ed.), *Power in the blood: A handbook on AIDS, politics, and communication* (pp. 121–132). Mahwah, NJ: Lawrence Erlbaum Associates, Inc.

Epstein, H., & Chen, L. (2002, March 14). Can AIDS be stopped? *New York Review of Books,* pp. 29–31.

Ernst, F. A., Francis, R. A., Perkins, J., Britton-Williams, Q., & Kang, A. S. (1998). The Meharry Questionnaire: The measurement of attitudes toward AIDS-related issues. In C. M. Davis, W. L. Yarber, R. Bauserman, G. Schreer, & S. L. Davis (Eds.), *Handbook of sexuality-related measures* (pp. 316–317). Thousand Oaks, CA: Sage.

Ezzy, D. (1998). Lived experience and interpretation in narrative theory: Experiences of living with HIV/AIDS. *Qualitative Sociology, 21,* 169–179.

Ezzy, D. (2000). Illness narratives: Time, hope, and HIV. *Social Science and Medicine, 50,* 605–617.

Festinger, L. A. (1954). A theory of social comparison processes. *Human Relations, 7,* 117–140.

Fife, B. L., & Wright, E. R. (2000). The dimensionality of stigma: A comparison of its impact on the self of persons with HIV/AIDS and cancer. *Journal of Health and Social Behavior, 41,* 50–67.

Finney, P. D., & Snell, W. E., Jr. (1989, April). *The AIDS anxiety scale: Components and correlates.* Paper presented at the annual meeting of the Southwestern Psychological Association, Houston, TX.

Fishbein, M. J., & Laird, J. D. (1979). Concealment and disclosure: Some effects of information control on the person who controls. *Journal of Experimental Social Psychology, 15,* 114–121.

Fisher, J. D., Kimble Willcutts, D. L., Misovich, S. J., & Weinstein, B. (1998). Dynamics of sexual risk behavior in HIV-infected men who have sex with men. *AIDS and Behavior, 2,* 101–113.

Fisher, L., Goldschmidt, R. H., Hays, R. B., & Catania, J. A. (1993). Families of homosexual men: Their knowledge and support regarding sexual orientation and HIV disease. *Journal of the American Board of Family Practice, 6,* 25–32.

Fisher, M. (1992). *A whisper of AIDS: Address to the Republican National Convention.* Retrieved December 2, 2002, from http://gos.sbc.edu/f/fisher/html.

Fiske, S. T. (1998). Stereotyping, prejudice, and discrimination. In D. T. Gilbert, S. T. Fiske, G. Lindzey (Eds.), *The handbook of social psychology* (Vol. II, 4th ed., pp. 357–411). Boston: McGraw-Hill.

Flaskerud, J. H., & Nyamathi, A. M. (2000). Attaining gender and ethnic diversity in health intervention research: Cultural responsiveness versus resource provision. *Advances in Nursing Science, 22*(4), 1–15.

Fleishman, J. A., & Fogel, B. (1994). Coping and depressive symptoms among people with AIDS. *Health Psychology, 13,* 156–169.

Folkman, S., Chesney, M. A., & Christopher-Richards, A. (1994). Stress and coping in caregiving partners of men with AIDS. *Psychiatric Clinics of North America, 17,* 35–53.

Fox, R., Odaka, N. J., Brookmeyer, R., & Polik, B. F. (1987). Effect of HIV antibody disclosure on subsequent sexual activity in homosexual men. *AIDS, 1,* 241–246.

Freimuth, V. S., Hammond, S. L., Edgar, T., & Monahan, J. L. (1990). Reaching those at risk: A content-analytic study of AIDS PSAs. *Communication Research, 17,* 775–791.

Frey, L. R., Query, J. L., Flint, L. J., & Adelman, M. B. (1998). Living together with AIDS: Social support processes in a residential facility. In V. J. Derlega & A. P. Barbee (Eds.), *HIV and social interaction* (pp. 129–146). Thousand Oaks, CA: Sage.

Friedman, S. R., Jose, B., Neaigus, A., Goldstein, M. F., Curtis, R., Ildefonso, G., et al. (1994). Consistent condom use in relationships between seropositive injecting drug users and sex partners who do not inject drugs. *AIDS, 8,* 357–361.

Fullilove, M. T., & Fullilove, R. E. (1999). Stigma as an obstacle to AIDS action: The case of the African American community. *American Behavioral Scientist, 42,* 1117–1129.

Gard, L. H. (1990). Patient disclosure of human immunodeficiency virus (HIV) status to parents: Clinical considerations. *Professional Psychology: Research and Practice, 21,* 252–256.

Gerbert, B., Maguire, B. T., Bleeker, T., Coates, T. J., & McPhee, S. J. (1991). Primary care physicians and AIDS: Attitudinal and structural barriers to care. *Journal of the American Medical Association, 266,* 2837–2842.

Gewirtz, A., & Gossart-Walker, S. (2000). Home-based treatment for children and families affected by HIV and AIDS. *Child and Adolescent Psychiatric Clinics of North America, 9,* 313–330.

Gielen, A. C., O'Campo, P., Faden, R. R., & Eke, A. (1997). Women's disclosure of HIV status: Experiences of mistreatment and violence in an urban setting. *Women & Health, 25,* 19–31.

Gilbert, S. J. (1976). Empirical and theoretical extensions of self-disclosure. In G. R. Miller (Ed.), *Explorations in interpersonal communication* (pp. 197–216). Beverly Hills, CA: Sage.

Gill, V. T., & Maynard, D. W. (1995). On "labeling" in actual intervention: Delivering and receiving diagnoses of developmental disabilities. *Social Problems, 42,* 11–31.

Glaser, B., & Strauss, A. (1967). *The discovery of grounded theory.* Chicago: Aldine.

Goffman, E. (1963). *Stigma: Notes on the management of spoiled identity.* Engelwood Cliffs, NJ: Prentice Hall.

Golden, M R. (2002). HIV partner notification: A neglected prevention intervention. *Sexually Transmitted Diseases, 29,* 472–475.

Goldsmith, D., & Parks, M. R. (1990). Communicative strategies for managing the risks of seeking social support. In S. Duck & R. C. Silver (Eds.), *Personal relationships and social support* (pp. 104–121). London: Sage.

Gouldner, A. W. (1960). The norm of reciprocity: A preliminary statement. *American Sociological Review, 25,* 161–178.

Graham, S., Weiner, B., Giuliano, T., & Williams, E. (1993). An attributional analysis of reactions to Magic Johnson. *Journal of Applied Social Psychology, 23,* 996–1010.

Gramling, L., Boyle, J. S., McCain, N., Ferrell, J., Hodnicki, D., & Muller, R. (1996). Reconstructing a woman's experiences with AIDS. *Family and Community Health, 19,* 49–56.

Gray, L. A., & Saracino, M. (1989). AIDS on campus: A preliminary study of college students' knowledge and behaviors. *Journal of Counseling and Development, 68,* 199–202.

Green, G. (1994). Positive sex: Sexual relationships following an HIV-positive diagnosis. In P. Aggleton, P. Davis, & G. Hart (Eds.), *AIDS: Foundations for the future* (pp. 136–146). London: Taylor & Francis.

Green, G., & Rademan, P. (1997). Evangelical leaders and people with HIV. *AIDS Care, 9,* 715–726.

Greene, K. (2000). Disclosure of chronic illness varies by topic and target: The role of stigma and boundaries in willingness to disclose. In S. Petronio (Ed.), *Balancing the secrets of private disclosures* (pp. 123–135). Mahwah, NJ: Lawrence Erlbaum Associates, Inc.

Greene, K. (2001). *The effects of relational quality on disclosure of HIV-infection.* Manuscript submitted for publication, Rutgers University, New Brunswick, NJ.

Greene, K., & Cassidy, B. (1999). Ethical choices regarding noncompliance: Prescribing protease inhibitors for HIV-infected adolescent females. In W. N. Elwood (Ed.), *Power in the blood: A handbook on AIDS, politics, and communication* (pp. 369–384). Mahwah, NJ: Lawrence Erlbaum Associates, Inc.

Greene, K., & Faulkner, S. L. (2002). Self-disclosure in relationships of HIV-positive African-American adolescent females. *Communication Studies, 53,* 297–317.

Greene, K., Frey, L. R., & Derlega, V. J. (2002). Interpersonalizing AIDS: Attending to the personal and social relationships of individuals living with HIV and/or AIDS. *Journal of Social and Personal Relationships, 19,* 5–17.

Greene, K., Parrott, R., & Serovich, J. M. (1993). Privacy, HIV testing, and AIDS: College students' versus parents' perspectives. *Health Communication, 5,* 59–74.

Greene, K., & Serovich, J. M. (1995, November). *Predictors of willingness to disclose HIV infection to nuclear family members.* Paper presented at the annual meeting of the Speech Communication Association, San Antonio, TX.

Greene, K., & Serovich, J. M. (1996). Appropriateness of disclosure of HIV testing information: The perspective of PLWAs. *Journal of Applied Communication Research, 24,* 50–65.

Greene, K., & Serovich, J. M. (1998). An eye to the future of HIV/AIDS and social relationships: An epilogue. In V. J. Derlega & A. P. Barbee (Eds.), *HIV and social interaction* (pp. 218–238). Thousand Oaks, CA: Sage.

Haas, S. M. (2002). Social support as relationship maintenance in gay male couples coping with HIV/AIDS. *Journal of Social and Personal Relationships, 19,* 87–111.

Hackl, K. L., Somlai, A. M., Kelly, J. A., & Kalichman, S. C. (1997). Women living with HIV/AIDS: The dual challenge of being a patient and caregiver. *Health and Social Work, 22,* 53–62.

Hammer, S. M. (2002). Increasing choices for HIV therapy. *New England Journal of Medicine, 346,* 2022–2023.

Haney, D. Q. (2002, February 27). High hopes in human tests of AIDS vaccine. *The Virginian-Pilot,* p. A8.

Harney, D. M. (1999). Lesbians on the frontline: Battling AIDS, gays, and they myth of community. In W. N. Elwood (Ed.), *Power in the blood: A handbook on AIDS, politics, and communication* (pp. 167–179). Mahwah, NJ: Lawrence Erlbaum Associates, Inc.

Hassin, J. (1994). Living a responsible life: The impact of AIDS on the social identity of intravenous drug users. *Social Science and Medicine, 39,* 391–400.

Hatala, M. N., Baack, D. W., & Parmenter, R. (1998). Dating with HIV: A content analysis of gay male HIV-positive and HIV-negative personal advertisements. *Journal of Social and Personal Relationships, 15,* 268–276.

Hays, R. B., Catania, J. A., McKusick, L., & Coates, T. J. (1990). Help-seeking for AIDS-related concerns: A comparison of gay men with various HIV diagnoses. *American Journal of Community Psychology, 18,* 743–755.

Hays, R. B., Chauncey, S., & Tobey, L. (1990). The social support networks of gay men with AIDS. *Journal of Community Psychology, 18,* 374–385.

Hays, R. B., Magee, R. H., & Chauncey, S. (1994). Identifying helpful and unhelpful behaviors of loved ones: The PWA's perspective. *AIDS Care, 6,* 379–392.

Hays, R. B., McKusick, L., Pollack, L., Hilliard, R., Hoff, C. C., & Coates, T. J. (1993). Disclosing HIV seropositivity to significant others. *AIDS, 7,* 425–431.

Hays, R. B., Turner, H., & Coates, T. J. (1992). Social support, AIDS-related symptoms, and depression among gay men. *Journal of Consulting and Clinical Psychology, 60,* 463–469.

Helgeson, V. S., & Mickelson, K. D. (1995). Motives for social comparison. *Personality and Social Psychology Bulletin, 21,* 1200–1209.

Herek, G. M. (1997). The HIV epidemic and public attitudes toward lesbians and gay men. In M. P. Levine, P. Nardi, & J. Gagnon (Eds.), *In changing times: Gay men and lesbians encounter HIV/AIDS* (pp. 191–218). Chicago: University of Chicago Press.

Herek, G. M. (1999a). AIDS and stigma. *American Behavioral Scientist, 42,* 1106–1116.

Herek, G. M. (Ed.). (1999b). AIDS and stigma in the United States. [Special issue]. *American Behavioral Scientist, 42.*

Herek, G. M., & Capitanio, J. P. (1993). Public reactions to AIDS in the United States: A second decade of stigma. *American Journal of Public Health, 83,* 574–577.

Herek, G. M., & Capitanio, J. P. (1999). AIDS and stigma and sexual prejudice. *American Behavioral Scientist, 42,* 1130–1147.

Herek, G. M., Capitanio, J. P., & Widaman, K. F. (2002). HIV-related stigma and knowledge in the United States: Prevalence and trends, 1991–1999. *American Journal of Public Health, 92,* 371–377.

Herek, G. M., & Cogan, J. (1995). *AIDS and stigma: A review of the scientific literature.* San Francisco: Public Media Center.

Hewes, D. E., Graham, M. K., Doelger, J., & Pavitt, C. (1985). "Second guessing": Message interpretation in social networks. *Human Communication Research, 11,* 299–334.

Hines, S. C. (2001). Coping with uncertainties in advance care planning. *Journal of Communication, 51,* 498–513.

HIV/AIDS Surveillance Report. (2002). 13(1). AIDS cases through June 2001.

Hoff, C. C., Coates, T. J., Barrett, D. C., Collette, L., & Ekstrand, M. (1996). Differences between gay men in primary relationships and single men: Implications for prevention. *AIDS Education and Prevention, 8,* 546–559.

Hoff, C. C., Stall, R., Paul, J., Acree, M., Daigle, D., & Phillips, K. (1997). Differences in sexual behavior among HIV discordant and concordant gay men in primary relationships. *Journal of Acquired Immune Deficiency Syndromes and Human Retrovirology, 14,* 72–78.

Hoffman, M. A. (1996). *Counseling clients with HIV disease: Assessment, intervention, and prevention*. New York: Guilford.

Holt, R., Court, P., Vedhara, K., Nott, K. H., Holmes, J., & Snow, M. H. (1998). The role of disclosure in coping with HIV infection. *AIDS Care, 10*, 49–60.

Ickovics, J. R., Thayaparan, B., & Ethier, K. A. (2001). Women and AIDS: A contextual analysis. In A. Baum, T. A. Revenson, & J. E. Singer (Eds.), *Handbook of health psychology* (pp. 817–839). Mahwah, NJ: Lawrence Erlbaum Associates, Inc.

Ingram, K. M., Jones, D. A., Fass, R. J., Neidig, J. L. & Song, Y. S. (1999). Social support and unsupportive social interactions: Their association with depression among people living with HIV. *AIDS Care, 11*, 313–329.

Jackson, L. A., Millson, M., Calzavara, L., Dtrathdee, S., Walmsley, S., Rachlis, A., et al. (1998–1999). Community HIV prevention: What can we learn from the perceptions and experiences of HIV-positive women living in metropolitan Toronto, Canada? *International Quarterly of Community Health Education, 18*, 307–330.

Jefferson, G. (1984). On stepwise transition from talk about a trouble to inappropriately next-positioned matters. In J. M. Atkinson & J. Heritage (Eds.), *Structures of social action: Studies in conversation analysis* (pp. 191–222). Cambridge, England: Cambridge University Press.

Jones, E. E., Farina, A., Hastorf, A. H., Markus, H., Miller, D. T., & Scott, R. A. (1984). *Social stigma: The psychology of marked relationships*. New York: Freeman.

Jones, E. E., & Gordon, E. M. (1972). Timing of self-disclosure and its effects on personal attraction. *Journal of Personality and Social Psychology, 24*, 358–365.

Jourard, S. M. (1971). *The transparent self* (Rev. ed.). New York: Van Nostrand Reinhold.

Julian, P. (1997). Prevention may be getting wiser: New study puts AIDS risk in the context of reality. *San Francisco Frontiers, 27*, 11–13.

Kahn, J. H., Achter, J. A., & Shambaugh, E. J. (2001). Client distress disclosure, characteristics at intake, and outcome in brief counseling. *Journal of Counseling Psychology, 48*, 203–211.

Kahn, J. H., & Hessling, R. M. (2001). Measuring the tendency to conceal versus disclose psychological distress. *Journal of Social and Clinical Psychology, 20*, 41–65.

Kalichman, S. C. (1995). *Understanding AIDS: A guide for mental health professionals*. Washington, DC: American Psychological Association.

Kalichman, S. C. (2000). Couples with HIV/AIDS. In K. B. Schmaling & T. G. Sher (Eds.), *The psychology of couples and illness: Theory, research, and practice* (pp. 171–190). Washington, DC: American Psychological Association.

Kalichman, S. C., Roffman, R. A., Picciano, J. F., & Bolan, M. (1998). Risk for HIV infection among bisexual men seeking HIV-prevention services and risks posed to their female partners. *Health Psychology, 17*, 320–327.

Kalichman, S. C., Rompa, D., & Cage, M. (2000). Distinguishing between overlapping somatic symptoms of depression and HIV disease in people living with HIV-AIDS. *The Journal of Nervous and Mental Disease, 188*, 662–670.

Kellerman, K. (1987). Information exchange in social interaction. In M. E. Roloff & G. E. Miller (Eds.), *Interpersonal processes: New directions in communication research* (pp. 188–219). Newbury Park, CA: Sage.

Kellerman, K., & Lim, T. (1990). The conversion MOP III: Timing of scenes in discourse. *Journal of Personality and Social Psychology, 59*, 1163–1179.

Kelley, J. E., Lumley, M. A., & Leisen, J. C. C. (1997). Health effects of emotional disclosure in rheumatoid arthritis patients. *Health Psychology, 16*, 331–340.

Kelly, A. E. (2002). *The psychology of secrets*. New York: Kluwer Academic/Plenum.

Kelly, A. E., Klusas, J. A., von Weiss, R. T., & Kenny, C. (2001). What is it about revealing secrets that is beneficial? *Personality and Social Psychology Bulletin, 27*, 651–665.

Kelly, A. E., & McKillop, K. J. (1996). Consequences of revealing personal secrets. *Psychological Bulletin, 120*, 450–465.

Kelly, A. E., Otto-Salaj, L. L., Sikkema, K. J., Pinkerton, S. D., & Bloom, F. R. (1998). Implications of HIV treatment advances for behavioral research on AIDS: Protease inhibitors and new challenges in HIV secondary prevention. *Health Psychology, 17*, 310–319.

Kelly, J. A., St. Lawrence, J. S., Smith, S., Hood, H. V., & Cook, D. J. (1987a). Medical students, attitudes towards AIDS and homosexual patients. *Journal of Medical Education, 62*, 549–556.

Kelly, J. A., St. Lawrence, J. S., Smith, S., Hood, H. V., & Cook, D. J. (1987b). Stigmatization of AIDS patients by physicians. *American Journal of Public Health, 77*, 789–791.

Kelvin, P. (1977). Predictability, power, and vulnerability in interpersonal attraction. In S. Duck (Ed.), *Theory and practice in interpersonal attraction* (pp. 355–378). New York: Academic.

Kennedy, R. E., & Fulton, R. (1998). The emerging third stage of the AIDS epidemic: The low-risk heterosexual. *Illness, Crisis and Loss, 6*, 45–61.

Kiesler, C., Kiesler, S., & Pallak, M. (1967). The effects of commitment to future interaction on reactions to norm violations. *Journal of Personality, 35*, 389–399.

Kimberly, J. A., & Serovich, J. M. (1996). Perceived social support among people living with HIV/AIDS. *The American Journal of Family Therapy, 24*, 41–53.

Kimberly, J. A., Serovich, J. M., & Greene, K. (1995). Disclosure of HIV-positive status: Five women's stories. *Family Relations, 44*, 316–322.

Kimerling, R., Armistead, L., & Forehand, R. (1999). Victimization experiences and HIV infection in women: Associations with serostatus, psychological symptoms, and health status. *Journal of Traumatic Stress, 12*, 41–58.

King, N. (1995). HIV and the gay male community: One clinician's reflections over the years. In G. M. Herek & B. Greene (Eds.), *AIDS, identity, and community: The HIV epidemic and lesbians and gay men* (pp. 1–18). Thousand Oaks, CA: Sage.

Kitzinger, J. (1991). Judging by appearances: Audience understandings of the look of someone with HIV. *Journal of Community and Applied Social Psychology, 1*, 155–163.

Kleiser, R. (Producer/Writer/Director), Knapp, H. (Producer), & Thurm, J. (Producer). (1996). *It's my party* [Motion Picture]. United States: MGM/United Artists.

Kline, A., & VanLandingham, M. (1994). HIV-infected women and sexual risk reduction: The relevance of existing models of behavior change. *AIDS Education and Prevention, 6*, 390–402.

Klitzman, R. L. (1999). Self-disclosure of HIV status to sexual partners: A qualitative study of issues faced by gay men. *Journal of the Gay and Lesbian Medical Association, 3*, 39–49.

Koopman, C., Rotheram-Borus, M. J., Henderson, R., Bradley, J. S., & Hunter, J. (1990). Assessment of knowledge of AIDS and beliefs about AIDS prevention among adolescents. *AIDS Education and Prevention, 2*, 58–69.

Kotchick, B. A., Forehand, R., Brody, G., Armistead, L., Morse, E., Simon, P., et al. (1997). The impact of maternal HIV infection on parenting in inner-city African American families. *Journal of Family Psychology, 11*, 447–461.

Kresge, K. (2002, July). International AIDS conference to focus on the epidemic's unchecked spread. Retrieved July 15, 2002, from http://www.amfar.prg/cgi-bin (Amfar News/Analysis).

Lane, J. D., & Wegner, D. M. (1995). The cognitive consequences of secrecy. *Journal of Personality and Social Psychology, 69*, 237–253.

Langer, E. J. (1978). Rethinking the role of thought in social interaction. In J. H. Harvey, W. Ickes, & R. F. Kidd (Eds.), *New directions in attribution research* (Vol. 2, pp. 35–58). Hillsdale, NJ: Lawrence Erlbaum Associates, Inc.

Larsen, K., Serra, M., & Long, E. (1990). AIDS victims and heterosexual attitudes. *Journal of Homosexuality, 19*, 103–116.

Larson, D. G., & Chastain, R. L. (1990). Self-concealment: Conceptualization, measurement, and health implications. *Journal of Social and Clinical Psychology, 9*, 439–455.

Larson, J. (Writer), Mardin, A. (Producer), & Grief, M. (Director). (1996). *Rent* [Play]. Broadway, NY.

Leary, M. R., & Schreindorfer, L. S. (1998). The stigmatization of HIV and AIDS: Rubbing salt in the wound. In V. J. Derlega & A. P. Barbee (Eds.), *HIV and social interaction* (pp. 12–29). Thousand Oaks, CA: Sage.

Lehman, D. R., Ellard, J. H., & Wortman, C. B. (1986). Social support for the bereaved: Recipients' and providers' perspectives on what is helpful. *Journal of Consulting and Clinical Psychology, 54,* 438–446.

Lemieux, R., Tighe, M. R., Daniels, M. J., Greene, K., Hocking, J. E., Cairns, A. B., et al. (1998). The persuasive effect of the AIDS NAMES quilt on behavioral intentions. *Communication Research Reports, 15,* 113–120.

Leone, C., & Wingate, C. (1991). A functional approach to understanding attitudes toward AIDS victims. *Journal of Social Psychology, 131,* 761–768.

Lepore, S. J., Greenberg, M. A., Brunjo, M., & Smyth, J. M. (2002). Expressive writing and health: Self-regulation of emotion-related experiences, physiology, and behavior. In S. J. Lepore & J. M. Smyth (Eds.), *The writing cure: How expressive writing promotes health and emotional well-being* (pp. 99–117). Washington, DC: American Psychological Association.

Lepore, S. J., Ragan, J. D., & Jones, S. (2000). Talking facilitates cognitive-emotional processes of adaptation to an acute stressor. *Journal of Personality and Social Psychology, 78,* 499–508.

Lepore, S. J., & Smyth, J. M. (Eds.). (2002). *The writing cure: How expressive writing promotes health and emotional well-being.* Washington, DC: American Psychological Association.

Leserman, J., Perkins, D. O., & Evans, D. L. (1992). Coping with the threat of AIDS: The role of social support. *American Journal of Psychiatry, 149,* 1514–1520.

Leserman, J., Petitto, J. M., Golden, R. N., Gaynes, B. N., Gu, H., Perkins, D. O., et al. (2000). Impact of stressful life events, depression, social support, coping and cortisol on progression to AIDS. *American Journal of Psychiatry, 157,* 1221–1228.

Leslie, M. B., Stein, J. A., & Rotheram-Borus, M. J. (2002). The impact of coping strategies, personal relationships, and emotional distress on health-related outcomes of parents living with HIV or AIDS. *Journal of Social and Personal Relationships, 19,* 45–66.

Lester, P., Partridge, J. C., Chesney, M. A., & Cooke, M. (1995). The consequences of a positive prenatal HIV antibody test for women. *Journal of Acquired Immune Deficiency Syndromes and Human Retrovirology, 10,* 341–349.

Levin, B. W., Krantz, D. H., Driscoll, J. M., & Fleischman, A. R. (1995). The treatment of non-HIV-related conditions in newborns at risk for HIV: A survey of neonatologists. *American Journal of Public Health, 85,* 1507–1513.

Levine, C. (1993). *Orphans of the HIV epidemic.* New York: United Hospital Fund of New York.

Levinger, G., & Snoek, D. J. (1972). *Attraction in relationship: A new look at interpersonal attraction.* Morristown, NJ: General Learning Press.

Limandri, B. J. (1989). Disclosure of stigmatizing conditions: The discloser's perspective. *Archives of Psychiatric Nursing, 3,* 69–78.

Lindhorst, T., & Mancoske, R. (1993). Structuring support for volunteer commitment: An AIDS services program study. *Journal of Sociology and Social Welfare, 20,* 175–188.

Lindsay, M. B., Grant, J., Peterson, H. B., Willis, S., Nelson, P., & Klein, L. (1995). The impact of knowledge of human immunodeficiency virus serostatus on contraceptive choice and repeat pregnancy. *Obstetrics and Gynecology, 85,* 675–679.

Louganis, G. (1996). *Breaking the surface.* New York: Penguin.

Lutgendorf, S. K., Antoni, M. H., Schneiderman, N., & Fletcher, M. A. (1994). Psychosocial counseling to improve quality of life in HIV infection. *Patient Education and Counseling, 24,* 217–235.

Lutgendorf, S. K., & Ullrich, P. (2002). Cognitive processing, disclosure, and health: Psychological and physiological mechanisms. In S. J. Lepore & J. M. Smyth (Eds.), *The writing cure: How expressive writing promotes health and emotional well-being* (pp. 177–196). Washington, DC: American Psychological Association.

Lyketsos, C. G., Hoover, D. R., Guccione, M., Senterfitt, W., Dew, M. A., Wesch, J., et al. (1993). Depressive symptoms as predictors of medical outcomes in HIV infection. *Journal of the American Medical Association, 270,* 2563–2567.

MMWR (Morbidity & Mortality Weekly Report). (2002, November 22). Notice to readers: Approval of a new rapid test for HIV anitbody. *MMWR, 51,* 1051–1052. Retrieved November 27, 2002, from http://www.cdc.gov/mmwr/preview/mmwrhtml/mm5146a5.htm.

MacFarlane, K., & Krebs, S. (1986). Techniques for interviewing and evidence gathering. In K. MacFarlane & J. Waterman (Eds.), *Sexual abuse of young children: Evaluation and treatment* (pp. 67–100). New York: Guilford.

MacKellar, D. (2002). Many HIV positive gays unaware they're infected. Presented at the XIV International AIDS Conference, Barcelona, Spain. Retrieved July 19, 2002, from http://www.cnn.com/2002/HEALTH/conditions/07/08/aids.awareness.ap/index.html.

Mansergh, G., Marks, G., & Simoni, J. M. (1995). Self-disclosure of HIV infection among men who vary in time since seropositive diagnosis and symptomatic status. *AIDS, 9,* 639–644.

Markova, I., & Power, K. (1992). Audience response to health messages about AIDS. In T. Edgar, M. A. Fitzpatrick, & V. S. Freimuth (Eds.), *AIDS: A communication perspective* (pp. 111–130). Hillsdale, NJ: Lawrence Erlbaum Associates, Inc.

Markova, I., Wilkie, P. A., Naji, S. A., & Forbes, C. D. (1990). Self- and other-awareness of the risk of HIV/AIDS in people with hemophilia and implications for behavioral change. *Social Science and Medicine, 31,* 73–79.

Markowitz, J. C., Rabkin, J. G., & Perry, S. W. (1994). Treating depression in HIV-positive patients. *AIDS, 8,* 403–412.

Marks, G., Bundek, N. I., Richardson, J. L., Ruiz, M. S., Maldonado, N., & Mason, H. R. (1992). Self-disclosure of HIV infection: Preliminary results from a sample of Hispanic men. *Health Psychology, 11,* 300–306.

Marks, G., Cantero, P. J., & Simoni, J. M. (1998). Is acculturation associated with sexual risk behaviours? An investigation of HIV-positive Latino men and women. *AIDS Care, 10,* 283–295.

Marks, G., Mason, H. R., & Simoni, J. M. (1995). The prevalence of patient disclosure of HIV infection to doctors. *American Journal of Public Health, 85,* 1018–1019.

Marks, G., Richardson, J. L., & Maldonado, N. (1991). Self-disclosure of HIV infection to sexual partners. *American Journal of Public Health, 81,* 1321–1322.

Marks, G., Ruiz, M. S., Richardson, J. L., Reed, D., Mason, H. R., Sotelo, M., et al. (1994). Anal intercourse and disclosure of HIV infection among seropositive gay and bisexual men. *Journal of Acquired Immune Deficiency Syndrome, 7,* 866–869.

Mason, H. R. C., Marks, G., Simoni, J. M., Ruiz, M. S., & Richardson, J. L. (1995). Culturally sanctioned secrets? Latino men's nondisclosure of HIV infection to family, friends, and lovers. *Health Psychology, 14,* 6–12.

Mattson, M. (1999). Toward a reconceptualization of communication cues to action in the health belief model: HIV Test counseling. *Communication Monographs, 66,* 240–265.

Mattson, M. (2000). Empowerment through agency-promoting dialogue: An explicit application of harm reduction theory to reframe HIV test counseling. *Journal of Health Communication, 5,* 333–347.

Mattson, M., & Roberts, F. (2001). Overcoming truth telling as an obstacle to initiating safer sex: Clients and health practitioners planning deception during HIV test counseling. *Health Communication, 13,* 343–362.

Mayes, S. D., Elsesser, V., Schaefer, J. H., Handford, H. A., & Michael-Good, L. (1992). Sexual practices and AIDS knowledge among women partners of HIV-infected hemophiliacs. *Public Health Reports, 107,* 504–514.

Maynard, D. W. (1997). The news delivery sequence: Bad news and good news in conversational interaction. *Research on Language and Social Interaction, 30,* 93–130.

Mays, V. M. (Ed.). (1996). The behavioral and social contexts of HIV infection risk in lesbians and other women who have sex with women. [Special issue]. *Women's Health: Research on Gender, Behavior, & Policy, 2*(1 & 2).

McAllister, M. P. (1992). AIDS, medicalization, and the news media. In T. Edgar, M. A. Fitzpatrick, & V. S. Freimuth (Eds.), *AIDS: A communication perspective* (pp. 195–221). Hillsdale, NJ: Lawrence Erlbaum Associates, Inc.

McCall, G. J., & Simmons, J. L. (1978). *Identities and interactions: An examination of human associations in everyday life.* New York: The Free Press.

McCusker, J., Stoddard, A. M., Mayer, K. H., Zapka, J., Morrison, C., & Saltzman, S. P. (1988). Effects of HIV antibody test knowledge on subsequent sexual behaviors in a cohort of homosexually active men. *American Journal of Public Health, 78,* 462–467.

Metts, S., & Fitzpatrick, M. A. (1992). Thinking about safe sex: The risky business of "know your partner" advice. In T. Edgar, M. A. Fitzpatrick, & V. S. Freimuth (Eds.), *AIDS: A communication perspective* (pp. 1–20). Hillsdale, NJ: Lawrence Erlbaum Associates, Inc.

Metts, S., & Manns, H. (1996). Coping with HIV and AIDS: The social and personal challenges. In E. B. Ray (Ed.), *Communication and disenfranchisement: Social health issues and implications* (pp. 347–364). Mahwah, NJ: Lawrence Erlbaum Associates, Inc.

Miell, D. E. (1984). *Cognitive and communicative strategies in developing relationships.* Unpublished doctoral dissertation, University of Lancaster, Lancaster, Lancashire, United Kingdom.

Miell, D. E., & Duck, S. W. (1986). Strategies in developing friendships. In V. J. Derlega & B. A. Winstead (Eds.), *Friendship and social interaction* (pp. 129–143). New York: Springer-Verlag.

Miles, M. S., Burchinal, P., Holditch-Davis, D., Wasilevski, Y., & Christian, B. (1997). Personal, family, and health-related correlates of depressive symptoms in mothers with HIV. *Journal of Family Psychology, 11,* 23–34.

Millar, F. E., & Rogers, L. E. (1987). Relational dimensions of interpersonal dynamics. In M. E. Roloff & G. E. Miller (Eds.), *Interpersonal processes: New directions in communication research* (pp. 117–139). Newbury Park, CA: Sage.

Miller, D. H. (1998). *Freedom to differ: The shaping of the gay and lesbian struggle for civil rights.* New York: New York University Press.

Miller, L. C., Berg, J. H., & Archer, R. L. (1983). Openers: Individuals who elicit intimate self-disclosure. *Journal of Personality and Social Psychology, 44,* 1234–1244.

Misener, T. R., & Sowell, R. L. (1998). HIV-infected women's decisions to take antiretrovirals. *Western Journal of Nursing Research, 20,* 431–447.

Mofenson, L. M. (2002). U.S. public health service task force recommendation for use of antiretroviral drugs in pregnant HIV-1 infected women for maternal health and interventions to reduce perinatal HIV-1 transmission in the United States. *MMWR, 51,* 1–38. Retrieved November 27, 2002, from http://www.cdc.gov/mmwr/preview/mmwrhtml/rr5118a1.htm.

Mondragon, D., Kirkman-Liff, B., & Schneller, E. S. (1991). Hostility to people with AIDS: Risk perception and demographic factors. *Social Science and Medicine, 32,* 1137–1142

Monette, P. (1988). *Borrowed time: An AIDS memoir.* San Diego: Harcourt Brace Jovanovich.

Moneyham, L., Seals, B., Demi, A., Sowell, R., Cohen, L., & Guillory, J. (1996). Experiences of disclosure in women infected with HIV. *Health Care for Women International, 17,* 209–221.

Moore, B. (1984). *Privacy: Studies in social and cultural history.* Armank, NY: Sharpe.

Morr, M. C. (2002). *Private disclosure in a family membership transition: In-laws' disclosures to newlyweds.* Unpublished doctoral dissertation, Arizona State University, Tempe.

Moulton, J. M., Sweet, D. M., Temoshok, L., & Mandel, J. S. (1987). Attributions of blame and responsibility in relation to distress and health behavior change in people with AIDS and AIDS-related complex. *Journal of Applied Social Psychology, 17,* 493–506.

Murphy, S. T., Monahan, J. L., & Miller, L. C. (1998). Inference under the influence: The impact of alcohol and inhibition conflict on women's sexual decision making. *Personality and Social Psychology Bulletin, 24,* 517–528.

Nimmons, D., & Folkman, S. (1999). Other-sensitive motivation for safer sex among gay men: Expanding paradigms for HIV prevention. *AIDS and Behavior, 3,* 313–324.

No Child Left Behind Act of 2001, Pub. L. No. 107-110, § 9525, 115, Stat. 1425, 1981. (2002).

Norman, L. R., Kennedy, M., & Parish, K. (1998). Close relationships and safer sex among HIV-infected men with hemophilia. *AIDS Care, 10,* 339–354.

North, R. L., & Rothenberg, K. H. (1993). Partner notification and the threat of domestic violence against women with HIV infection. *New England Journal of Medicine, 329,* 1194–1196.

Nott, K. H., & Vedhara, K. (1999). Nature and consequences of stressful life events in homosexual HIV-positive men: A review. *AIDS Care, 11,* 235–243.

Nyanjom, D., Greaves, W., Delapenha, R., Barnes, S., Boynes, F., & Frederick, W. R. (1988). Sexual behavior change among HIV-seropositive individuals. *AIDS and Public Policy Journal, 3,* 71–73.

Oddi, L. F. (1994). Disclosure of human immunodeficiency virus status in health care settings: Ethical concerns. *Journal of Intravenous Nursing, 17,* 93–102.

O'Donnell, L., O'Donnell, C., Pleck, J. H., Snarey, J., & Rose, R. (1987). Psychological responses of hospital workers to acquired immune deficiency syndrome (AIDS). *Journal of Applied Sociology, 17,* 269–285.

Omarzu, J. (2000). A disclosure decision model: Determining how and when individuals will disclose. *Personality and Social Psychology Review, 4,* 174–185.

Omoto, A. M., Gunn, D. O., & Crain, A. L. (1998). Helping in hard times: Relationship closeness and the AIDS volunteer experience. In V. J. Derlega & A. P. Barbee (Eds.), *HIV and social interaction* (pp. 106–128). Thousand Oaks, CA: Sage.

Omoto, A. M., Snyder, M., & Berghuis, J. P. (1993). The psychology of volunteerism: A conceptual analysis and a program of action research. In J. B. Pryor & G. D. Reeder (Eds.), *The social psychology of HIV infection* (pp. 263–286). Hillsdale, NJ: Lawrence Erlbaum Associates, Inc.

Pakenham, K. I., Dadds, M. R., & Terry, D. J. (1994). Relationships between adjustment to HIV and both social support and coping. *Journal of Consulting and Clinical Psychology, 62,* 1194–1203.

Pakenham, K. I., Dadds, M. R., & Terry, D. J. (1996). Adaptive demands along HIV disease continuum. *Social Science and Medicine, 42,* 245–256.

Pearce, W. B., & Sharp, S. M. (1973). Self-disclosing communication. *Journal of Communication, 23,* 409–425.

Pennebaker, J. W. (1988). Confession, inhibition, and disease. In L. Berkowitz (Ed.), *Advances in experimental social psychology* (Vol. 22, pp. 211–242). Orlando, FL: Academic.

Pennebaker, J. W. (1990). *Opening up: The healing power of confiding in others.* New York: Morrow.

Pennebaker, J. W. (Ed.). (1995). *Emotion, disclosure, and health.* Washington, DC: American Psychological Association.

Pennebaker, J. W., Colder, M., & Sharp, L. K. (1990). Accelerating the coping process. *Journal of Personality and Social Psychology, 58,* 528–537.

Pequegnat, W., & Bray, J. H. (1997). Families and HIV / AIDS: Introduction to the special section. *Journal of Family Psychology, 11,* 3–10.

Pequegnat, W., & Szapocznik, J. (Eds.). (2000). *Working with families in the era of HIV/AIDS.* Thousands Oaks, CA: Sage.

Perry, S. W., Mofatt, M. J., Card, C. A., Fishman, B., Azima-Heller, R., & Jacobsberg, L. B. (1993). Self-disclosure of HIV infection to dentists and physicians. *Journal of the American Dental Association, 124,* 51–54.

Perry, S., Ryan, J., Ashman, T., & Jacobsberg, L. (1992). Refusal of zidouvine by HIV-positive patients. *AIDS, 6,* 514–515.

Perry, S., Ryan, J., Fogel, K., Fishman, B., & Jacobsberg, L. (1990). Voluntarily informing others of positive HIV test results: Patterns of notification by infected gay men. *Hospital and Community Psychiatry, 41,* 549–551.

Peters, L., den Boer, D. J., Kok, G., & Schaalma, H. P. (1994). Public reactions towards people with AIDS: An attributional analysis. *Patient Education and Counseling, 24,* 323–335.

Peterson, J. L., Coates, T. J., Catania, J. A., Hilliard, B., Middleton, L., & Hearst, N. (1995). Help-seeking for AIDS high-risk sexual behavior among gay and bisexual African-American men. *AIDS Education and Prevention, 7,* 1–9.

Petronio, S. (1991). Communication boundary management: A theoretical model of managing disclosure of private information between marital couples. *Communication Theory, 1,* 311–335.

Petronio, S. (2000a). The boundaries of privacy: Praxis of everyday life. In S. Petronio (Ed.), *Balancing the secrets of private disclosures* (pp. 37–49). Mahwah, NJ: Lawrence Erlbaum Associates, Inc.

Petronio, S. (2000b). The ramifications of a reluctant confidant. In A. C. Richards & T. Schumrum (Eds.), *Invitations to dialogue: The legacy of Sidney Jourard* (pp. 113–132). Dubuque, IA: Kendell/Hunt.

Petronio, S. (2002). *Boundaries of privacy: Dialectics of disclosure.* Albany: State University of New York Press.

Petronio, S., & Bantz, C. (1991). Controlling the ramifications of disclosure: "Don't tell anybody but...." *Journal of Language and Social Psychology, 10,* 263–269.

Petronio, S., Flores, L., & Hecht, M. (1997). Locating the voice of logic: Disclosure discourse of sexual abuse. *Western Journal of Communication, 61,* 101–113.

Petronio, S., Jones, S., & Morr, M. C. (2003). Family privacy dilemmas: A communication boundary management perspective. In L. R. Frey (Ed.), *Group communication in context: Studies of bona fide groups* (2nd ed., pp. 23–56). Mahwah, NJ: Lawrence Erlbaum Associates, Inc.

Petronio, S., & Magni, J. (1996, November). *Being gay and HIV positive: Boundary regulation of disclosure discourse.* Paper presented at the annual meeting of the Speech Communication Association, San Diego, CA.

Petronio, S., & Martin, J. N. (1986). Ramifications of revealing private information. *Journal of Clinical Psychology, 42,* 499–506.

Petronio, S., Martin, J., & Littlefield, R. (1984). Prerequisite conditions for self-disclosure: A gender issue. *Communication Monographs, 51,* 268–273.

Petronio, S., Reeder, H. M., Hecht, M. L., & Mon't Ros-Mendoza, T. M. (1996). Disclosure of sexual abuse by children and adolescents. *Journal of Applied Communication Research, 24,* 181–199.

Pilowsky, D. J., Sohler, N., & Susser, E. (1999). The parent disclosure interview. *AIDS Care, 11,* 447–452.

Pingree, S., Hawkins, R. P., Gustafson, D. H., Boberg, E., Bricker, E., Wse, M., et al. (1996). Will the disadvantaged ride the information highway? Hopeful answers from a computer-based health crisis system. *Journal of Broadcasting and Electronic Media, 40,* 331–353.

Pleck, J. H., O'Donnell, L., O'Donnell, C., & Snarey, J. (1988). AIDS-phobia, contact with AIDS, and AIDS-related job stress in hospital workers. *Journal of Homosexuality, 15,* 41–54.

Pliskin, M., Farrell, K., Crandles, S., & DeHovitz, J. (1993). Factors influencing HIV positive mothers' disclosure to their non-infected children. *International Conference on AIDS, 9,* 898.

Plummer, K. (1995). *Telling sexual stories: Power, change and social worlds.* London: Routledge.

Powell-Cope, G. M. (1995). The experience of gay couples affected by HIV infection. *Qualitative Health Research, 5,* 36–62.

Powell-Cope, G. M. (1998). Heterosexism and gay couples with HIV infection. *Western Journal of Nursing Research, 20,* 478–496.

Powell-Cope, G. M., & Brown, M. A. (1992). Going public as an AIDS family caregiver. *Social Science Medicine, 34,* 571–580.

Prager, K. J. (1995). *The psychology of intimacy.* New York: Guilford.

Price, J. H., Desmond, S., & Kukulka, G. (1985). High school students' perceptions and misperceptions of AIDS. *Journal of School Health, 55,* 107–109.

Pryor, J. B., Reeder, G. D., & Landau, S. (1999). A social-psychological analysis of HIV-related stigma: A two-factor theory. *American Behavioral Scientist, 42,* 1193–1211.

Pryor, J. B., Reeder, G. D., & McManus, J. (1991). Fear and loathing in the workplace: Reaction to AIDS-infected co-workers. *Personality and Social Psychology Bulletin, 17,* 133–139.

Pryor, J. B., Reeder, G. D., Vinacco, R., & Kott, T. L. (1989). The instrumental and symbolic functions of attitudes towards persons with AIDS. *Journal of Applied Social Psychology, 19,* 377–404.

Rada, R. (2002). *HIPAA@IT Essentials: Health information transactions, privacy, and security.* Baltimore, MD: Hypermedia Solutions Ltd. (see also http://www.hypermediasol.com)

Radloff, L. S. (1977). The CES-D scale: A self-report depression scale for research in the general population. *Applied Psychological Measurement, 1,* 385–401.

Rawlins, W. K. (1983). Openness as problematic in ongoing friendships: Two conversational dilemmas. *Communication Monographs, 50,* 1–13.

Reel, B. W., & Thompson, T. L. (1994). A test of the effectiveness of strategies for talking about AIDS and condom use. *Journal of Applied Communication Research, 22,* 127–140.

Reeves, P. M. (2000). Coping in cyberspace: The impact of Internet use on the ability of HIV-positive individuals to deal with their illness. *Journal of Health Communication, 5*(Suppl. V5), 47–59.

Reis, H. T., & Shaver, P. (1988). Intimacy as an interpersonal process. In S. W. Duck (Ed.), *Handbook of personal relationships: Theory, research and interventions* (pp. 367–389). Chichester, NY: Wiley.

Remien, R. H., & Rabkin, J. G. (1995). Long-term survival with AIDS and the role of community. In G. M. Herek & B. Greene (Eds.), *AIDS, identity, and community: The HIV epidemic and lesbians and gay men* (pp. 169–186). Thousand Oaks, CA: Sage.

Remien, R. H., Rabkin, J. G., Williams, J. B., & Katoff, L. (1992). Coping strategies and health beliefs of AIDS longterm survivors. *Psychology and Health, 6,* 335–345.

Rice, R. E., & Katz, J. E. (Eds.). (2001). *The Internet and health communication: Experiences and expectations.* Thousand Oaks, CA: Sage.

Rich, J. D., Back, A., Tuomala, R. E., & Kazanjian, P. H. (1993). Transmission of human immunodeficiency virus presumed to have occurred via female homosexual contact. *Clinical Infectious Disease, 17,* 1003–1005.

Robinson, B. E., Walters, L. H., & Skeen, P. (1989). Response of parents to learning that their child is homosexual and concern over AIDS: A national study. *Journal of Homosexuality, 18,* 59–80.

Roscoe, B., & Kruger, T. L. (1990). AIDS: Late adolescents' knowledge and its influence on sexual behavior. *Adolescence, 25,* 39–48.

Rose, S. (1998). Searching for the meaning of AIDS: Issues affecting seropositive black gay men. In V. J. Derlega & A. P. Barbee (Eds.), *HIV and social interaction* (pp. 56–82). Thousand Oaks, CA: Sage.

Rosenblatt, P., & Meyer, C. (1986). Imagined interactions and the family. *Family Relations, 35,* 319–324.

Rosengard, C., & Folkman, S. (1997). Suicidal ideation, bereavement, HIV serostatus and psychosocial variables in partners of men with AIDS. *AIDS Care, 9,* 373–384.

Roth, N., & Fuller, L. K. (Eds.). (1998). *Women and AIDS: Negotiating safer practices, care, and representation.* New York: Harrington Park Press.

Roth, N. L., & Nelson, M. S. (1997). HIV diagnosis rituals and identity narratives. *AIDS Care, 9,* 161–179.

Rothenberg, K. H., & Paskey, S. J. (1995). The risk of domestic violence and women with HIV infection: Implications for partner notification, public policy, and the law. *American Journal of Public Health, 85,* 1569–1576.

Rotheram, M. J. (1995, February). *Interventions for parents with AIDS with their adolescents.* Paper presented at the Role of Families in Preventing and Adapting to HIV/AIDS conference, Washington, DC.

Rotheram-Borus, M. J., Draimin, B. H., Reid, H. M., & Murphy, D. A. (1997). The impact of ill-ness disclosure and custody plans on adolescents whose parents live with AIDS. *AIDS, 11,* 1159–1164.

Rotheram-Borus, M. J., & Lightfoot, M. (2000). Helping adolescents and parents with AIDS to cope effectively with life. In W. Pequegnat & J. Szapocznik (Eds.), *Working with families in the era of HIV/AIDS* (pp. 189–211). Thousand Oaks, CA: Sage.

Rozin, P., Markwith, M., & McCauley, C. (1994). Sensitivity to indirect contacts with other per-sons: AIDS aversion as a composite of aversion to strangers, infection, moral taint, and mis-fortune. *Journal of Abnormal Psychology, 103,* 495–504.

Russell, D. E. H. (1986). *The secret trauma.* New York: Basic Books.

Sarason, B. R., Sarason, I. G., & Gurung, R. A. R. (1997). Close personal relationships and health outcomes: A key to the role of social support. In S. Duck (Ed.), *Handbook of personal relation-ships: Theory, research and interventions* (2nd ed., pp. 547–573). Chichester, NY: Wiley.

Sarason, I. G., Levine, H. M., Basham, R. B., & Sarason, B. R. (1983). Assessing social support: The social support questionnaire. *Journal of Personality and Social Psychology, 44,* 127–139.

Sarason, I. G., Sarason, B. R., Shearin, E. N., & Pierce, G. R. (1987). A brief measure of social sup-port: Practical and theoretical implications. *Journal of Social and Personal Relationships, 4,* 497–510.

Schaefer, S., & Coleman, E. (1992). Shifts in meaning, purpose, and values following a diagnosis of human immunodeficiency virus (HIV) infection among gay men. *Journal of Psychology and Human Sexuality, 5,* 13–29.

Schechter, M. T., Craib, K. J., Willoughby, B., Douglas, B., Mcleod, A., Maynard, M., et al. (1988). Patterns of sexual behavior and condom use in a cohort of homosexual men. *American Jour-nal of Public Health, 78,* 1535–1538.

Schegloff, E. A. (1986). The routine as achievement. *Human Studies, 9,* 111–151

Schegloff, E. A., & Sacks, H. (1973). Opening up closings. *Semiotica, 7,* 289–327. (Reprinted in *Ethnomethodology,* pp. 233–264 by R. Turner, Ed., Harmondsworth: Penguin).

Schnell, D. J., Higgins, D. L., Wilson, R. M., Goldbaum, G., Cohn, D. L., & Wolitski, R. J. (1992). Men's disclosure of HIV test results to male primary sex partners. *American Journal of Public Health, 82,* 1675–1676.

School Board of Nassau County, Fla. v. Arline (1987). 480 US 273.

Schrimshaw, E. W., & Siegel, K. (2002). HIV-infected mothers' disclosures to their uninfected children: Rates, reasons, and reactions. *Journal of Social and Personal Relationships, 19,* 19–43.

Scully, C., & Porter, S. (2000). HIV topic update: Oro-genital transmission of HIV. *Oral Diseases, 6,* 92–98.

Selwyn, P. A., Carter, R. J., Schoenbaum, E. E., Robertson, V. J., Klein, R. S., & Rogers, M. F. (1989). Knowledge of HIV antibody status and decisions to continue or terminate pregnancy among intravenous drug users. *Journal of the American Medical Association, 216,* 3567–3571.

Semple, S. J., Patterson, T. L., Temoshok, L. R., Straits-Troster, K., Hampton Atkinson, J., Koch, W., et al. (1997). Family conflict and depressive symptoms: A study of HIV-seropositive men. *AIDS Care, 1,* 53–60.

Sepkowitz, K. A. (2001). AIDS—The first 20 years. *New England Journal of Medicine, 344,* 1764–1772.

Serovich, J. M., Brucker, P. S., & Kimberly, J. A. (2000). Barriers to social support for persons liv-ing with HIV/AIDS. *AIDS Care, 12,* 651–662.

Serovich, J. M., & Greene, K. (1993). Perceptions of family boundaries: The case of disclosure of HIV testing information. *Family Relations, 42,* 193–197.

Serovich, J. M., Greene, K., & Parrott, R. (1992). Boundaries and AIDS testing: Privacy and the family system. *Family Relations, 41,* 104–109.

Serovich, J. M., Kimberly, J. A., & Greene, K. (1998). Perceived family member reaction to women's disclosure of HIV-positive information. *Family Relations, 47,* 15–22.

Shilts, R. (1987). *And the band played on: Politics, people, and the AIDS epidemic.* New York: Penguin.

Siegel, K., & Gorey, E. (1994). Childhood bereavement due to parental death from acquired immunodeficiency syndrome. *Journal of Developmental and Behavioral Pediatrics, 15,* S66–S70.

Siegel, K., & Gorey, E. (1997). HIV-infected women: Barriers to AZT use. *Social Science and Medicine, 45,* 15–22.

Siegel, K., Karus, D., Epstein, J., & Raveis, V. (1996). Psychological and psychosocial adjustment of HIV-infected gay/bisexual men: Disease stage comparisons. *Journal of Community Psychology, 24,* 229–243.

Siegel, K., Lune, H., & Meyer, I. (1998). Stigma management among gay/bisexual men with HIV/AIDS. *Qualitative Sociology, 21,* 3–24.

Siegel, K., & Raveis, V. (1997). Perceptions of access to HIV-related information, care, and services among infected minority men. *Qualitative Health Research, 7,* 9–31.

Simmel, G. (1964/1950). *The sociology of Georg Simmel* (K. H. Wolff, Trans.). New York: Free Press.

Simoni, J. M., Mason, H. R. C., & Marks, G. (1997). Disclosing HIV status and sexual orientation to employers. *AIDS Care, 9,* 589–599.

Simoni, J. M., Mason, H. R. C., Marks, G., Ruiz, M. S., Reed, D., & Richardson, J. L. (1995). Women's self-disclosure of HIV infection: Rates, reasons, and reactions. *Journal of Consulting and Clinical Psychology, 63,* 474–478.

Simoni, J. M., Walters, K. L., & Nero, D. K. (2000). Safer sex among HIV+ women: The role of relationships. *Sex Roles, 42,* 691–708.

Singleton, D. C. (1993). Nonconsensual HIV testing in the health care setting: The case for extending the occupational protections of California Proposition 96 to health care workers. *Loyola of Los Angeles Law Review, 26,* 1251–1290.

Skurnick, J. H., Abrams, J., Kennedy, C. A., Valentine, S. N., & Cordell, J. R. (1998). Maintenance of safe sex behavior by HIV-serodiscordant heterosexual couples. *AIDS Education and Prevention, 10,* 493–505.

Smaglik, P., Hawkins, R. P., Pingree, S., Gustafson, D. H., Boberg, E., & Bricker, E. (1998). The quality of interactive computer use among HIV-infected individuals. *Journal of Health Communication, 3*(1), 53–67.

Smart, L., & Wegner, D. M. (1999). Covering up what can't be seen: Concealable stigma and mental control. *Journal of Personality and Social Psychology, 77,* 474–486.

Smyth, J. M. (1998). Written emotional expression: Effect sizes, outcome types, and moderating variables. *Journal of Consulting and Clinical Psychology, 66,* 174–184.

Snell, W. E., Jr., & Finney, P. D. (1990). Interpersonal strategies associated with the discussion of AIDS. *Annals of Sex Research, 3,* 425–451.

Snell, W. E., Jr., & Finney, P. D. (1996). *The multidimensional AIDS anxiety questionnaire.* Unpublished manuscript. Department of Psychology, Southeast Missouri State University.

Snell, W. E., Jr., Fisher, T. D., & Miller, R. (1991). Development of the sexual awareness questionnaire: Components, reliability, and validity. *Annals of Sex Research, 4,* 65–92.

Snyder, M., Omoto, A. M., & Crain, A. L. (1999). Punished for their good deeds: Stigmatization of AIDS volunteers. *American Behavioral Scientist, 42,* 1175–1192.

Sobo, E. J. (1997). Self-disclosure and self-construction among HIV-positive people: The rhetorical uses of stereotypes and sex. *Anthropology and Medicine, 4,* 67–87.

Song, Y. S., & Ingram, K. M. (2002). Unsupportive social interactions, availability of social support, and coping: Their relationship to mood disturbance among African Americans living with HIV. *Journal of Social and Personal Relationships, 19,* 67–85.

Sontag, S. (1989). *AIDS and its metaphors.* New York: Doubleday.

Sorensen, T., & Snow, B. (1991). How children tell: The process of disclosure of child sexual abuse. *Journal of the Child Welfare League of America, 70,* 3–15.

Sowell, R. L., Lowenstein, A., Moneyham, L., Demi, A., Mizuno, Y., & Seals, B. F. (1997). Resources, stigma, and patterns of disclosure in rural women with HIV infection. *Public Health Nursing, 14,* 302–312.

Sowell, R. L., Phillips, K. D., & Grier, J. (1998). Restructuring life to face the future: The perspective of men after a positive response to protease inhibitor therapy. *AIDS Patient Care and STDs, 12,* 33–42.

Spencer, T. (1994). Transforming relationships through ordinary talk. In S. Duck (Ed.), *Understanding relationship process IV: Dynamics of relationships* (pp. 58–85). Thousand Oaks, CA: Sage.

Spencer, T., & Derlega, V. J. (1995, February). *Important self-disclosure decisions: Coming out to family and HIV-positive disclosures.* Paper presented to the annual meeting of the Western States Communication Association, Portland, OR.

Spiro, H. (1971). Privacy in comparative perspectives. In J. R. Pennock & J. W. Chapman (Eds.), *Privacy* (pp. 121–148). New York: Atherton.

Squire, C. (1999). "Neighbors who might become friends": Selves, genres, and citizenship in narratives of HIV. *Sociological Quarterly, 40*(1), 109–137.

Stall, R., & McKusick, L. (1988). *AIDS survey instrument.* Unpublished manuscript, University of California, San Francisco, Center for AIDS Prevention Studies.

Stanton, A. L., Danoff-Burg, S., Cameron, C. L., & Snider, P. R. (1999). Social comparison and adjustment to breast cancer: An experimental examination of upward affiliation and downward evaluation. *Health Psychology, 18,* 151–158.

Starace, F., & Sherr, L. (1998). Suicidal behaviours, euthanasia and AIDS. *AIDS, 12,* 339–347.

Stein, M. D., Freedberg, A., Sullivan, L. M., Savetsky, J., Levenson, S. M., Hingson, R., et al. (1998). Sexual ethics: Disclosure of HIV-positive status to partners. *Archives of Internal Medicine, 158,* 253–257.

Stempel, R., Moulton, J., Bachetti, P., & Moss, A. R. (1989, June). *Disclosure of HIV-antibody tests results and reactions of sexual partners, friends, family, and health professionals.* Paper presented at the 5th International Conference on AIDS, Montreal, Quebec, Canada.

Stempel, R. R., Moulton, J. M., & Moss, A. R. (1995). Self-disclosure of HIV-1 antibody test results: The San Francisco General Hospital cohort. *AIDS Education and Prevention, 7,* 116–123.

Stephenson, J. (2002). Cheaper HIV drugs for poor nations bring a new challenge: Monitoring treatment. *Journal of the American Medical Association, 288*(2).

Stevens, P. E., & Tighe Doerr, B. (1997). Trauma of discovery: Women's narratives of being informed they are HIV-infected. *AIDS Care, 9,* 523–538.

Stiles, W. B. (1987). "I have to talk to somebody." A fever model of disclosure. In V. J. Derlega & J. H. Berg (Eds.), *Self-disclosure: Theory, research, and therapy* (pp. 257–282). New York: Plenum.

Stiles, W. B. (1995). Disclosure as a speech act: Is it psychotherapeutic to disclose? In J. W. Pennebaker (Ed.), *Emotion, disclosure, and health* (pp. 71–91). Washington, DC: American Psychological Association.

Stiles, W. B., Shuster, P. L., & Harrigan, J. A. (1992). Disclosure and anxiety: A test of the fever model. *Journal of Personality and Social Psychology, 63,* 980–988.

St. Lawrence, J. S., Husfeldt, B. A., Kelly, J. A., Hood, H. V., & Smith, S. (1990). The stigma of AIDS: Fear of disease and prejudice toward gay men. *Journal of Homosexuality, 19,* 85–99.

Stokes, J. P. (1983). Predicting satisfaction with social support from social network structure. *American Journal of Community Psychology, 11,* 141–152.

Stokes, J., Fuehrer, A., & Childs, L. (1980). Gender differences in self-disclosure to various target persons. *Journal of Counseling Psychology, 27,* 192–198.

Stolberg, S. G. (2002, June 20). Bush offers plan to help mothers avoid passing HIV to babies. *New York Times.* Retrieved June 20, 2002, from http://www.nytimes.com/2002/06/20/health/20AIDS.html.

Summit, R. C. (1983). The child sexual abuse accommodation syndrome. *Child Abuse and Neglect, 7,* 177–193.

Sunderland, A., Minkoff, H. L., Handte, J., Moroso, G., & Landesman, S. (1992). The impact of human immunodeficiency virus serostatus on reproductive decisions of women. *Obstetrics and Gynecology, 79,* 1027–1031.

Sunenblick, M. B. (1988). The AIDS epidemic: Sexual behaviors of adolescents. *Smith College Studies in Social Work, 59,* 21–37.

Sunnafrank, M. (1986). Predicted outcome value during initial interactions: A reformation of uncertainty reduction theory. *Human Communication Research, 13,* 3–33.

Tardy, C. H., Hosman, L. A., & Bradac, J. J. (1981). Disclosing self to friends and family: A reexamination of initial questions. *Communication Quarterly, 29,* 263–268.

Taylor, D. A., & Altman, I. (1987). Communication in interpersonal relationships: Social penetration processes. In M. E. Roloff & G. E. Miller (Eds.), *Interpersonal processes: New directions in communication research* (pp. 257–277). Newbury Park, CA: Sage.

Taylor, S. F., & Lobel, M. (1989). Social comparison activity under threat: Downward evaluation and upward contacts. *Psychological Review, 96,* 569–575.

Thompson, S. C., Nanni, C., & Levine, A. (1996). The stressors and stress of being HIV-positive. *AIDS Care, 8,* 5–14.

Tracy, K. (1985). Conversational coherence: A cognitively grounded rules approach. In R. L. Street & J. N. Cappella (Eds.), *Sequence and pattern in communication behavior* (pp. 30–49). London: Edward Arnold.

Trainor, A., & Ezer, H. (2000). Rebuilding life: The experience of living with AIDS after facing imminent death. *Qualitative Health Research, 10,* 646–660.

Treichler, P. A. (1988). AIDS, gender, and biomedical discourse: Current contests for meaning. In E. Fee & D. M. Fox (Eds.), *AIDS: The burdens of history* (pp. 190–266). Berkeley: University of California Press.

Troncoso, A. P., Romani, A., Carranza, C. M., Macias, J. R., & Masini, R. (1995). Probable HIV transmission by female homosexual contact. *Medicina, 55,* 334–336.

UNAIDS. (2001). *Joint United Nations Programme on HIV/AIDS.* Retrieved June 15, 2002, from http://www.unaids.org.

UNAIDS/WHO Global AIDS Statistics. (2001). *AIDS Care, 13,* 263–272.

van der Straten, A., King, R., Grinstead, O., Vittinghoff, E., Serufilira, A., & Allen, S. (1998). Sexual coercion, physical violence, and HIV infection among women in steady relationships in Kigali, Rwanda. *AIDS and Behavior, 2,* 61–73.

van der Straten, A., Vernon, K. A., Knight, K. R., Gomez, C. A., & Padian, N. S. (1998). Managing HIV among serodiscordant heterosexual couples: Serostatus, stigma, and sex. *AIDS Care, 10,* 533–548.

Van Devanter, N., Thacker, A., Bass, G., & Arnold, M. (1999). Heterosexual couples confronting the challenges of HIV infection. *AIDS Care, 11,* 181–193.

Vangelisti, A. L. (1994). Family secrets: Forms, functions, and correlates. *Journal of Social and Personal Relationships, 11,* 113–135.

Vangelisti, A. L., & Caughlin, J. P. (1997). Revealing family secrets: The influence of topic, function, and relationships. *Journal of Social and Personal Relationships, 14,* 679–705.

Vangelisti, A. L., Caughlin, J. P., & Timmerman, L. (2001). Criteria for revealing family secrets. *Communication Monographs, 68,* 1–27.

Vázquez-Pacheco, R. (2000). A code of silence. *Body Positive, 13*(5), 22–26.

Vlahov, D., Wientge, D., Moore, J., Flynn, C., Schuman, P., Schoenbaum, E., et al. (1998). Violence among women with or at risk for HIV infection. *AIDS and Behavior, 2,* 53–60.

Wallack, J. (1989). AIDS anxiety among health care professionals. *Hospital and Community Psychiatry, 40,* 507–510.

Wallston, K. A., Stein, M. J., & Smith, C. A. (1994). Form C of the MHLC scales: A condition-specific measure of locus of control. *Journal of Personality Assessment, 63,* 534–553.

Wang, J., Rodés, A., Blanch, C., & Casabona, J. (1997). HIV testing history among gay/bisexual men recruited in Barcelona: Evidence of high levels of risk behavior among self-reported HIV+ men. *Social Science and Medicine, 44,* 469–477.

Warren, C., & Laslett, B. (1977). Privacy and secrecy: A conceptual comparison. *Journal of Social Issues, 33*(3), 43–51.

Watney, S. (1987). *Policing desire: Pornography, AIDS, and the media.* Minneapolis: University of Minnesota Press.

Weatherburn, P., Hickson, F., Reid, D. S., Davies, P. M., & Crosier, A. (1998). Sexual HIV risk behavior among men who have sex with both men and women. *AIDS Care, 10*, 463–471.

Weeks, M. R., Grier, M., Radda, K., & McKinley, D. (1999). AIDS and social relations of power: Urban African-American women's discourse on the contexts of risk and prevention. In W. N. Elwood (Ed.), *Power in the blood: A handbook on AIDS, politics, and communication* (pp. 181–197). Mahwah, NJ: Lawrence Erlbaum Associates, Inc.

Wegner, D. M. (1989). *White bears and other unwanted thoughts: Suppression, obsession, and the psychology of mental control.* New York: Viking.

Wegner, D. M. (1994). Ironic processes of mental control. *Psychological Review, 101*, 34–52.

Wegner, D. M., & Lane, J. D. (1995). From secrecy to pathology. In J. W. Pennebaker (Ed.), *Emotion, disclosure, and health* (pp. 11–46). Washington, DC: American Psychological Association.

Wegner, D. M., Lane, J. D., & Dimitri, S. (1994). The allure of secret relationships. *Journal of Personality and Social Psychology, 66*, 287–300.

Weiner, B. (1993). On sin versus sickness: A theory of perceived responsibility and social motivation. *American Psychologist, 48*, 957–965.

Weiner, B., Perry, R. P., & Magnusson, J. (1988). An attributional analysis of reactions to stigmas. *Journal of Personality and Social Psychology, 55*, 738–748.

Werner, C. M., Altman, I., & Brown, B. B. (1992). A transactional approach to interpersonal relations: Physical environment, social context and temporal qualities. *Journal of Social and Personal Relationships, 9*, 297–323.

Wheeless, L. R. (1976). Self-disclosure and interpersonal solidarity: Measurement, validation, and relationships. *Human Communication Research, 3*, 47–61.

Wheeless, L. R., & Grotz, J. (1977). The measurement of trust and its relationship to self-disclosure. *Human Communication Research, 3*, 250–257.

White, R., & Cunningham, A. M. (1991). *Ryan White, my own story.* New York: Dial Books.

Wiener, L. S., Battles, H. B., & Heilman, N. E. (1998). Factors associated with parents' decision to disclose their HIV diagnosis to their children. *Child Welfare League of America, 77*, 115–135.

Wiener, L. S., & Figueroa, V. (1998). Children speaking with children and families about HIV infection. In P. A. Pizzo & C. M. Wilfert (Eds.), *Pediatric AIDS: The challenge of HIV infection in infants, children, and adolescents* (3rd ed., pp. 729–758). Philadelphia: Lippincott, Williams, & Wilkins.

Wiener, L. S., Heilman, N., & Battles, H. B. (1998). Public disclosure of HIV: Psychosocial considerations. In V. J. Derlega & A. P. Barbee (Eds.), *HIV and social interaction* (pp. 193–217). Thousand Oaks, CA: Sage.

Wiener, L. S., Septimus, A., & Grady, C. (1998). Psychological support and ethical issues for the child and family. In P. A. Pizzo & C. M. Wilfert (Eds.), *Pediatric AIDS: The challenge of HIV infection in infants, children, and adolescents* (3rd ed., pp. 703–727). Philadelphia: Lippincott, Williams, & Wilkins.

Williams, A. B. (1997). New horizons: Antiretroviral therapy in 1997. *Journal of the Association of Nurses in AIDS Care, 8*, 26–42.

Wilson, H. S., Hutchinson, S. A., & Holzemer, W. L. (1997). Salvaging quality of life in ethnically diverse patients with advanced HIV / AIDS. *Qualitative Health Research, 7*, 75–97.

Wilson, L. L., Roloff, M. E., & Carey, C. M. (1998). Boundary rules: Factors that inhibit expressing concerns about another's romantic relationship. *Communication Research, 25*, 618–640.

Wilson, T. E., Massad, L. S., Riester, K. A., Barkan, S., Richardson, J., Young, M., et al. (1999). Sexual, contraceptive, and drug use behaviors of women with HIV and those at high risk for infection: Results from the women's interagency HIV study. *AIDS, 13*, 591–598.

Winstead, B. A., Derlega, V. J., Barbee, A., Sachdev, M., Antle, B., & Greene, K. (2002). Close relationships as sources of strength or obstacles for mothers coping with HIV. *Journal of Loss and Trauma, 7*, 157–184.

Winston, B. V. (1992, April 9). I have AIDS. *The Virginian-Pilot*, pp. A1–A2.

Wolitski, R. J., Rietmeijer, C. A. M., Goldbaum, G. M., & Wilson, R. M. (1998). HIV serostatus disclosure among gay and bisexual men in four American cities: General patterns and relation to sexual practices. *AIDS Care, 10,* 599–610.

Wortman, C. B., Adesman, P., Herman, E., & Greenberg, R. (1976). Self-disclosure: An attributional perspective. *Journal of Personality and Social Psychology, 33,* 184–191.

Wright, K. B. (1999). AIDS, the status quo, and the elite media: An analysis of the guest lists of "The MacNeil/Lehrer News Hour" and "Nightline." In W. N. Elwood (Ed.), *Power in the blood: A handbook on AIDS, politics, and communication* (pp. 281–292). Mahwah, NJ: Lawrence Erlbaum Associates, Inc.

Wrubel, J., & Folkman, S. (1997). What informal caregivers actually do: The caregiving skills of partners of men with AIDS. *AIDS Care, 9,* 691–706.

Yarber, W. L., & Torabi, M. R. (1990-91). HIV prevention knowledge test for teenagers. *SIECUS Report, 19,* 28–32.

Yarber, W. L., & Torabi, M. R. (1998). HIV prevention knowledge test for teenagers. In C. M. Davis, W. L. Yarber, R. Bauserman, G. Schreer, & S. L. Davis (Eds.), *Handbook of sexuality-related measures* (pp. 361–364). Thousand Oaks, CA: Sage.

Yep, G. A. (1992). Communicating the HIV/AIDS risk to Hispanic populations: A review and integration. *Hispanic Journal of Behavioral Sciences, 14,* 403–420.

Yep, G. A. (1993). Health beliefs and HIV prevention: Do they predict monogamy and condom use? *Journal of Social Behavior and Personality, 8,* 507–520.

Yep, G. A. (1995). Healthy desires/unhealthy practices: Interpersonal influence strategies for the prevention of HIV/AIDS among Hispanics. In L. K. Fuller & L. McPherson Shilling (Eds.), *Communicating about communicable diseases* (pp. 139–154). Amherst, MA: Human Resource Development Press.

Yep, G. A. (2000). Disclosure of HIV infection in interpersonal relationships: A communication boundary management approach. In S. Petronio (Ed.), *Balancing the secrets of private disclosures* (pp. 83–96). Mahwah, NJ: Lawrence Erlbaum Associates, Inc.

Yep, G. A., Lovaas, K. E., & Pagonis, A. V. (2002). Sexual practices and the paradoxes of identity in the era of AIDS: The case of "Riding Bareback." *Journal of Homosexuality, 42,* 1–14.

Yep, G. A., Merrigan, G., Martin, J. B., Lovaas, K. E., & Cetron, A. B. (2002). *HIV/AIDS in Asian and Pacific Islander communities in the Unites States: A follow-up review and analysis with recommendations for researchers and practitioners.* Manuscript submitted for publication.

Yep, G. A., & Pietri, M. (1999). In their own words: Communication and the politics of HIV education for transgenders and transsexuals in Los Angeles. In W. N. Elwood (Ed.), *Power in the blood: Handbook on AIDS, politics, and communication* (pp. 199–213). Mahwah, NJ: Lawrence Erlbaum Associates, Inc.

Yep, G. A., Reece, S., & Negrón, E. L. (2003). Culture and stigma in a bona fide group: An analysis of boundaries and context in a closed support group for Asian Americans living with HIV infection. In L. R. Frey (Ed.), *Group communication in context: Studies of bona fide groups* (2nd ed., pp. 157–180). Mahwah, NJ: Lawrence Erlbaum Associates, Inc.

Author Index

A

Abbott, D. W., 38
Abrams, J., 156
Achter, J. A., 192
Adam, B. D., 66, 69, 80, 98, 101, 111, 114,
    158, 177
Adelman, M. B., 64, 135
Adesman, P., 106
Afifi, W. A., 64
Agne, R. R., 48, 49, 54, 58, 63, 76, 111, 112,
    113, 114
Albert, E., 43, 44
Albrecht, T. L., 64
All, A., 139
Allen, J. E., 148, 172
Allen, M., 82
Allman, J., 46
Alonzo, A. A., 13, 39, 41, 83, 138, 140, 174
Altman, I., 5, 21, 53, 64, 94, 95, 97, 173, 178
Altman, L. K., 173
Andrews, S., 102
Antoni, M. H., 131
Archer, R. L., 106, 193
Argyle, M., 36, 74, 93
Armistead, L., 58, 61, 72, 82, 99, 102, 142,
    147, 150
Arnold, M., 36
Asch, A., 146
Aschenbach, A. N., 148
Ashe, A., 5
Ashman, T., 148
Atkinson, J. M., 109
Austin, S. B., 178

B

Baack, D. W., 159
Bachetti, P., 68
Back, A., 177
Baltimore, D., 173
Bantz, C., 94
Barbee, A. P., 1, 2, 6, 15, 26, 36, 128, 129,
    130, 175, 176, 219
Bargh, J. A., 104
Barnes, D. B., 76
Barrett, D. C., 137
Barroso, J., 137
Bartlett, J. G., 1, 6, 7, 36, 100, 108, 149, 156,
    162, 164, 172, 219
Basham, R. B., 201
Bass, G., 36
Battles, H. B., 51, 72, 150
Bauer, G. R., 177, 178
Bauman, L. J., 39, 40, 58, 72, 102
Baxter, L. A., 118
Bayer, R., 154
Beardsley, M., 155
Beck, A. T., 204
Beland, F., 76
Bem, D., 146
Benotsch, E. G., 148
Berg, J. H., 193
Berger, C., 112
Berger, C. R., 64, 90, 106
Berghuis, J. P., 135
Blanch, C., 155
Blau, P., 38
Bleeker, T., 76

Blendon, R. J., 174
Bloom, F. R., 47, 101
Blower, S. M., 148
Boberg, E., 134
Bocarnea, M. C., 213
Boerum, S. J., 101
Bogart, L. M., 148
Bok, S., 4, 5
Bolan, M., 115
Booth, R. J., 8
Bor, R., 36
Borrill, J., 36
Bradac, J. J., 67
Bradley, J. S., 214
Braithwaite, D. O., 44, 50, 145
Brashers, D. E., 64, 134, 135, 162, 210
Bray, J. H., 73
Britton-Williams, Q., 213
Brookmeyer, R., 155
Brouwer, D. C., 118, 119
Brown, B. B., 94, 95
Brown, M. A., 77
Brown, P., 106
Brown, V. B., 147, 171, 176
Brown, W. J., 213
Brucker, P. S., 7
Brunjo, M., 47
Burchinal, P., 36
Burleson, J. A., 106
Burris, S., 4, 39, 58, 154
Button, G., 106
Buunk, B. P., 55

C

Cage, M., 136
Camacho, S., 39
Cameron, C. L., 55
Cameron, L. D., 169, 183
Cantero, P. J., 9
Capitanio, J. P., 1, 22, 38, 43, 60, 140
Cappella, J. N., 106
Carballo-Diéguez, A., 158
Carey, C. M., 56
Carey, M. P., 212, 214
Caron, S. L., 69, 146
Carpenter, C. C. J., 147
Carranza, C. M., 177
Carter, K. K., 158
Casabona, J., 155

Casey, N., 106
Cassidy, B., 147, 148
Castro, R., 36
Catania, J. A., 99, 133
Catz, S. L., 1, 148
Caughlin, J. P., 57, 64, 78, 144, 168
Cetron, A. B., 81
Chaikin, A. L., 19, 56, 97, 133
Chandler, K., 220
Charbonneau, A., 76
Chartrand, T. L., 104
Chastain, R. L., 194
Chauncey, S., 66, 128, 172
Chelune, G. J., 64, 97
Chen, L., 1, 172, 173
Chesney, M. A., 1, 39, 73, 149
Chidwick, A., 36
Childs, L., 67
Christian, B., 36
Christopher-Richards, A., 149
Chuang, H. T., 137
Chung, J. Y., 71
Ciesla, J. A., 137
Clark, K. A., 75, 76, 107
Clark, L., 99
Clement, U., 39
Cline, R. J. W., 23, 64, 76, 107, 108, 133
Coates, T. J., 47, 76, 133, 137
Cogan, J., 43
Cohen, S., 203
Colder, M., 183
Cole, S. W., 8, 168, 169
Coleman, E., 43
Coleman, R., 138
Collette, L., 137
Collins, E., 164
Collins, N. L., 78
Collins, R. L., 21, 156
Cook, D. J., 38
Cooke, M., 73
Cordell, J. R., 156
Couch, L. L., 146
Cowles, K. V., 67, 149
Coyne, J. C., 190
Cozby, P., 78
Crain, A. L., 135
Crandall, C. S., 138
Crandles, S., 71
Cranson, D. A., 69, 146
Crawford, A. M., 41, 138, 143

Crawford, I., 76, 139
Crespo-Fierro, M., 148
Crocker, J., 37, 83
Crosby, G. M., 69, 99, 116, 118, 147
Crosier, A., 146
Crossley, M. L., 100, 136
Cunningham, A. M., 153
Cunningham, M. R., 26, 130
Cusella, L. P., 48

D

D'Angelo, R. J., 38, 39
Dadds, M. R., 36, 130
Danoff-Burg, S., 55
Davies, M. L., 136
Davies, P. M., 146
Davison, K. P., 133
Dawson, J. M., 155
DeHovitz, J., 71
DeJong, W., 178
De Vincenzi, I., 157, 158
de Wit, J. B., 8
Demi, A., 195, 205
Demme, J., 163
den Boer, D. J., 38
Deren, S., 155
Derlega, V. J., 1, 2, 4, 5, 6, 8, 9, 13, 15, 19, 24,
    26, 36, 37, 38, 39, 40, 43, 46, 49,
    50, 51, 53, 54, 56, 57, 61, 62, 67,
    78, 84, 85, 97, 98, 105, 106, 111,
    124, 130, 133, 140, 141, 161, 174,
    175, 176, 189, 219
Derse, A. R., 76
Desmond, S., 214
Devine, P. G., 22, 38, 43, 44, 138, 140
Devins, G. M., 137
de Vroome, E. M., 8, 137
Diaz, R. M., 61, 81
Dickerson, S. S., 133
DiClemente, R. J., 214
Dimitri, S., 144
Dindia, K., 5, 64, 65, 67, 73, 77, 78, 82, 101,
    178
Doelger, J., 90
Doll, L. S., 76
Donelan, K., 174
Dorman, S. M., 214
Draimin, B., 72
Draimin, B. H., 150

Driscoll, J. M., 153
Druley, J. A., 190
Duck, S. W., 64

E

Edgar, T., 178
Eke, A., 58
Ekstrand, M., 137
Ellard, J. H., 130
Elsesser, V., 155
Elwood, W. N., 8, 154, 158, 161, 189, 219
Epstein, H., 1, 172, 173
Epstein, J., 36
Ernst, F. A., 213
Ethier, K. A., 63
Evans, D. L., 136
Ezer, H., 162
Ezzy, D., 100

F

Faden, R. R., 58
Fahey, J. L., 8
Farrell, K., 71
Fass, R. J., 132, 199
Faulkner, S. L., 8, 9, 13, 15, 17, 23, 36, 39, 41,
    45, 47, 50, 54, 56, 57, 60, 61, 65,
    66, 69, 70, 71, 73, 78, 79, 81, 82,
    85, 88, 89, 90, 91, 93, 98, 99, 100,
    102, 111, 125, 126, 133, 138, 140,
    142, 143, 150, 160, 161, 162, 164,
    177, 213
Festinger, L. A., 55
Fife, B. L., 13, 138, 196, 197, 206, 207
Figueroa, V., 72, 150, 151, 152, 153, 183
Fine, M., 146
Finney, P. D., 213, 214
Fishbein, M. J., 146
Fisher, J. D., 69, 79, 155
Fisher, L., 99
Fisher, M., 5
Fisher, T. D., 214
Fishman, B., 73
Fiske, S. T., 37
Fitzpatrick, M. A., 5, 117, 119
Flaskerud, J. H., 81
Fleischman, A. R., 153
Fleishman, J. A., 130
Fletcher, M. A., 131

Flint, L. J., 135
Flores, L., 24
Fogel, B., 130
Fogel, K., 73
Folk-Barron, L., 46
Folkman, S., 49, 149, 150, 154
Forbes, C. D., 39, 69
Forbes-Jones, E., 39
Forehand, R., 58, 61, 99
Fox, R., 155
Francis, R. A., 213
Freimuth, V. S., 178
Frey, L. R., 1, 135
Friedman, S. R., 155
Fuehrer, A., 67
Fuller, L. K., 81, 82
Fullilove, M. T., 81
Fullilove, R. E., 81
Fulton, R., 174
Furnham, A., 37

G

Gallant, J. E., 1, 6, 7, 36, 100, 108, 149, 156, 162, 164, 172, 219
Gard, L. H., 70, 114
Gerbert, B., 76, 139
Gershengorn, H. B., 148
Gewirtz, A., 72, 73, 150, 151, 152, 153
Gibbons, F. X., 55
Gielen, A. C., 58, 98, 147, 171, 176
Gilbert, S. J., 4, 54
Gill, M. J., 137
Gill, V. T., 39
Giuliano, T., 44
Glaser, B., 126
Goffman, E., 37, 138, 141, 145
Goldbaum, G. M., 67
Golden, M. R., 147
Goldman, E., 36
Goldschmidt, R. H., 99
Goldsmith, D., 73
Goldsmith, D. J., 64
Goldstein, M. F., 155
Gomez, C. A., 39
Gordon, E. M., 106, 161
Gorey, E., 72, 148, 157
Gossart-Walker, S., 72, 73, 150, 151, 152, 152
Gouldner, A. W., 38, 105
Grady, C., 72
Graham, M. K., 90

Graham, S., 44
Gramling, L., 81
Gray, L. A., 214
Green, G., 43, 59, 69, 155, 158
Greenberg, M. A., 47
Greenberg, R., 106
Greenblatt, R. M., 76
Greene, K., 1, 2, 6, 7, 8, 9, 13, 15, 17, 23, 36, 37, 39, 41, 43, 45, 47, 50, 54, 56, 57, 60, 61, 63, 64, 65, 66, 67, 69, 70, 71, 73, 77, 78, 79, 81, 82, 85, 88, 89, 90, 91, 93, 97, 98, 99, 100, 102, 104, 111, 125, 126, 133, 138, 140, 142, 143, 147, 148, 150, 158, 160, 161, 162, 163, 164, 168, 175, 177, 187, 189, 213
Greenspan, M., 46
Griensven, G. J., 8
Grier, J., 162
Grier, M., 23
Grimshaw, A., 15
Grotz, J., 78
Grzelak, J., 84, 124
Gunn, D. O., 135
Gurung, R.A. R., 127

H

Haas, S. M., 134, 135, 145, 149, 210
Hackl, K. L., 39
Hammer, S. M., 1, 172
Hammond, S. L., 178
Hampton Crockett, P., 219
Handford, H. A., 155
Handte, J., 157
Haney, D. Q., 1, 173
Harney, D. M., 22
Harrigan, J. A., 107
Harrison, K., 22
Hassin, J., 101, 114
Hatala, M. N., 159, 177
Haynes, K. M., 64
Hays, R. B., 9, 47, 55, 61, 66, 69, 70, 71, 72, 73, 75, 85, 99, 100, 114, 127, 128, 131, 132, 133, 172
Hecht, M., 24
Hecht, M. L., 17
Heilman, N., 51, 52, 72, 136, 153
Helgeson, V. S., 55
Henderson, M., 36, 74, 93
Henderson, R., 214

Herek, G. M., 14, 22, 36, 38, 39, 41, 43, 60, 138, 140, 174
Heritage, J., 109
Herman, E., 106
Hessling, R. M., 192
Hewes, D. E., 90
Hickson, F., 146
Hines, S. C., 64
Ho, F. C., 76
Hoff, C. C., 137, 154, 156, 158, 159
Hoffman, M. A., 36, 38, 41, 47
Holditch-Davis, D., 36
Holmes, J.
Holt, R., 1, 2, 9, 46, 47, 48, 49, 77, 98, 104
Holzemer, W. L., 136
Hood, H. V., 38
Hosman, L. A., 67
Hsieh, E., 64
Huba, G. J., 58
Hudis, J., 72
Humfleet, G., 76
Hunsley, J., 137
Hunter, J., 214
Husfeldt, B. A., 38
Hutchinson, S. A., 136

I

Ickovics, J. R., 63, 97
Ingram, K. M., 131, 132, 176, 198, 199

J

Jackson, L. A., 81
Jacobsberg, L., 73, 148
Jefferson, G., 109
Johnson, B. T., 212
Jones, D. A., 132, 199
Jones, E. E., 106, 138, 161
Jones, S., 28, 47
Jones, W. H., 146
Jourard, S. M., 5
Julian, P., 116, 118

K

Kahn, J. H., 192
Kahn, J. O., 148
Kalichman, S. C., 6, 7, 36, 38, 39, 47, 68, 115, 128, 136, 137, 146, 154, 156, 164, 175, 204, 219

Kang, A. S., 213
Karus, D., 36
Katoff, L., 7
Katz, J. E., 86, 134
Kazanjian, P. H., 177
Kellerman, K., 79, 95, 97, 106, 112
Kelley, J. E., 184
Kelly, A. E., 4, 5, 6, 8, 46, 47, 64, 160, 162, 169, 175, 180, 219
Kelly, J. A., 1, 38, 39, 76, 139, 148
Kelvin, P., 56
Kemeny, M. E., 8, 168, 169
Kennedy, C. A., 156
Kennedy, M., 39
Kennedy, R. E., 174
Kenny, C., 169
Kenny, D. A., 5
Kiesler, C., 97
Kiesler, S., 97
Kimberly, J. A., 7, 9, 23, 57, 65, 66, 69, 70, 71, 98, 100, 102, 125, 127, 150, 152
Kimble Willcutts, D. L., 69
Kimerling, R., 58, 60, 147, 176
King, N., 101
King, R., 13, 58, 60, 147, 154, 176
Kirkman-Liff, B., 41
Kitzinger, J., 119
Klein, K., 61
Kleiser, R., 137
Kline, A., 156
Klingle, R. S., 134
Klitzman, R. L., 39, 45, 46, 48, 49, 54, 58, 61, 68, 69, 92, 95, 98, 99, 103, 109, 111, 112, 113, 116, 118, 119, 154, 158, 159, 177
Klusas, J. A., 169
Knight, K. R., 39
Kok, G., 38
Kommor, M. J., 64
Koopman, C., 214
Kotchick, B. A., 142
Kott, T. L., 38
Krantz, D. H., 153
Krebs, S., 98
Kresge, K., X., xii, 172
Kruger, T. L., 214
Kukulka, G., 214

L

Laird, J. D., 146

Landau, S., 98
Landesman, S., 157
Lane, J. D., 46, 47, 144, 169, 170, 175
Langer, E. J., 104
Larsen, K., 43
Larson, D. G., 194
Larson, J., 105, 135
Laslett, B., 160, 169
Leary, M. R., 8, 22, 39, 40, 41, 42, 43, 44, 60,
       138, 141, 174
Lehman, D. R., 130, 176
Leisen, J. C. C., 184
Lemieux, R., 38, 43
Leone, C., 39
Lepore, S. J., 8, 46, 47, 168, 169, 183, 219
Leserman, J., 127, 130, 132, 136
Leslie, M. B., 130
Lester, P., 73, 131, 137, 157
Levin, B. W., 153
Levine, A., 36, 203
Levine, C., 72, 152
Levine, H. M., 201
Levinger, G., 53
Levinson, S., 106
Lewis, R. J., 38
Lightfoot, M., 72
Lim, T., 106
Limandri, B. J., 2, 39, 46, 62, 65, 75, 98, 118,
       125, 133, 178
Lindhorst, T., 135
Lindsay, M. B., 157
Littlefield, R., 64
Lobel, M., 55
Long, E., 43
Louganis, G., 76, 107
Lovaas, K. E., 81, 156
Lovejoy, D., 8, 50, 51, 54, 57, 61, 85, 98
Lowenstein, A., 195, 205
Lumley, M. A., 184
Lune, H., 38
Lutgendorf, S. K., 8, 131, 134
Lyketsos, C. G., 137

M

MacFarlane, K., 98
Macias, J. R., 177
MacKellar, D., xii
Magee, R. H., 128
Magni, J., 85
Magnusson, J., 44

Magraw, M. M., 71
Maguire, B., 76
Maheux, B., 76
Major, B., 37, 83
Maldonado, N., 68
Mancoske, R., 135
Mandel, J. S., 39
Manns, H., 39, 98, 126, 135, 137
Mansergh, G., 65, 68, 71, 72, 80, 85, 126
Margulis, S. T., 4
Markova, I., 69, 79, 117, 119
Markowitz, J. C., 137
Marks, G., 9, 17, 21, 54, 55, 65, 67, 68, 69, 70,
       71, 72, 73, 74, 75, 76, 78, 79, 81,
       85, 100, 115, 155, 159
Markwith, M., 40
Martin, J., 64
Martin, J. B., 81
Martin, J. N., 64, 95, 125
Masini, R., 178
Mason, H. R., 55, 75
Mason, H. R. C., 54, 61, 68, 70, 71, 73, 74,
       81, 82, 85
Mattson, M., 135, 155, 158
Mayes, S. D., 155
Maynard, D. W., 39, 113
Mays, V. M., 22, 177
McAllister, M. P., 44
McAuliffe, T. L., 148
McCall, G. J., 95
McCauley, C., 40
McCusker, J., 155
McGuire, J. M., 38
McKenzie, N. J., 23, 76, 107, 108, 133
McKillop, K. J., 64
McKinley, D., 23
McKusick, L., 133, 214
McManus, J., 38
McMaster, J. R., 76
McPhee, S. J., 76
Melchior, L. A., 58
Merrigan, G., 81, 85
Metts, S., 4, 39, 98, 117, 119, 126, 135, 137
Meyer, C., 182
Meyer, I., 38
Michael-Good, L., 155
Mickelson, K. D., 55
Miell, D. E., 53, 64, 101
Miles, M. S., 36
Millar, F. E., 64
Miller, D. H., 39

Miller, L. C., 78, 119, 193
Miller, R., 36, 214
Minkoff, H. L., 157
Misener, T. R., 148
Misovich, S. J., 69
Mizuno, Y., 195, 205
Mofenson, L. M., 148, 156, 176
Mon't Ros-Mendoza, T. M., 17
Monahan, J. L., 119, 178
Mondragon, D., 41, 174
Monette, P., 83, 219
Moneyham, L., 39, 57, 65, 69, 76, 79, 81, 85, 102, 104, 158, 195, 205
Moore, B., 21
Moore, D. S., 146
Moroso, G., 157
Morr, M. C., 28, 141
Morrison-Beedy, D., 212
Morse, E., 99
Morse, P., 99
Moss, A. R., 68, 69
Moulton, J., 39, 68, 69
Moulton, J. M., 39
Murphy, D. A., 150
Murphy, S. T., 119

N

Naji, S. A., 69
Nanni, C., 36, 203
Negrón, E. L., 66
Neidig, J. L., 132, 134, 135, 162, 199, 210
Neil, K., 102
Nelson, M. S., 101
Nero, D. K., 155
Nicholls, G., 169, 183
Nimmons, D., 49, 154
Norman, L. R., 39, 69, 79
North, R. L., 147, 177
Nott, K. H., 36
Nyamathi, A. M., 81
Nyanjom, D., 158

O

O'Campo, P., 58
O'Donnell, C., 139, 214
O'Donnell, L., 139, 214
Odaka, N. J., 155
Oddi, L. F., 76
Oldfield, E. C., 26

Omarzu, J., 5, 37, 38, 104
Omoto, A. M., 135
Otto-Salaj, L. L., 47

P

Padian, N. S., 39
Pagonis, A. V., 156
Pakenham, K. I., 36, 130
Pallak, M., 97
Parish, K., 39
Parks, M. R., 73
Parmenter, R., 159
Parrott, R., 7, 67, 187
Partridge, J. C., 73
Paskey, S. J., 4, 58, 60, 147, 157, 171, 176
Patterson, T. L.
Pavitt, C., 90
Pearce, W. B., 78, 94
Pennebaker, J. W., 8, 46, 47, 133, 168, 169, 183
Pequegnat, W., 71, 72, 73, 131
Perkins, D. O., 136
Perkins, J., 213
Perry, R. P., 44
Perry, S., 73, 76, 148
Perry, S.W., 137
Peters, L., 38, 138
Peterson, J. L., 133
Petrie, K. J., 8
Petronio, S., 2, 4, 5, 6, 8, 9, 16, 17, 18, 19, 20, 21, 23, 24, 25, 26, 27, 28, 29, 30, 32, 33, 34, 36, 37, 40, 48, 51, 56, 61, 62, 64, 65, 66, 67, 84, 85, 90, 92, 93, 94, 95, 96, 97, 98, 99, 100, 101, 102, 105, 106, 108, 110, 111, 114, 121, 124, 125, 127, 133, 141, 143, 144, 145, 146, 147, 149, 160, 161, 178
Phillips, K. D., 162
Picciano, J. F., 115
Pierce, G. R., 201
Pietri, M., 21
Pilowsky, D. J., 191
Pingree, S., 134
Pinkerton, S. D., 47
Plant, E. A., 22
Pleck, J. H., 139, 214
Pliskin, M., 71
Plummer, K., 21
Polik, B. F., 155

Porter, S., 154
Powell, J., 219
Powell-Cope, G. M., 77, 83, 145
Power, K., 117, 119
Prager, K. J., 64
Price, J. H., 214
Pryor, J. B., 38, 42, 98

Q

Query, J. L., 135

R

Rabkin, J. G., 7, 101, 137
Rada, R., 58, 175
Radda, K., 23
Rademan, P., 43
Radloff, L. S., 204
Ragan, J. D., 47
Rampersad, A., 5
Raveis, V., 36, 81
Rawlins, W. K., 56
Reback, C. J., 58
Reece, S., 66
Reeder, G. D., 17, 38, 98
Reeder, H. M., 17
Reel, B. W., 158
Reeves, P. M., 134
Reid, D. S., 146
Reid, H. M., 150
Reis, H. T., 64
Remien, R. H., 7, 101
Reynolds, N. R., 13, 39, 41, 83, 134, 138, 140,
          174
Ribordy, S. C., 76
Rice, R. E., 86, 134
Rich, J. D., 177
Richardson, J. L., 54, 68
Rienzo, B. R., 214
Rietmeijer, C. A. M., 67
Rintamaki, L. S., 135
Roberts, F., 158
Roberts, J. E., 137
Robinson, B. E., 61
Robinson, J. T., 64
Rodés, A., 155
Rodgers, B. L., 67, 150
Roffman, R. A., 115
Rogers, L. E., 64
Roloff, M. E., 56

Romani, A., 177
Rompa, D., 136
Roscoe, B., 214
Rose, R., 214
Rose, S., 43, 60, 81, 100
Rosenblatt, P., 182
Rosengard, C., 149, 150
Roth, N., 81, 82
Roth, N. L., 101
Rothenberg, K. H., 4, 58, 60, 147, 157, 171,
          176, 177
Rotheram, M. J., 102
Rotheram-Borus, M. J., 72, 130, 150, 214
Rozin, P., 40, 41, 42, 43
Ruiz, M. S., 54
Russell, D. E. H., 38
Ryan, J., 73, 148

S

Sacks, H., 110
Sandfort, T. G., 8
Saracino, M., 214
Sarason, B. R., 127, 176, 201
Sarason, I. G., 127, 201
Schaalma, H. P., 38
Schaefer, J. H., 155
Schaefer, S., 43
Schechter, M. T., 155
Schegloff, E. A., 86, 106, 108, 110, 125
Schneiderman, N., 131
Schnell, D. J., 80, 154
Schneller, E. S., 41
Schonnesson, N., 39
Schoub, B. D., 220
Schreindorfer, L. S., 8, 22, 39, 40, 41, 42, 43,
          44, 60, 138, 141, 174
Schrimshaw, E. W., 71, 100, 102, 150
Scully, C., 154
Seals, B. F., 195, 205
Sears, A., 66, 69, 80, 98, 101, 111, 114, 158,
          177
Selwyn, P. A., 157
Semple, S. J., 143
Sepkowitz, K. A., 1, 2, 3, 150, 172, 173
Septimus, A., 72, 73, 150, 151, 152, 153, 154
Serovich, J. M., 2, 7, 8, 9, 17, 23, 37, 41, 50,
          56, 62, 63, 64, 65, 66, 67, 70, 73,
          77, 78, 81, 85, 98, 104, 126, 127,
          131, 132, 133, 142, 160, 187, 189,
          213

Serra, M., 43
Shambaugh, E. J., 192
Sharp, L. K., 183
Sharp, S. M., 78, 94
Shaver, P., 64
Shearin, E. N., 201
Sherburne, S. P., 15, 38, 43, 140, 141
Sheridan, K., 38
Sherr, L., 137
Shilts, R., 41
Shuster, P. L., 107
Siegel, K., 36, 38, 39, 41, 51, 71, 72, 81, 83,
        100, 102, 111, 130, 135, 138, 148,
        150, 157
Sikkema, K. J., 47
Simmel, G., 64, 160
Simmons, J. L., 95
Simoni, J. M., 9, 39, 54, 55, 57, 61, 65, 67, 68,
        70, 71, 72, 73, 74, 76, 81, 82, 85,
        98, 100, 126, 155
Singleton, D. C., 76
Skeen, P., 61
Skurnick, J. H., 156
Smaglik, P., 86, 134
Smart, L., 169, 170
Smith, A. W., 1, 39
Smith, C. A., 208, 209
Smith, S., 38
Smyth, J. M., 8, 46, 47, 168, 169, 183, 219
Snarey, J., 139, 214
Snell, W. E., Jr., 213, 214
Snider, P. R., 55
Snoek, D. J., 53
Snow, B., 101
Snyder, M., 135
Sobo, E. J., 158
Sohler, N., 191
Somlai, A. M., 39
Song, Y. S., 131, 132, 199
Sontag, S., 41
Sorenson, T., 101
Sowell, R. L., 36, 148, 162, 195, 205
Spencer, T., 78, 110, 111
Spiro, H., 21
Squire, C., 28, 79, 80, 101
St. Lawrence, J. S., 38, 140, 141
Stall, R., 214
Stanton, A. L., 55
Staples, B., 94
Starace, F., 137

Steele, C., 37
Steer, R. A., 204
Stein, J. A., 130
Stein, M. D., 69, 79, 81, 82, 154, 155
Stein, M. J., 208, 209
Stempel, R., 68
Stempel, R. R., 69, 70, 71, 73, 75, 76, 79, 104,
        127, 138
Stephens, M. A. P., 190
Stephenson, J., 173
Stevens, P. E., 47, 98, 100, 136
Stiles, W. B., 107, 170
Stokes, J., 67
Stokes, J. P., 127
Stolberg, S. G., 174
Strauss, A., 126
Stroebe, W., 8
Sultan, R. F., 97
Summit, R. C., 101
Sunderland, A., 157
Sunenblick, M. B., 214
Sunnafrank, M., 106
Susser, E., 191
Sweet, D. M., 39
Szapocznik, J., 71, 72, 73, 131

T

Tardy, C. H., 67
Taylor, D. A., 5, 53, 64, 97, 178
Taylor, S. E., 8, 168, 169
Taylor, S. F., 55
Temoshok, L., 39, 214
Terry, D. J., 36, 130
Thacker, A., 36
Thayaparan, B., 63
Thompson, S. C., 36, 203
Thompson, T. L., 44, 48, 145, 158
Tieu, T., 78
Tighe Doerr, B., 47, 98, 100, 136
Timmerman, L., 64
Tobey, L., 66
Torabi, M. R., 214
Tortu, S., 155
Tracy, K., 106
Trainor, A., 162
Treichler, P. A., 43
Troncoso, A. P., 177
Tuomala, R. E., 177

Turner, H., 47

U

Ullrich, P., 8

V

Valentine, S. N., 156
van der Straten, A., 13, 39, 58, 60, 83, 147,
    154, 171, 176
Van Devanter, N., 36, 83, 154
Vangelisti, A. L., 57, 64, 73, 78, 99, 144, 168
VanLandingham, M., 156
Vázquez-Pacheco, R., 1, 2, 8, 69, 103, 134,
    158, 180
Vedhara, K., 36
Vernon, K. A., 39, 83, 171
Vickers, V. L., 76
Vinacco, R., 38
Visscher, B. R., 8, 168, 169
Vlahov, D., 13, 60, 147, 176
von Weiss, R. T., 169

W

Wagner, C., 164
Wallack, J., 139
Wallston, K. A., 208, 209
Walmsley, S., 164
Walters, K. L., 155
Walters, L. H., 61
Wang, J., 155
Warren, C., 160, 169
Wasilevski, Y., 36
Watney, S., 43, 220
Watstein, S. B., 220
Weatherburn, P., 146
Weeks, M. R., 23
Wegner, D. M., 46, 47, 144, 169, 170, 175
Weiner, B., 44
Weiner, J. L., 64
Weinstein, B., 69
Welles, S. L., 177, 178

Werner, C. M., 94, 95
Westbrook, L., 39
Wheeless, L. R., 78
White, R., 153
Widaman, K. F., 1
Wiener, L. S., 51, 52, 72, 73, 136, 150, 151,
    152, 153, 154, 183
Wierson, M., 61
Wilkie, P. A., 69
Williams, A. B., 102, 147, 148
Williams, C. L., 97
Williams, E., 44
Williams, J. B., 7
Williams, M. L., 158, 161
Williamson, G. M., 203
Wilmot, W., 118
Wilson, H. S., 136
Wilson, L. L., 56, 106
Wilson, R. M., 67
Wilson, T. E., 155
Wingate, C., 39
Winstead, B. A., 1, 6, 8, 9, 15, 26, 36, 39, 40,
    46, 50, 51, 53, 54, 56, 61, 71, 72,
    145, 148, 150, 152, 174, 177, 189
Winston, B. V., 5
Wolf, R. C., 178
Wolitski, R. J., 67, 69, 73, 76, 154
Wong, P. T. P., 46
Wortman, C. B., 106, 130
Wright, E. R., 13, 138, 196, 197, 206, 207
Wright, K. B., 5
Wrubel, J., 149

Y

Yarber, W. L., 214
Yep, G. A., 17, 21, 56, 66, 81, 85, 90, 103, 133,
    156

Z

Zapka, J., 240
Zorn, J., 214

Subject Index

A

Accidental disclosure, *see* Unintentional disclosure
ACT UP, *see* Proactive behaviors
Adherence, 99, 147–149, 176
Alcohol, 157–158
Alternative disclosure messages, *see also* Vernacular tactics, 12, 116–119
Anger, 59, 190
Anticipated response to disclosure, *see* Reactions
Assault, *see* Sexual abuse and Violence
AZT, *see* Medical advances

B

Benefits, *see* Consequences
Betrayal, *see* Third party and Gossip
Blaming, *see also* Stigma, 44, 198
Body image, *see also* Eating disorders, 117, 164, 196
Boundary management, *see also* Communication Privacy Management
    linkages, 17, 27, 84, 92, 100
    ownership, 19, 20, 26, 28–30, 41, 57, 94, 168
    permeability, 27, 160
Breakdown in informational control, 163–168

C

Caregiving, *see also* Social support, 147–150
Catharsis, *see* Self-gain

Celebrities, *see* Public Disclosure
Channel, *see* Mode
Children and disclosure, 71–72, 150–153, 191
    plans for children's future, 72, 151–152, 154, 191
Closeness and relationships, *see also* Relationships, 53, 54
Communication difficulties, 189, 213
Communication Privacy Management, CPM, 2, 9–11, 17–35, 36, 178–180
    boundary coordination, 25–30, 84, 124, 133, 162, *see also* Boundary management
    boundary turbulence, 30–34, 93, 143
    privacy rule development, 20–25
    rule management system, 20–34
    suppositions, 18–20
Condom, *see also* Sexual behavior, 7, 154–156, 157, 158, 211–212
Confidants, *see also* CPM and Social support, 27, 61, 127
Consequences, 9, 121–171
    of disclosure, 125–160
    of nondisclosure, 161–171
Content of disclosure message, *see also* Length and Directness, 110–116
Context, *see* Setting and Timing
Coping, 130–133
Courtesy stigma, *see* Stigma
Coworkers, disclosure to, *see* Relationships
Culture, 21, 74, 81–82, 177

D

Dating, *see* Relationships
Deception, 113, 130, 158, 162–163, 167

Decisions to disclose or not disclose, 36–83
Denial, 32, 45, 59, 72, 98, 113, 122, 124, 131,
        152, 166
Dependence, 48, 54, 56, 145
Depression, 131, 132, 137, 182, 204
        and physical symptoms, 131–132, 137
        and social support, 131
Directness of disclosure, 66, 96, 110–112,
        117, 121
        direct questions about HIV diagnosis,
                51, 70, 76, 77, 89–90, 96–97,
                104, 105, 112–113, 163
Disabilities, 44, 50, 145–146
Disapproval, of infected person, *see* Stigma
Disclosure
        definition, 4–6, 178
        importance of, 7–8
        measures, 192, 193, 194, 213
Disclosure messages, 12, 84–120
        direct/explicit, 110–112, 117, 121
        indirect/equivocality, 110–112, 116, 119
        see Content, Directness, Length, Setting,
                Sexual orientation, and Timing
Disease
        cancer, 44, 45, 138, 163
        mental illness, 44
        progression of HIV/AIDS, 99, 127, 130,
                137, 162, 163, 168, 172
Distress, *see also* Catharsis, 8, 9, 170, 192
Divorce, *see* Relationship, disruption
Drugs/drug use, *see also* Stigma, 114,
        157–158
Duty to inform, *see* Other-gain

E

Eating disorders, 169–170
Electronic privacy, 57–58, 76
Employer, disclosure to, *see* Relationships
Ethnicity, *see* Culture
Explicit, *see* Directness

F

Face-to-face disclosure, *see also* Mode, 89–90,
        96
Failure to contribute to society, *see* Stigma
Family, disclosure to, *see* Relationships
Fear, *see also* Stigma, 53, 58–59, 66, 123, 138,
        151, 152, 189, 195
Fever model, 107, 170

Friends, *see* Relationships

G

Gender and disclosure, 21, 70, 71, 73, 82, 177
Gossip, *see also* Third-party disclosure, 57,
        93, 102, 162
Gradual, *see* Disclosure messages

H

Health, *see also* Adherence, Medical Ad-
        vances, and Psychological health,
        208, 211–212
        effects from disclosure, 7, 8, 99–100
        physical, 8, 100, 117, 118, 127, 190, 206
Help seeking, *see* Information seeking
Hemophilia, 55, 153, 155, 178, 217
Highly Active Antiretroviral Therapy,
        HAART, *see also* Medical Ad-
        vances, xii, 147–148, 162, 172
HIV symptoms, 100, 130, 204, 206
HIV testing, xi–xii, 6, 8, 31, 49, 64, 92, 156, 187

I

Identity and disclosure, 58, 101, 136–137
Implicit disclosure, *see also* Directness, 66
Income, xii, 22, 173, 196, 202, 205
Incremental disclosure, 23, 50, 100–102, 106
Indirect disclosure, *see* Directness and
        Third-party
Infant, *see* Perinatal and Children
Information seeking, 64, 119, 133–134
Internet, 86, 133–134
Interpersonal-gain,
        reasons for disclosure, 52–55, 188
                common experiences or similarity,
                        54–55, 73, 105, 188
                establishing emotionally close and
                        supportive relationships,
                        53–54, 188
                testing others' reactions, 53, 100,
                        101, 188
        reasons for nondisclosure, 62, 188–189
                superficial relationship, *see also* Rela-
                        tionship quality, 62, 189
Informational control, 13, 162–168

K

Knowledge of HIV, 211–212, 214

L

Length of disclosure message, 113–114
Lovers, *see* Relationships and Significant
    others

M

Measures, 186–214
Medical advances
    drugs, 14, 118, 148, 157
    medication adherence, *see also* Adher-
        ence, 1, 147–149
    therapies, xii, 1, 3, 6, 14, 172
    antiretroviral therapies, *see* HAART
    protease inhibitors, 1, 6, 172
    see Vaccine and Treatments
Message, *see* Disclosure message
Mode of communication, 12, 85–94
    face-to-face disclosure, 89–90
    non-face-to-face disclosure, 86–88
    see also Third-party disclosure
Motivation, *see also* Interpersonal-, Other-,
        and Self-Gain
    for disclosure, 11, 45–55, 188
    for nondisclosure, 11, 55–63, 188–189

N

Non-face-to-face disclosure, 86–88
Nonverbal disclosure, *see* Vernacular or Al-
    ternative disclosure messages

O

Other-gain
    reasons for disclosure, 49–52, 188
        duty to inform, 49–50, 89, 99, 160,
            188
        educating others, 50–52, 134, 188
    reasons for nondisclosure, 61–62,
            188–189
        protect others, 61–62, 66, 108, 112,
            189
Others' right to know, conflicted feelings,
        32, 49–50, 88, 160–162, 164

P

Parent, *see* Relationships
Partner, *see* Relationships and Significant
    Others

Partner notification, 4, 147, 171
Past discussion of HIV/AIDS, 42, 77
Past experience with disclosing, 79–80
Perinatal, *see also* Children, 4, 148, 153,
        156–157, 174
Planning, *see* Timing
Prevalence of HIV and AIDS, xii, 2–4,
        172–173
Pregnancy, *see* Reproductive decisions
Privacy, *see also* CPM, 6, 40, 56, 67, 94, 163,
        165, 187, 188
    maintaining, 4–5, 18–19, 160–170
    see also Threats
Proactive behaviors, 133–135, 208, 210,
        215–222
    ACT UP, 134, 142
    HIV/AIDS groups, 133–135
    speaking to groups, 51–52, 134
Protection, *see also* Other-gain, 39, 40, 42, 47,
        50, 59, 66, 107, 112, 118, 141, 151,
        154, 158, 160, 163, 189
Psychological health, 136–138
    and HIV disclosure, 101, 137, 168–169,
        183
    and HIV progression, 100, 130
Psychological inhibition, 13, 168–170
    concealing sexual identity, 168–169, *see*
        also Sexual orientation
Public disclosure, 5, 44, 51–52, 62, 76, 107,
        114, 153

R

Reactions to HIV disclosure and
        nondisclosure (also Responses),
        86, 93, 121–171
    actual, 13, 62, 65, 68, 77, 80, 125–127
    expected or anticipated, 32, 64–66, 121,
        123, 125
    unanticipated, 65–66, 121
Reasons for disclosure or nondisclosure, *see*
        Motivations
Reciprocity, 105, 106
Rehabilitation, *see also* Drug use and Stigma,
        152–153
Rejection, 53, 55, 58–60, 70, 81, 88, 133, 138,
        158, 177, 196
Relational ties, 67–77, 142
Relationships and disclosure
    and commitment, 69, 79
    change in after diagnosis/disclosure, 8,
        59–60, 123, 143–146

dating, 53, 79, 80, 101, 103, 118–119,
        146, 159, 177
disclosure and risk behaviors, 7, 53,
        154–156
disclosure to children, 62, 71–72, 102,
        150–153, 191
disclosure to coworkers, 74–75
disclosure to employer, 55, 74–75
disclosure to family, 33, 57, 61, 72–73,
        93, 99, 122, 141
disclosure to friends, 55, 73–74, 159, 193
disclosure to health care workers, 6, 21,
        31, 48, 49, 54, 58, 75–77, 107
disclosure to parents, 32, 69–70
disclosure to partners, 7, 49, 59, 68–69,
        88, 103, 118, 154–159
disclosure to siblings, 71
disruption of, 59, 88, 109, 126, 145–146,
        158, 177
effect on children, *see also* Children,
        71–72, 102, 131, 150–153
effect on close relationships, 59, 142–159
effect on couples, 33, 144–146, 154–157
perceived relational quality, 62, 64, 71,
        78–79, 122, 142, 189
relational development, 53, 59, 64
relational violations, 161–162
short term vs long term, 69, 79
significant others as caregivers, *see also*
        Significant others, 147–150
strength of relational ties, 67–77
Religion (also Faith, Spirituality), 32, 43
Reproductive decisions, 156–157, 176
abortion, 157
pregnancy, 148, 156
Resources, *see* Income
Responses to disclosure, *see* Reactions

S

Safer sex, *see* Sexual behavior
Secrets, 4–5, 19, 20, 46–47, 73, 146, 160,
        169–170, 194
Secret test, 118
Seeking help, *see* Information seeking and
        Self-gain
Self-advocacy, *see* Proactive behaviors
Self-esteem, *see also* Self-gain, 58, 164, 189,
        196
Self-gain,
        reasons for disclosure, 46–49, 188

catharsis, 46–47, 107, 124, 170, 183,
        188
seeking help, *see also* Information
        seeking, 48–49
reasons for nondisclosure, 56–60,
        188–189
fear of rejection or being misunder-
        stood, 58–60, 103, 126,
        140, 189
self-blame and self-concept difficul-
        ties, *see also* Stigma, 58, 189
third-party leakage, *see also* Gossip
        and Third party, 56–58
Setting and disclosure, 12, 24, 94–97, 108
Sexual abuse and disclosure, 38, 62, 98
childhood, 23, 61, 95, 100, 108
Sexual behavior, 154
after disclosure, 68, 158
and condom use, *see also* Condoms, 7,
        154–158
practicing safer sex, 7, 59, 68, 118,
        154–158, 161, 177
unprotected, 154–156, 158
Sexual orientation and disclosure, 21–22, 55,
        146, 177
disclosing sexual identity, 21, 70, 74, 80,
        114, 168–169
gay men (also MSM), 21–22, 144, 146,
        218
lesbian (also WSW), 22, 157, 177–178
Siblings, *see* Relationships
Significant others, disclosure to, *see also* Re-
        lationships
ex-partner, 49, 79, 86
need for safer sex, 49, 59, 68, 103,
        154–158
partner, also lover, 49, 59, 68–69, 103,
        119, 154–159
Similarity, *see* Interpersonal-gain
Social support, 7, 13, 48, 126, 127–136,
        148–150, 159, 200–201
and activism groups, 133–135
and coping, 130, 131–133, 134, 136
emotional support, 7, 49
helpful support, 90, 128–130, 133, 1760
informational support, 48, 131–132
practical support, 7, 48, 149
satisfaction with, 127, 131–132, 200–201
unhelpful support, 32, 128–131, 132,
        143–144, 165–166, 176,
        198–199

Source of infection, *see also* Stigma, 51, 70, 144, 145, 153

Spirituality, *see* Religion

Stigma, xii–xiii, 1, 7, 13, 36, 37–45, 58, 76, 80, 101, 115, 138–142, 153, 166, 174–175, 177, 195, 196, 198

types of stigma, 40–45

disapproval, 43–44

failure to contribute, 44–45

fear of infection and contagion, 42–43, 139

negative emotional reactions, 41–42, 126

and attitudes, 38, 43

changes in, 7, 14, 39, 51, 175–175

courtesy stigma, 41, 62, 135, 141

discrimination, 8, 38, 58, 74, 138, 164, 174

and group bias, 51, 101, 140–141

HIV association with homosexuality, 1, 21–22, 38, 43, 101, 115, 140, 144

influence on disclosure, 39–40

injection drug use, *see also* Drug use, 1, 23, 38, 43, 101, 114, 140, 152

and misinformation, 1, 39, 42, 50, 58, 138–140

perceived risk for disclosure, 11, 40

prevalence of, 38–39

Stressors for HIV, 2, 46–47, 66, 98, 149, 202–203

Support providers, *see* Social support

T

Testing others' reactions, *see* Incremental disclosure and Interpersonal-gain

Third-party disclosure, *see also* Gossip and Mode of disclosure, 70, 90–94, 123

as support, 91–92

role of intention, 57, 92–94

Threats, 60, 164–166

Timing and disclosure, 2, 24, 80, 97–110, 121

after HIV diagnosis, 47, 98

in conversation, 105–110

planned, 92, 95, 103–105, 108

spontaneous, 89, 95, 104–105

in relationship, 53, 99, 102–103

Treatments, *see also* Medical advances and HAART, xi, 1, 7, 172, 190

U

Uncertainty, 55, 64, 86–87, 110–111, 119, 134

Unintentional disclosure, 92, 95–96, 102, 105, 150, 166–167

V

Vaccine, xi, 1, 14, 173–174

Venting, *see* Self-gain, catharsis

Vernacular tactics of disclosure and discovery, 118–119

trick examinations and intuitions, 119

Victim continuum, *see also* Stigma, 43

Violence, *see also* Threats and Sexual abuse, 41, 60, 147, 176–177

physical, 58, 60, 146–147

sexual, 60

Volunteer, 135

W

Withdrawal after disclosure, *see also* Reactions, 42, 70, 126, 133

Printed in the United States
by Baker & Taylor Publisher Services